T0259360

Sports Cardiology

Editor

ROBERT W. BATTLE

CLINICS IN
SPORTS MEDICINE

www.sportsmed.theclinics.com

Consulting Editor
MARK D. MILLER

July 2015 • Volume 34 • Number 3

ELSEVIER

1600 John F. Kennedy Boulevard • Suite 1800 • Philadelphia, Pennsylvania, 19103-2899

http://www.theclinics.com

CLINICS IN SPORTS MEDICINE Volume 34, Number 3
July 2015 ISSN 0278-5919, ISBN-13: 978-0-323-39119-1

Editor: Jennifer Flynn-Briggs
Developmental Editor: Donald Mumford

Clinics in Sports Medicine (ISSN 0278-5919) is published quarterly by Elsevier Inc., 360 Park Avenue South, New York, NY 10010-1710. Months of issue are January, April, July, and October. Business and Editorial Offices: 1600 John F. Kennedy Blvd., Ste. 1800, Philadelphia, PA 19103-2899. Customer Service Office: 3251 Riverport Lane, Maryland Heights, MO 63043. Periodicals postage paid at New York, NY and additional mailing offices. Subscription prices are $340.00 per year (US individuals), $540.00 per year (US institutions), $165.00 per year (US students), $385.00 per year (Canadian individuals), $666.00 per year (Canadian institutions), $235.00 (Canadian students), $470.00 per year (foreign individuals), $666.00 per year (foreign institutions), and $235.00 per year (foreign students). Foreign air speed delivery is included in all *Clinics* subscription prices. All prices are subject to change without notice. **POSTMASTER:** Send address changes to *Clinics in Sports Medicine*, Elsevier Health Sciences Division, Subscription Customer Service, 3251 Riverport Lane, Maryland Heights, MO 63043. Customer Service (orders, claims, online, change of address): Elsevier Health Sciences Division, Subscription Customer Service, 3251 Riverport Lane, Maryland Heights, MO 63043. **Tel: 1-800-654-2452 (U.S. and Canada); 314-447-8871 (outside U.S. and Canada). Fax: 314-447-8029. E-mail: journalscustomerservice-usa@elsevier.com (for print support); journalsonlinesupport-usa@ elsevier.com (for online support).**

Reprints. For copies of 100 or more of articles in this publication, please contact the Commercial Reprints Department, Elsevier Inc., 360 Park Avenue South, New York, NY 10010-1710. Tel.: 212-633-3874; Fax: 212-633-3820; E-mail: reprints@elsevier.com.

Clinics in Sports Medicine is covered in *MEDLINE/PubMed (Index Medicus) Current Contents/Clinical Medicine, Excerpta Medica,* and *ISI/Biomed.*

Contributors

CONSULTING EDITOR

MARK D. MILLER, MD
S. Ward Casscells Professor, Head, Division of Sports Medicine, Department of
Orthopaedic Surgery, University of Virginia, Charlottesville, Virginia; Team Physician,
James Madison University, Harrisonburg, Virginia

EDITOR

ROBERT W. BATTLE, MD, FACC
Director, Adult Congenital Heart Disease Clinic and Sports Cardiology Clinic; Professor,
Division of Cardiology, Departments of Medicine and Pediatrics, University of Virginia
Health System; Team Cardiologist, UVA Division I Athletic Programs; Department of
Athletics, University of Virginia, Sports Medicine, McCue Center, Charlottesville, Virginia

AUTHORS

MICHAEL J. ACKERMAN, MD, PhD
Division of Cardiovascular Medicine, Mayo Clinic; Professor of Medicine, Pediatrics, and
Pharmacology, Mayo Clinic Windland Smith Rice Sudden Death Genomics Laboratory,
Rochester, Minnesota

CRAIG ALPERT, MD
Division of Cardiovascular Medicine, Department of Internal Medicine, Frankel
Cardiovascular Center, University of Michigan School of Medicine, Ann Arbor, Michigan

AARON L. BAGGISH, MD
Cardiovascular Performance Program, Massachusetts General Hospital, Boston,
Massachusetts

ROBERT W. BATTLE, MD, FACC
Director, Adult Congenital Heart Disease Clinic and Sports Cardiology Clinic; Professor,
Division of Cardiology, Departments of Medicine and Pediatrics, University of Virginia
Health System; Team Cardiologist, UVA Division I Athletic Programs; Department of
Athletics, University of Virginia, Sports Medicine, McCue Center, Charlottesville, Virginia

ALFRED A. BOVE, MD, PhD, MACC
Emeritus Professor of Medicine, Cardiology Section, Temple University School of
Medicine, Philadelphia, Pennsylvania

SHARLENE M. DAY, MD
Associate Professor, Division of Cardiovascular Medicine, Department of Internal
Medicine, Frankel Cardiovascular Center, University of Michigan School of Medicine,
Ann Arbor, Michigan

PETER N. DEAN, MD
Assistant Professor of Pediatrics, Department of Pediatric Cardiology, University of Virginia, Charlottesville, Virginia

CHRISTOPHER V. DESIMONE, MD, PhD
Assistant Professor of Medicine, Cardiovascular Fellow, Division of Cardiovascular Medicine, Mayo Clinic, Rochester, Minnesota

MICHAEL S. EMERY, MD, FACC
Medical Director, Sports Cardiology Program, Greenville Health System; Clinical Assistant Professor, Department of Medicine, University of South Carolina School of Medicine Greenville, Greenville, South Carolina

MICHELLE GRENIER, MD
Pediatric Cardiologist, Pediatrix Cardiology Associates of New Mexico, Albuquerque, New Mexico

WALTER J. HOYT Jr, MD
Fellow of Pediatric Cardiology, Department of Pediatric Cardiology, University of Virginia, Charlottesville, Virginia

ALINE ISKANDAR, MD
Division of Cardiovascular Medicine, Cardiology, UMass Memorial Medical Center, Worcester, Massachusetts

CHRISTINE E. LAWLESS, MD, MBA, FACC, FACSM
President, Sports Cardiology Consultants LLC, Chicago, Illinois; Adjunct Professor, Department of Nutrition and Health Sciences, University of Nebraska, Lincoln, Lincoln, Nebraska

BENJAMIN D. LEVINE, MD, FACC, FAHA, FACSM
Professor of Medicine and Cardiology, Distinguished Professorship in Exercise Science, Department of Internal Medicine, University of Texas Southwestern Medical Center; Director, Institute for Exercise and Environmental Medicine; Harry S. Moss Heart Chair for Cardiovascular Research, S. Finley Ewing Jr Chair for Wellness, Texas Health Presbyterian Hospital Dallas, Dallas, Texas

MATTHEW W. MARTINEZ, MD
Associate Professor of Medicine, Medical Director, Cardiac Imaging, Division of Cardiology, Lehigh Valley Health Network, Allentown, Pennsylvania

DILAAWAR J. MISTRY, MD, MS, ATC
Primary Care Team Physician, USA Swimming; Primary Care Team Physician, Colorado Rockies; Department of Physical Medicine and Rehabilitation, Western Orthopedics and Sports Medicine, Grand Junction, Colorado; Visiting Associate Professor, Department of Physical Medicine and Rehabilitation, University of Virginia Health System, Charlottesville, Virginia

SILVANA MOLOSSI, MD, PhD
Associate Professor, Section of Pediatric Cardiology, Department of Pediatrics, Texas Children's Hospital, Baylor College of Medicine, Houston, Texas

MILDRED A. OPONDO, MD
Post-doctoral Research Fellow-Cardiovascular Physiology, Department of Internal Medicine, University of Texas Southwestern Medical Center; Institute for Exercise and Environmental Medicine; Texas Health Presbyterian Hospital Dallas, Dallas, Texas

SHIVA P. PONAMGI, MD
Hospitalist, Division of Hospital Internal Medicine, Mayo Clinic Health System–Austin, Austin, Minnesota

KEERTHI PRAKASH, BSc (Hons), MBChB, MRCP
Cardiology Speciality Registrar and Cardiology Research Fellow, Department of Cardiovascular Sciences, St. George's University of London, London, United Kingdom

ERIC F. QUANDT, JD
Partner, Scharf Banks Marmor LLC, Chicago, Illinois

SARA SABERI, MD, MS
Clinical Lecturer, Division of Cardiovascular Medicine, Department of Internal Medicine, Frankel Cardiovascular Center, University of Michigan School of Medicine, Ann Arbor, Michigan

SATYAM SARMA, MD
Assistant Professor of Cardiology, Department of Internal Medicine, University of Texas Southwestern Medical Center; Institute for Exercise and Environmental Medicine; Texas Health Presbyterian Hospital Dallas, Dallas, Texas

SANJAY SHARMA, BSc (Hons), MD, FRCP, FESC
Professor of Inherited Cardiac Diseases and Sports Cardiology, Department of Cardiovascular Sciences, St. George's University of London, London, United Kingdom

SIOBHAN STATUTA, MD, CAQSM
Assistant Professor of Family Medicine and Physical Medicine and Rehabilitation; Director, Primary Care Sports Medicine Fellowship; Team Physician, UVA Division I Athletic Programs, University of Virginia Health System, Charlottesville, Virginia

MATTHEW J. THOMAS, ScM, CGC
Genetic Counselor, Clinical Lecturer, Division of Genetics, Department of Pediatrics, University of Virginia Health System, Charlottesville, Virginia

PAUL D. THOMPSON, MD
Division of Cardiology, Hartford Hospital, Hartford, Connecticut

RORY B. WEINER, MD
Cardiovascular Performance Program, Massachusetts General Hospital, Boston, Massachusetts

Contents

remains an incompletely understood area. Ongoing and future work are required to further understand this process and ultimately to determine where the boundary lies between adaptive physiology and maladaptive disease.

Regular intensive exercise is associated with a constellation of several structural and functional adaptations within the heart that permit the generation of a large and sustained increase in cardiac output and/or increase in blood pressure. The magnitude with which these markers of physiological remodeling manifest on the surface electrocardiogram is governed by several factors and some athletes show electrical and structural changes that overlap with those observed in cardiomyopathy and in ion channel diseases, which are recognized causes of sudden cardiac death in young athletes. This article provides a critical appraisal of the athlete's ECG.

 Videos of a steady state free precession (SSFP – white blood) cine image of hypertrophic cardiomyopathy with an apical aneurysm and a contrast enhanced gated computed tomography image illustrating a bicuspid aortic valve in short axis accompany this article

Cardiac magnetic resonance imaging and cardiac computed tomographic angiography have become important parts of the armamentarium for noninvasive diagnosis of cardiovascular disease. Emerging technologies have produced faster imaging, lower radiation dose, improved spatial and temporal resolution, as well as a wealth of prognostic data to support usage. Investigating true pathologic disease as well as distinguishing normal from potentially dangerous is now increasingly more routine for the cardiologist in practice. This article investigates how advanced imaging technologies can assist the clinician when evaluating all athletes for pathologic disease that may put them at risk.

The cardiac effects of aquatic sports have increased in interest with the experience of cardiac responses to swimming and diving. The syndrome of swimming-induced pulmonary edema is likely caused by a combination of central blood shifts, sudden onset of high exercise demands, and impaired diastolic relaxation of the left ventricle. Divers also develop venous gas emboli caused by nitrogen supersaturation in blood and tissues during ascent from depth. The physiology and physics of water immersion and diving are unique. Knowledge of pressure effects, gas solubility, and changes in gas volumes with depth is needed to understand the disorders related to these activities.

Sudden cardiovascular deaths in athletes are rare and only a fraction are due to aortic events. There has been concern that the hemodynamic load during exercise may lead to aortic dilation, but aortic dimensions in endurance and strength-trained athletes are only slightly larger than those in sedentary comparison subjects. The presence of a bicuspid aortic valve without significant valvular dysfunction and normal aortic dimensions should not influence eligibility to practice sport. Patients with genetic syndromes associated with aortopathy generally should be restricted from vigorous sports participation. This article reviews the diagnosis and management of diseases of the aorta in athletes.

Athletes with an implantable cardioverter defibrillator (ICD) represent a diverse group of individuals who may be at an increased risk of sudden cardiac death when engaging in vigorous physical activity. Therefore, they are excluded by the current guidelines from participating in most competitive sports except those classified as low intensity, such as bowling and golf. The lack of substantial data on the natural history of the cardiac diseases affecting these athletes as well as the unknown efficacy of ICDs in terminating life-threatening arrhythmias occurring during intense exercise has resulted in the restrictive nature of these now decade old guidelines.

Hypertrophic cardiomyopathy (HCM) is the most common genetic cardiovascular disease and one of the most common causes of sudden cardiac death (SCD). Current guidelines restrict the participation of patients with HCM in competitive sports, limiting the health benefits of exercise. However, many individuals with HCM have safely participated in sports, with a low incidence of SCD. Improved stratification of patients and desired activity may allow most individuals with HCM to engage in physical activity safely. Therefore, physicians should create an individualized approach in guiding each patient with HCM eager to enjoy the benefits of physical activity in a safe manner.

This article presents an overview of the legal and ethical issues in the cardiovascular care of elite athletes. An important distinction between the assessment and care of elite athletes and the general population necessitates an understanding of the applicable legal standard and the limitation of potential exposures. Important recommendations and pertinent case law is presented that can assist the medical provider in comprehending important considerations with regard to preparticipation evaluations, return-to-play decisions, and second opinions in elite athletes.

Sports cardiology has evolved as a result of these tragedies, which high-lighted a need for safer play and more programmatic protection of the athlete in play. In this article, athletic sudden death is analyzed from a historical and literary perspective and the development of modern initiatives to protect athletes from sudden death is reviewed.

CLINICS IN SPORTS MEDICINE

RELATED INTEREST

Cardiology Clinics, November 2014 (Vol. 32, Issue 4)
Atrial Fibrillation
Hakan Oral, *Editor*
Available at: http://www.cardiology.theclinics.com/

THE CLINICS ARE AVAILABLE ONLINE!
Access your subscription at:
www.theclinics.com

Foreword

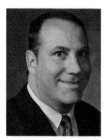

Mark D. Miller, MD
Consulting Editor

Dr Battle and his distinguished group of authors really put their hearts into this issue! It has been said that one comes both into the world via the pelvis (childbirth) and out of the world via the pelvis (hip fracture). However, it is far more likely that I, as an aging male, will come out of the world via the heart (MI). It is for that reason that I have developed a deep respect for cardiologists and am routinely seen by a preventative cardiologist (let's hope he lives up to his title!).

As sports medicine physicians for two major Division I colleges, my colleagues and I have consulted with Dr Robert Battle on numerous occasions and have always benefited from his excellent insight and wisdom. It is for that reason that I asked him to put together this issue of *Clinics in Sports Medicine*. It is certainly no surprise to me that he has completed an absolutely superb treatise on sports cardiology.

The issue begins with an overview of the importance of this topic and then addresses physiology, adaptation, and evaluation. High-interest topics, such as sudden death, congenital heart disease, and genetic testing, and a variety of other topics are also included. In sum, this issue doesn't miss a beat! I am deeply grateful that Dr Robert Battle agreed to take on this labor of love.

Mark D. Miller, MD
Division of Sports Medicine
Department of Orthopaedic Surgery
University of Virginia
400 Ray C. Hunt Drive, Suite 330
Charlottesville, VA 22908-0159, USA

James Madison University
Harrisonburg, VA 22807, USA

E-mail address:
MDM3P@hscmail.mcc.virginia.edu

Clin Sports Med 34 (2015) xiii
http://dx.doi.org/10.1016/j.csm.2015.04.003
0278-5919/15/$ – see front matter © 2015 Published by Elsevier Inc.

sportsmed.theclinics.com

Preface

Sports Cardiology: A Discipline Emerged

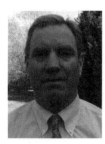

Robert W. Battle, MD, FACC
Editor

The first description of athletic remodeling ("athletic heart") was published over 125 years ago when a Swedish physician diagnosed an enlarged heart in a Nordic skier using only the most basic skills of auscultation and percussion.[1] In the century that followed, a large accrual of data emerged, furthering our understanding of exercise physiology, the training-related effects on the cardiovascular system, and the overall salutary effects of exercise on individual and population health. In recent years, the discipline of sports cardiology has emerged and evolved with growing numbers of specialists within the field with the expertise to both understand and assist athletes with any cardiovascular issue. However, there continues to be a significant provider gap both nationally and internationally, and the opportunity to push our knowledge forward through clinical practice and research must be seized. Accordingly, our field is deeply indebted to Mark Miller, MD, who, as consulting editor to *Clinics in Sports Medicine*, had the vision to include sports cardiology. This entire issue of *Clinics in Sports Medicine* is dedicated to a thorough exploration of our discipline and will allow an accessible portal for all providers to explore a wide range of topics within the field. From water sports to medical genetics, electrocardiogram (ECG) to MRI, anomalous coronaries to implantable defibrillators, medical-legal to psychosocial: it is all here. The debate over screening athletes with ECG/echocardiography has been so widely debated in the literature and at national and international meetings it would be redundant to revisit it here. Therefore, that topic is not addressed by design.

The medical home for the cardiovascular care of the athlete comprises athletic trainers, team medical doctors and nurses, exercise physiologists, and sports cardiologists. You have all been kept in mind for this issue, and there should be ample here for all to consider. We have arrived to a time where athletes deserve specialized cardiovascular care, and the challenge is to develop learning pathways within fellowship training for sports medicine and cardiology to allow that provider gap to be bridged. This issue of *Clinics in Sports Medicine* will also push the boundaries of

Clin Sports Med 34 (2015) xv–xvi
http://dx.doi.org/10.1016/j.csm.2015.04.002
sportsmed.theclinics.com
0278-5919/15/$ – see front matter © 2015 Published by Elsevier Inc.

current guidelines with regard to restriction of athletes with known cardiovascular diagnoses and explore the concept of shared decision-making with our athlete/patients and allow for a more thorough understanding of risk, therefore placing the assumption of that risk back on the athlete and not solely on the shoulders of the physician in counsel. I thank and salute all of the authors in this issue for dedicating their time and expertise to advance the field.

Robert W. Battle, MD, FACC
University of Virginia Health System
1215 Lee Street
Charlottesville, VA 22903, USA

E-mail address:
battle@virginia.edu

REFERENCE

1. Henschen S. Skidlauf und skidwerrlauf: eine medizinishce sports studie. Mitt Med Klin Upsala 1899;2.

The Impact of Sports Cardiology on the Practice of Primary Care Sports Medicine

Where Were We, Where Are We, Where Are We Headed?

Siobhan Statuta, MD, CAQSM[a], Dilaawar J. Mistry, MD, MS, ATC[b,c,*], Robert W. Battle, MD[d]

KEYWORDS

- Sports cardiology • Primary care team physician • Preparticipation evaluation
- Collaboration • Sudden cardiac arrest • Heart disease
- Preparticipation cardiovascular screening • Primary prevention
- Secondary prevention

KEY POINTS

- The cardiovascular care of competitive athletes is complex and demands a team effort between primary care team physicians and sports cardiologists.
- Training for competitive athletics induces several physiologic changes in the cardiovascular system that may mimic heart disease (HD) during cardiac testing (athlete's heart).
- Several cardiovascular pathologies can mimic athlete's heart, and primary care team physicians may not have the appropriate training necessary to fully understand the characteristics of this condition.
- The integration of sports cardiologists into sports medicine teams is beneficial to the practice of primary care sports medicine as well as the safety and well-being of athletes.

There was no funding needed to support this work and the authors have no financial disclosures.
[a] UVA Division I Athletic Programs, University of Virginia Health System, 1215 Lee Street, Charlottesville, VA 22908-0158, USA; [b] Department of Physical Medicine and Rehabilitation, Western Orthopedics and Sports Medicine, 2373 G Road, Suite 100, Grand Junction, CO 81505, USA; [c] Department of Physical Medicine and Rehabilitation, University of Virginia Health System, 1215 Lee Street, Charlottesville, VA 22908-0158, USA; [d] UVA Division I Athletic Programs, Division of Cardiology, University of Virginia Health System, PO Box 800158, Charlottesville, VA 22908-0158, USA
* Corresponding author. Department of Physical Medicine and Rehabilitation, Western Orthopedics and Sports Medicine, 2373 G Road, Suite 100, Grand Junction, CO 81505.
E-mail address: dannym@westernortho.com

INTRODUCTION

Sports participation in the United States has amplified rapidly over the past several years. Although exercise has been proved to provide health benefits due to physiologic adaptations, competitive athletes with undiagnosed HD remain at risk for sudden cardiac arrest (SCA). The various nuances of modern-era competitive athletics, the expectation for excellence both on and off the playing field, and the devastating effects of the loss of an athlete due to undiagnosed HD dictates an overwhelming need for a team approach. Sports cardiologists and primary care team physicians must collaborate to effectively diagnose masked HD, to potentially prevent SCA, and to provide ongoing care for athletes with HD. Fortunately, SCA is a rarity,[1,2] yet the tragic consequences of the demise of any such afflicted athlete leaves a distressing void for several generations. The memories of SCA in athletes has spanned centuries—from Pheidippides (legendary Greek Olympic champion) to Hank Gathers (Loyola Marymount basketball player) to Marc-Vivien Foé (Cameroon national soccer player) to Fabrice Muamba (English Premier League soccer player).[3] And although primary prevention of SCA is a multifaceted process in which there is no single absolute method to prevent SCA, modern medicine is better equipped today to try to prevent further tragedies on the playing field and to accomplish better outcomes if SCA does occur.

Aside from the vital importance of SCA prevention, if deemed safe by a capable sports cardiologist, athletes should be considered for athletic participation even in the presence of diagnosed HD. As such, special attention must be directed toward the intricacies and rigors of the specific sport. The medical disqualification of an athlete from the athletic arena is fraught with implications beyond imagination. The psychological effects of a lost passion after countless hours of hard work on the practice "field of dreams" and commitment to excellence are immeasurable. Long gone are the days when a primary care team physician could solely care for and make prudent decisions about the cardiovascular health of athletes. Primary care team physicians who have not had the good fortune of working closely with cardiologists knowledgeable about sports and exercise cardiology lack the necessary experience and education and thus are at a distinct disadvantage to make independent medical recommendations on the activity or disqualification status of athletes with HD.

Primary care sports medicine practitioners must understand that the specialty of sports medicine has evolved to the point where a thoroughness, a commitment to excellence, and a team approach to cardiovascular care of competitive athletes are imperative and no longer a choice. Meticulous preparticipation cardiovascular screening programs that have a sports cardiology consultant to decipher the challenging cases undoubtedly provide a level of comfort for primary care team physicians. Cardiologists prove an invaluable resource for reviewing any questionable components of the history suggestive of underlying HD as, with extremes of training, cardiovascular symptoms emerge in competitive athletes with otherwise seemingly normal hearts. Although preparticipation cardiovascular screening programs may aid in the diagnosis of HD and thus hypothetically help prevent SCA, physicians must also consider the expected normal physiologic adaptations to training—athlete's heart—that lead to a high rate of false-positive electrocardiogram (ECG) tests.[4–6] Athlete's heart may prove misleading to primary care team physicians who are either unfamiliar or inexperienced with such adaptations. Consequently, athletes may be incorrectly disqualified from athletic participation, resulting in numerous potential negative consequences. Furthermore, studies have revealed insufficient evidence to show that routine ECGs obtained as part of a PPE followed by activity restriction in at-risk individuals are decisive in reducing the risk of athletic-induced sudden death.[7]

Therefore, prior to implementation of primary prevention programs on a large-scale basis in the United States, more trials on long-term outcomes data are imperative.

Current strategies for secondary prevention of SCA include comprehensive education on resuscitation and thorough emergency action plans for those on the front line of athletic care, including the potential use of automated external defibrillators (AEDs). Additionally, the advent of cutting-edge cardiovascular technology, such as a new smartphone application, will help identify rhythm abnormalities in athletes with palpitations. Variables, such as the diverse degrees of basic training in sports cardiology among primary care team physicians, the challenges associated with implementing thorough preparticipation cardiovascular screening programs, and the crucial nature of solid, secondary prevention educational programs on athlete safety, mandate the need for meaningful collaborations between sports cardiologists and primary care team physicians. This partnership will undoubtedly provide a degree of comfort and ongoing education to primary care team physicians and make the practice and competition fields safer for athletes.

The present environment proves ripe, as cardiologists with a passion for sports medicine are beginning to subspecialize and demonstrate a commitment to safe participation in sports. The benefits of a reliable collaboration are infinite and the true impact of sports cardiology on sports medicine will be judged not today and not tomorrow but by future generations who will be fortunate enough to have reaped the benefits of a thoughtful process that is still evolving today.

THE PREPARTICIPATION EVALUATION—WHERE WERE WE, WHERE ARE WE?

From a primary care sports medicine viewpoint, with the exception of systematic, progressive, meaningful modifications in the content of the preparticipation evaluation (PPE) over the past decade, "Where were we?" and "Where are we?" today are comparable with one exception. Before the advent of the field of sports cardiology, primary care team physicians referred athletes to cardiologists versed in their various subspecialties within cardiology. For example, an athlete with an accessory pathway was referred to a cardiac electrophysiologist, an athlete with structural HD to a structural or congenital heart specialist, and an athlete with exercise-induced syncope to a general cardiologist. Through the years, primary care sports medicine physicians have been mostly responsible for preparticipation medical clearance—relying solely on the PPE, which has been the fundamental gold standard toward safe participation in organized sports. A thorough PPE, usually performed by primary care team physicians, can uncover subtle clues and red flags that hint at HD, may help identify correctable medical problems, maintain health and safety during training and competition, educate athletes and parents about the impact of medical conditions on athletic performance, and, foremost, prevent unnecessary disqualification of athletes from training and/or competition.[8] Yet, a concerning question becomes, Do primary care team physicians have the training and experience in cardiovascular medicine to thoroughly and appropriately assess the cardiac history portion of the PPE to pick up on these vital clues? Although the PPE is not a substitute for an annual comprehensive evaluation as detailed by the American Medical Association, the PPE had been noted to substitute for the annual examination in up to 78% of adolescents.[9] The PPE should, therefore, be methodical and the goals, at all costs, should be to permit safe participation, while avoiding unnecessary restriction from sports participation. In a population of seventh to ninth graders thought to have occult cardiovascular disease during the PPE process, 80% were noted free of cardiovascular disease, yet 40% of these individuals had various activity restrictions unnecessarily imposed.[10] This observation illustrates the need for collective efforts between primary care team physicians and sports cardiologists at the outset of any meaningful PPE process, to both appropriately and expeditiously diagnose occult HD while minimizing needless activity restrictions.

As defined in the *Preparticipation Physical Evaluation, Fourth Edition*,[11] which endorses the recommendations by the 2007 American Heart Association (AHA) consensus statement on preparticipation cardiovascular screening,[12] key elements of clinical history and cardiovascular examination include the following.

History

1. Have you ever passed out or nearly passed out DURING or AFTER exercise?
2. Have you ever had discomfort, pain, tightness, or pressure in your chest during exercise?
3. Does your heart ever race or skip beats during exercise?
4. Has a doctor ever told you that you have any heart problems?
5. Has a doctor ever ordered a test for your heart?
6. Do you get lightheaded or feel more short of breath than expected during exercise?
7. Have you ever had an unexplained seizure?
8. Do you get more tired or short of breath more quickly than your friends during exercise?
9. Has any family member or relative died of heart problems or had any unexpected or unexplained sudden death before age 50?
10. Does anyone in your family have hypertrophic cardiomyopathy (HCM), Marfan syndrome, arrhythmogenic right ventricular cardiomyopathy (ARVC), long QT syndrome, Brugada syndrome, or catecholaminergic polymorphic ventricular tachycardia?
11. Does anyone in your family have a heart problem, pacemaker, or implanted defibrillator?
12. Has anyone in your family had unexplained fainting, unexplained seizures, or near drowning?

Cardiovascular Examination

1. Auscultation for heart murmurs (performed in a seated position and with Valsalva or squatting maneuvers, to accentuate potentially pathologic murmurs related to aortic stenosis or HCM)
2. Femoral pulses to exclude aortic coarctation
3. Physical stigmata of Marfan syndrome
4. Brachial artery blood pressure measured in the sitting position

Based on current recommendations, most primary care team physicians rely solely on key elements of history and cardiovascular examination during the PPE to help uncover silent HD. The current debate among primary care team physicians and sports cardiologists, however, regarding the adequacy of the PPE to help identify HD and prevent SCA is based on 2 questions:

1. Is the PPE an adequate clinical instrument for the identification of silent HD and the primary prevention of SCA?
2. Do a majority of primary care team physicians have the necessary experience and training to identify red flags of undiagnosed HD using the PPE without any additional cardiology consultation or supportive cardiovascular tests?

Both questions should be addressed today for a better tomorrow for competitive athletes.

Currently in the United States, the AHA—based on pragmatic issues, cost-efficiency, and the obvious implications of false-positive screening tests—does not support the routine use of a 12-lead ECG, echocardiography, and/or exercise testing for primary prevention of SCA.[12] Conversely, the European Society of Cardiology (ESC) and other sporting bodies, including Fédération Internationale de Football Association and Union of European Football Associations, recommend ECG as an essential component of the PPE.[13] The AHA panel is, however, not opposed to smaller-scale screening programs that include noninvasive tests and are "well designed and prudently implemented."[12] As a result, several universities and professional organizations that are fortunate to have the fiscal resources and help from cardiologists versed in the care of competitive athletes have devised thorough preparticipation cardiovascular screening programs as a component of the PPE.[14,15] Yet, herein lies the crux of challenges faced by most primary care team physicians empowered with the care of competitive athletes: realistically, there is no common ground for the implementation of thorough, cost-effective preparticipation cardiovascular screening programs for the primary prevention of SCA.

Other prominent issues that hamper the development of systematic preparticipation cardiovascular screening programs include

1. The prohibitive volume of competitive athletes, including 4 million high school athletes; 500,000 intercollegiate athletes; and more than 5000 professional athletes
2. Low specificity of ECG[16] and expensive diagnostic testing for large number of cardiovascular diseases that can potentially induce SCA, including coronary artery disease, electrical conduction disorders and channelopathies, cardiomyopathic pathologies such as HCM, dilated cardiomyopathy, ARVC, myocarditis, and congenital HD (CHD) inclusive of coronary artery anomalies and disorders of the aorta and vascular system[17]
3. Low incidence of SCA[16] and low prevalence of CHD: 0.3% of the athletic population[12]
4. Skepticism about whether restriction of athletic activity in individuals with HD actually reduces risk for SCA
5. Although HCM is the leading cause of SCA in competitive athletic adolescents,[2] there is no dominant cause for SCA between the ages of 3 and 24.[17] Furthermore, only 70% of individuals with occult HD may have warning signs, including chest pain, near syncope, fatigue, dyspnea, and lightheadedness. Additionally, a wide range of individuals (25%–61%) report a family history of premature sudden death.[18] Notably, the clinical manifestations of these cardiovascular conditions during the PPE can be subtle at best and often manifest as lethal arrhythmias during exercise.[17,19]
6. Some primary care team physicians do not have the expertise or training to manage the subtle, concerning clinical features of occult HD. They may not be adept at interpreting the various distinctions of ECGs in athletes or may not have easy access to cardiologists versed in the various subtleties of athlete's heart.
7. Many primary care team physicians, universities, and clubs do not have the fiscal resources to implement preparticipation screening programs and/or prompt access to sports cardiologists for consultation or cardiovascular testing.

Therefore, the current guidelines for the PPE and historical questions, outlined previously, are adequate to a point. Despite these notable challenges and limitations, there may prove to be an undefined value in incorporating preparticipation cardiovascular screening as part the PPE in the future. The success of preparticipation cardiovascular screening programs will depend, however, on including sports cardiologists adequately trained in the various nuances of athlete's heart.

A PRACTICAL APPROACH TO A COMPLEX PROBLEM—WHERE ARE WE HEADED?

Year after year, athletes with undiagnosed HD perish unexpectedly on their fields of dreams. Several who passed prematurely underwent PPEs as currently recommended; therefore, can and should more be done to prevent unnecessary loss of precious lives? Can thinking outside the box lead to attempts to implement programs that are pragmatic and cost-effective yet simple and thorough? The questions are simple; the answers are complex. All these and more may be resolved by an open team approach fostered between primary care team physicians and sports cardiologists.

The Sports Cardiologist Role on the Sports Medicine Team

Sports cardiology is increasingly recognized as an indispensable component of the practice of sports medicine, both in the United States and Europe. The escalation in knowledge and mounting necessity for expertise in the field of sports cardiology dictate the need for a systematic sports cardiology curriculum. In a 2008 publication by the ESC for general cardiologists, sports cardiology was merged with rehabilitation and exercise physiology to facilitate homogenous training of health care providers to create a level of expertise in the evaluation of competitive athletes or individuals engaging in recreational sports activities.[20]

More recently, after the implementation of the Sports and Exercise Cardiology Section by the American College of Cardiology in 2011, there has been a mounting interest among cardiologists in assimilating sports cardiology into routine cardiovascular care, as evidenced by a vast increase in membership from 150 to 4000 between 2011 and 2013. Moreover, an innovative paradigm for thorough cardiovascular care for athletes has been detailed in the thoughtful work of Lawless and colleagues[21] to enhance the care of all athletes by promoting safe participation in sports.

Four key opinions of Lawless and colleagues[21] define the significant impact of sports cardiologists as pivotal members of the sports medicine team providing comprehensive care for competitive athletes.

1. Primary care team physicians will benefit substantially by incorporating the expertise of knowledgeable sports cardiologists from the outset during the PPE and to help diagnose silent HD and identify athletes at risk. Specifically, if additional cardiovascular testing is deemed necessary, sports cardiologists can help guide the work-up and weed out the false-positive results.
2. Sports cardiologists are vital for the ongoing care of competitive athletes with HD. By working in partnership with primary care team physicians to assess and make recommendations, athletes, in turn, maximize their chances to attain their dreams while preventing unnecessary disqualification.
3. Sports cardiologists, in concert with primary care team physicians, can help in the development of "well designed and prudently implemented" preparticipation screening programs.
4. Sports cardiologists can be key participants in the implementation of educational programs that detail the importance of secondary prevention of SCA and the appropriate treatment of SCA ideally with a predesigned EAP.

Debate on the Development of "Well-Designed and Prudently Implemented" Preparticipation Cardiovascular Screening Programs

There is nothing more comforting to a primary care team physician or athletic trainer covering a sideline than the knowledge that their athletes' cardiovascular status has been thoroughly vetted by a skilled sports cardiologist. The concept of leaving no stone unturned from a cardiovascular viewpoint is easier stated than accomplished globally. The undecided debate regarding differing recommendations between the ESC and AHA for mass preparticipation cardiovascular screening is perhaps interminable yet bears a brief discussion.

In 2005, the ESC recommended guidelines for preparticipation screening.[22] Although a direct evaluation comparing the efficacy of ESC and AHA guidelines is lacking, 3 key differences are noted:

1. ESC guidelines recommend a 12-lead ECG with the goal of looking for suggestions of specific abnormalities, followed by a detailed ECG review for a suspicion of undiagnosed HD.
2. ESC guidelines recommend that evaluation be performed by a trained clinician in specific health care settings,[23] whereas the AHA guidelines recommend evaluation by a trained health care worker.
3. ESC guidelines recommend repeat evaluation every 2 years.

AHA recommendations are rooted in concerns regarding practicality, cost, and the obvious implications of false-positive screening tests. Yet, from a comfort level for primary care team physician and athletic trainers, several crucial facts suggest the need for further discussion on the development of detailed preparticipation cardiovascular screening programs to identify HD and thus potentially prevent SCA. Key elements include the following:

1. The overwhelming, emotional suffering of family, friends, and teammates after the loss of an athlete to undiagnosed HD is incomprehensible—especially knowing that there are tools to make a difference, despite current recommendations to the contrary.
2. During athletic competition and/or exercise, studies have shown a 2- to 2.5-times higher risk of SCA.[13,24]
3. Twenty-five percent of SCAs occur within 1 hour of the commencement of exercise in selected cases.[17]
4. In the United States, the Centers for Disease Control and Prevention estimates that approximately 2000 individuals younger than 25 years of age will die of SCA annually.[25]
5. In a retrospective analysis of SCA in high school and college athletes in the United States (N = 134), standard PPE (history and physical examination) was effective in suggesting potential cardiovascular abnormalities in only 3%.[26]
6. Acquisition of ECG during the PPE and evaluation by a trained clinician in specific health care settings, as recommended by the ESC, improves sensitivity for detection of life-threatening HD.[6]
7. Although ECG acquisition during PPE has shown to have a high false-positive rate,[4-6] secondary to inherent physiologic adaptations to conditioning (athlete's heart), a skilled sports cardiologist can help determine the need for additional expensive testing, thereby reducing cost.
8. The ECG is of value but not completely reliable in the exclusion of HCM. It may be abnormal in up to 95% of patients with HCM,[27] but by contrast, may be normal in up to 15% of patients with HCM.[28] This may be particularly relevant to large athletes with broad torsos who may not reflect same changes in voltage and repolarization seen in athletes with a normal chest configuration.
9. In 33,735 athletes screened over a 17-year period in Italy, the most common causes of cardiovascular abnormalities were arrhythmias and conduction abnormalities (38%), and of the 22 patients diagnosed with HCM, although only 5 had abnormalities on the initial PPE, 18 had ECG abnormalities.

10. ECG can have considerable value when evaluated by experienced sports cardiologists who understand physiologic adaptations to training and[29,30] the effects of race and gender[31,32] and augmented by readily available high-quality transthoracic echocardiogram performed shortly after ECG acquisition. This thorough approach can limit the number of false-positive results, especially for HCM, which can minimize either unwarranted, temporary withdrawal or permanent disqualification from participation.[3,33]

Because of the stalemate regarding conflicting viewpoints between the ESC and AHA on this fundamental issue of preparticipation cardiovascular screening, however, it may be acceptable to perhaps screen specific high-risk athletes. Such programs may be viable and may serve as the seed for future growth of preparticipation cardiovascular screening programs.[16] Regardless, any preparticipation cardiovascular screening programs for competitive athletes should be deliberate, well-designed, prudently implemented, and, perhaps most importantly, be directed by highly trained, experienced sports cardiologists with a comprehensive understanding of the world of the athlete inclusive of athlete's heart.

Secondary Prevention of Sudden Cardiac Arrest

Current strategies for the secondary prevention and successful treatment of SCA include comprehensive education on cardiopulmonary resuscitation (CPR) and thorough emergency action plans for those on the front line of athletic care, including the adequate use of AEDs. This is especially true for primary care team physicians who do not have the luxury and reassurance of a proficient sports cardiologist on their sports medicine team. The value of thorough education for primary care team physicians by sports cardiologists, preferably supplemented by practicing resuscitative measures during mimicked life-threatening scenarios on the sidelines, cannot be overstated.

Between 2000 and 2010, Race Associated Cardiac Event Registry (RACER) investigators have shown that bystander CPR is a predictor of survival, and mortality declined to 71% during athletic sudden death.[34] The extraordinary resuscitation of Fabrice Muamba after a sudden death event during a soccer match—which lasted for 78 minutes and included CPR and numerous defibrillation attempts[35]—is an encouraging example of the critical importance of preparedness using a meaningful team approach for secondary prevention of SCA. Thus, ensuring the availability and education on appropriate operation of AEDs, on all playing fields, is a goal to be accomplished sooner rather than later. An inspiring story from Grand Junction, Colorado, is an example of this attainable goal. A mother of a girl with ARVC founded the nonprofit foundation, ARVD Heart for Hope. In partnership with Western Orthopedics and Sports Medicine and Community Hospital, both of Grand Junction, Colorado, she was able to raise enough capital to provide 54 AEDs for all local schools.[36] A well-prepared athletic venue should strive to be the safest place to suffer an out-of-hospital SCA.

Finally, sports cardiologists can help train primary care team physicians and athletic trainers on the advent of cutting-edge cardiovascular technologies, including a smartphone application that may help identify rhythm abnormalities in athletes with infrequent, yet sustained palpitations.

ACKNOWLEDGMENTS

This article is dedicated to the memory of athletes who have passed unexpectedly on their fields of dreams. We honor and respect their passion and voice a commitment to meaningful discussions with the experts to help mitigate untimely demise in the future.

REFERENCES

1. Harmon KG, Asif IM, Klossner D, et al. Incidence of sudden cardiac death in National Collegiate Athletic Association athletes. Circulation 2011;123(15): 1594–600.
2. Maron BJ, Doerer JJ, Haas TS, et al. Sudden deaths in young competitive athletes: analysis of 1866 deaths in the United States, 1980–2006. Circulation 2009;119(8):1085–92.
3. Battle RW, Mistry DJ, Malhotra R, et al. Cardiovascular screening and the elite athlete: advances, concepts, controversies, and a view of the future. Clin Sports Med 2011;30(3):503–24.
4. Lawless CE, Best TM. Electrocardiograms in athletes: interpretation and diagnostic accuracy. Med Sci Sports Exerc 2008;40(5):787–98.
5. Sanchez LD, Pereira J, Berkoff DJ. The evaluation of cardiac complaints in marathon runners. J Emerg Med 2009;36(4):369–76.
6. Sharma S, Merghani A, Gati S. Cardiac screening of young athletes prior to participation in sports: difficulties in detecting the fatally flawed among the fabulously fit. JAMA Intern Med 2015;175:125–7.
7. Estes NA 3rd, Link MS. Preparticipation athletic screening including an electrocardiogram: an unproven strategy for prevention of sudden cardiac death in the athlete. Prog Cardiovasc Dis 2012;54(5):451–4.
8. Available at: https://www.acsm.org/docs/brochures/pre-participation-physical-examinations.pdf. Accessed January 3, 2015.
9. Krowchuk DP, Krowchuk HV, Hunter DM, et al. Parents' knowledge of the purposes and content of preparticipation physical examinations. Arch Pediatr Adolesc Med 1995;149(6):653–7.
10. Bergman AB, Stamm SJ. The morbidity of cardiac nondisease in schoolchildren. N Engl J Med 1967;276(18):1008–13.
11. Bernhardt D, Roberts W, editors. Preparticipation physical evaluation. 4th edition. Elk Grove Village (IL): American Academy of Pediatrics; 2010.
12. Maron BJ, Thompson PD, Ackerman MJ, et al. Recommendations and considerations related to preparticipation screening for cardiovascular abnormalities in competitive athletes: 2007 update: a scientific statement from the american heart association council on nutrition, physical activity, and metabolism: endorsed by the american college of cardiology foundation. Circulation 2007;115(12):1643–55.
13. Borjesson M, Dellborg M. Is there evidence for mandating electrocardiogram as part of the pre-participation examination? Clin J Sport Med 2011;21(1):13–7.
14. Le VV, Wheeler MT, Mandic S, et al. Addition of the electrocardiogram to the preparticipation examination of college athletes. Clin J Sport Med 2010;20(2):98–105.
15. Malhotra R, West JJ, Dent J, et al. Cost and yield of adding electrocardiography to history and physical in screening Division I intercollegiate athletes: a 5-year experience. Heart Rhythm 2011;8(5):721–7.
16. Bar-Cohen Y, Silka MJ. The pre-sports cardiovascular evaluation: should it depend on the level of competition, the sport, or the state? Pediatr Cardiol 2012;33(3):417–27.
17. Meyer L, Stubbs B, Fahrenbruch C, et al. Incidence, causes, and survival trends from cardiovascular-related sudden cardiac arrest in children and young adults 0 to 35 years of age: a 30-year review. Circulation 2012;126(11):1363–72.
18. Drezner JA, Fudge J, Harmon KG, et al. Warning symptoms and family history in children and young adults with sudden cardiac arrest. J Am Board Fam Med 2012;25(4):408–15.

19. Section on Cardiology and Cardiac Surgery. Pediatric sudden cardiac arrest. Pediatrics 2012;129:e1094–102.
20. Heidbuchel H, Papadakis M, Panhuyzen-Goedkoop N, et al. Position paper: proposal for a core curriculum for a European sports cardiology qualification. Eur J Prev Cardiol 2013;20(5):889–903.
21. Lawless CE, Olshansky B, Washington RL, et al. Sports and exercise cardiology in the United States: cardiovascular specialists as members of the athlete healthcare team. J Am Coll Cardiol 2014;63(15):1461–72.
22. Corrado D, Pelliccia A, Bjørnstad HH, et al. Cardiovascular pre-participation screening of young competitive athletes for prevention of sudden death: proposal for a common European protocol. Consensus Statement of the Study Group of Sport Cardiology of the Working Group of Cardiac Rehabilitation and Exercise Physiology and the Working Group of Myocardial and Pericardial Diseases of the European Society of Cardiology. Eur Heart J 2005;26(5):516–24.
23. Pelliccia A, Maron BJ. Preparticipation cardiovascular evaluation of the competitive athlete: perspectives from the 30-year Italian experience. Am J Cardiol 1995;75(12):827–9.
24. Corrado D, Basso C, Schiavon M, et al. Does sports activity enhance the risk of sudden cardiac death? J Cardiovasc Med (Hagerstown) 2006;7(4):228–33.
25. Kung HC, Hoyert DL, Xu J, et al. Deaths: final data for 2005. Natl Vital Stat Rep 2008;56(10):1–120.
26. Maron BJ, Shirani J, Poliac LC, et al. Sudden death in young competitive athletes. Clinical, demographic, and pathological profiles. JAMA 1996;276(3):199–204.
27. Maron BJ. Hypertrophic cardiomyopathy: a systematic review. JAMA 2002;287(10):1308–20.
28. Maron BJ, Ommen SR, Semsarian C, et al. Hypertrophic cardiomyopathy: present and future, with translation into contemporary cardiovascular medicine. J Am Coll Cardiol 2014;64(1):83–99.
29. D'Silva A, Sharma S. Exercise, the athlete's heart, and sudden cardiac death. Phys Sportsmed 2014;42(2):100–13.
30. Sharma S, Whyte G, Elliott P, et al. Electrocardiographic changes in 1000 highly trained junior elite athletes. Br J Sports Med 1999;33(5):319–24.
31. Rawlins J, Carre F, Kervio G, et al. Ethnic differences in physiological cardiac adaptation to intense physical exercise in highly trained female athletes. Circulation 2010;121(9):1078–85.
32. Fagard RH. Impact of different sports and training on cardiac structure and function. Cardiol Clin 1997;15(3):397–412.
33. Baggish AL, Hutter AM Jr, Wang F, et al. Cardiovascular screening in college athletes with and without electrocardiography: a cross-sectional study. Ann Intern Med 2010;152(5):269–75.
34. Weisfeldt ML, Sitlani CM, Ornato JP, et al. Survival after application of automatic external defibrillators before arrival of the emergency medical system: evaluation in the resuscitation outcomes consortium population of 21 million. J Am Coll Cardiol 2010;55(16):1713–20.
35. "Fabrice Muamba was 'dead' for 78 minutes – Bolton doctor". BBC Sport. 2012-03-21. Available at: http://www.bbc.co.uk/sport/0/football/17460781. Accessed January 5, 2015.
36. A drive to buy AED devices for local schools a success. Available at: http://www.postindependent.com/article/20121207/COMMUNITY_NEWS/121209964. Accessed January 5, 2015.

The Cardiovascular Physiology of Sports and Exercise

Mildred A. Opondo, MD[a,b,c], Satyam Sarma, MD[a,b,c],
Benjamin D. Levine, MD[a,b,c],*

KEYWORDS

- Exercise • Physiology • Athlete • $\dot{V}O_2$

KEY POINTS

- Exercise and sports performance are influenced by the ability of the cardiovascular system to meet the increased metabolic demand for oxygen by the working muscles.
- The 'athlete's' heart phenomenon involving physiologic hypertrophy and resting sinus bradycardia is among the mechanisms that facilitate a high stroke volume and cardiac output during exercise.
- Graded exercise tests are used to assess peak $\dot{V}O_2$. Other aspects of exercise testing may also be relevant for evaluating sports performance.
- When testing of athletes, it is critical to use a test that closely matches the demands of the sport, including training and competition.
- The level of supervision needed during an exercise test should be determined by the clinician before test and depends on the underlying cardiovascular risk of the individual being tested.

INTRODUCTION

Elite athletes are paragons of physical fitness in our society, and an entire "sports–industrial complex" has developed from playing, watching, and marketing sports.[1] A better understanding of the physiologic factors underlying the human body's ability to perform and sustain high workloads has helped to push sports science into a prominent role in athletic training.

Disclosures: The authors have no conflicts to disclose.
[a] Institute for Exercise and Environmental Medicine, 7232 Greenville Avenue, Suite 435, Dallas, TX 75231, USA; [b] Texas Health Presbyterian Hospital Dallas, 8200 Walnut Hill Lane, Dallas, TX 75231, USA; [c] Department of Internal Medicine, University of Texas Southwestern Medical Center, 5323 Harry Hines Boulevard, Dallas, TX 75390, USA
* Corresponding author. Institute of Exercise and Environmental Medicine, 7232 Greenville Avenue, Suite 435, Dallas, TX 75321.
E-mail address: BenjaminLevine@Texashealth.org

Clin Sports Med 34 (2015) 391–404
http://dx.doi.org/10.1016/j.csm.2015.03.004
0278-5919/15/$ – see front matter © 2015 Elsevier Inc. All rights reserved.
sportsmed.theclinics.com

Exercise and sports performance depend greatly on the ability of the cardiovascular system to respond to a wide range of metabolic demands and physical exertion. Certain sports, in particular endurance activities, place high demands on the heart and blood vessels to adequately deliver oxygen, remove carbon dioxide, and dissipate heat from exercising muscle. Analogous to a race car engine, the heart forms the core of the response, supplying circulatory power to generate hydraulic pressure. The greater the circulatory power, the more work that can be expended by the body. The regulation of cardiac output in turn is under the control of a complex system of feedback and feedforward signals originating from skeletal muscle metaboreceptors and mechanoreceptors, as well as coming directly from higher order centers in the brain, largely occurring under autonomic control. The integration of these neural reflexes with the cardiovascular system is controlled tightly, yet allows for flexibility such that the body can respond rapidly to changes in exercise intensity.

With habitual endurance exercise training, the cardiovascular system remodels and can undergo a number of changes, leading to improvements in internal cardiac efficiency (lower heart rate for a given cardiac output) and overall exercise capacity or fitness. The remarkable ability of the human body to increase aerobic fitness highlights the plasticity and trainability of the system. This article reviews the basic principles of exercise physiology, cardiovascular adaptations unique to the "athlete's heart," and utility of exercise testing in athletes.

PRINCIPLES OF EXERCISE PHYSIOLOGY

At the most basic level, the primary purpose of the cardiovascular system during physical exertion is to deliver oxygen to exercising muscle to support the metabolic demands of respiring mitochondria. Different sports or activities have different degrees of aerobic and strength requirements and forms the basis for categorization of recreational and competitive sports by the 36th Bethesda conference, which has been updated recently (**Fig. 1**).[2]

Physical activities can be characterized by their degree of dynamic (aerobic) or static (strength) requirements. Indeed, the cardiovascular and skeletal muscle adaptations of an endurance trained athlete are quite different compared with a sprinter and highlight the unique metabolic machinery necessary for each activity. Endurance activities typically place more demand on aerobic respiration and require large increases in cardiac output and a higher density of "slow twitch" skeletal muscle fibers. In contrast, short bursts of explosive activity place significant demands on substrate level phosphorylation to rapidly supply adenosine triphosphate for maximal power generation and rely less on bulk delivery of oxygen to the exercising muscle.

THE OXYGEN CASCADE AND QUANTIFYING AEROBIC FITNESS

The ability to absorb, deliver, and metabolize oxygen determines aerobic fitness. Oxygen uptake ($\dot{V}o_2$) is a direct measure of aerobic capacity and a fundamental concept in sports science. The V denotes "volume" and the dot over the V reflects "rate" and is expressed as liters per minute, but is often scaled by adjusting to body weight as milliliters per minute per kilogram to account for differences in body size. Measuring an individual's maximum $\dot{V}o_2$ provides a useful assessment of cardiorespiratory fitness by integrating the various organ systems (lung, heart, and muscle) involved in generating aerobic power into what is effectively a single variable. The determinants of oxygen uptake can be understood by following the "oxygen cascade," the steps in the respiratory chain that start with oxygen absorption within the lungs to oxidation within the mitochondria.

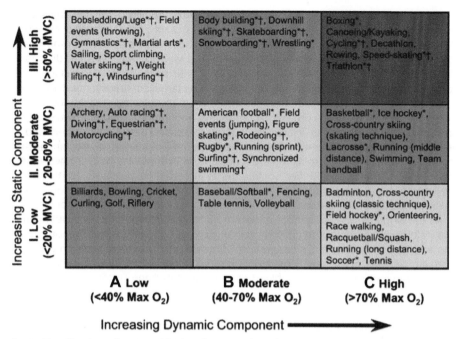

Fig. 1. Classification of sports. This classification is based on peak static and dynamic components achieved during competition. It should be noted, however, that higher values may be reached during training. The increasing dynamic component is defined in terms of the estimated percent of maximal oxygen uptake (Max O_2) achieved and results in an increasing cardiac output. The increasing static component is related to the estimated percent of maximal voluntary contraction (MVC) reached and results in an increasing blood pressure load. The lowest total cardiovascular demands (cardiac output and blood pressure) are shown in the bottom left and the highest in the top right. * Danger of bodily collision. † Increased risk if syncope occurs. (*From* Mitchell JH, Haskell W, Snell P, et al. Task Force 8: Classification of Sports. J Am Coll Cardiol 2005;45(8):1366; with permission.)

Gas exchange and oxygen consumption occur through two main processes, namely, external and internal respiration.

External respiration involves:

i. The movement of air in and out of the lungs; and
ii. The diffusion of oxygen into the pulmonary vasculature as carbon dioxide diffuses out of the blood.

Internal respiration involves:

i. Transportation of oxygen and carbon dioxide within the circulatory system; and
ii. The exchange of oxygen and carbon dioxide between the capillary vasculature and respiring mitochondria.[2,3]

External respiration requires intact alveoli to ensure sufficient oxygenation and ventilation (VE) at the atmospheric interface, and also requires adequate perfusion of aerated lung zones to allow for circulatory uptake. Internal respiration depends greatly on the arterial oxygen carrying capacity as well as the ability of the heart and blood vessels to deliver oxygen to the mitochondria.

At rest, the metabolic requirements of the body are dominated by the brain, liver, and kidneys. In general, most individuals have a resting metabolic rate of about 3.5 mL/min/kg, which is termed 1 MET or "metabolic equivalent." During exercise, there is an increased demand for oxygen by the working muscle such that more than 80% of blood flow during exercise is directed toward exercising muscle. This large increase in muscle blood flow is supported by large increases in cardiac output (heart rate × stroke volume) that at maximal aerobic exercise can reach levels 4 to 6 times that at rest, and even greater in competitive endurance athletes.[4,5] The increase in cardiac output is driven initially by a large increase in stroke volume owing to increased venous return as the skeletal muscle pump is engaged, as well as redistribution of blood from the splanchnic circulation. As exercise intensity increases, the heart rate increases and further contributes to increases in cardiac output. A large, well-conditioned, long-distance athlete, such as cross-country skier or rower, can augment cardiac output to more than 40 L/min.

As the working muscles extract oxygen from the capillaries, there is a widening of the difference between arterial and venous oxygen concentrations. This is termed the arterial venous oxygen difference (AV-O_2 difference) and depends on both the carrying capacity of oxygen by the blood and the oxidative potential of mitochondria. The oxygen carrying capacity of blood can be calculated as:

$$CaO_2(mL/dL) = [Hgb] \times 1.36 \times SaO_2 + (0.0031) \times Pao_2$$

Where [Hgb] is hemoglobin concentration (g/dL), SaO_2 is percent Hgb saturated with oxygen, and Pao_2 is the partial pressure of oxygen within the blood stream. As an example, if the [Hgb] is 14 g/dL and Pao_2 is 100 mm Hg, the oxygen content of arterial blood is 19 mL/dL or 190 mL per liter of blood. Because the vast majority of oxygen in blood is bound to Hgb, the latter part of the equation accounting for dissolved O_2 can be mostly ignored, except perhaps under hyperbaric conditions. As exercise intensity increases, the venous [Hgb] saturation of blood decreases as oxygen is extracted and can reach as low as 25% at maximal exercise. Using the same example, venous oxygen concentration decreases to 5 mL/dL yielding an AV-O_2 difference of 14 mL/dL.

Low Hgb mass decreases the AV-O_2 difference by lowering arterial oxygen content. Conversely, high Hgb mass can increase oxygen carrying capacity such that a 1 g/dL increase in Hgb concentration can increase arterial oxygen content by 7% to 10%, depending on the starting Hgb. The effectiveness of increasing [Hgb] in improving aerobic capacity forms the rationale behind red blood cell or erythropoietin doping, as well as most altitude training concepts.[6]

Exercise training can also improve the peripheral extraction of oxygen from the bloodstream, independent of any changes in Hgb mass. Indeed, the earliest improvements in aerobic fitness with training, particularly in previously sedentary individuals, occur largely owing to improvements in mitochondrial and capillary density, changes in oxidative fiber types, and increased muscle mass.[7] These adaptations occur early in the training response, well before changes within the central cardiac system.

Knowing the cardiac output (Qc), that is, delivery of oxygen, and AV-O_2 difference, that is, oxygen utilization, the rate of oxygen uptake ($\dot{V}o_2$) can be determined by the Fick equation:

$$\dot{V}o_2 = Q_C \times (AV-O_2)$$

$\dot{V}o_2$ is rarely calculated by the Fick equation owing to the difficulty of measuring cardiac output during exercise and the need for catheters to sample arterial and mixed venous blood directly. Instead, $\dot{V}O_2$ is measured most commonly using metabolic carts to assess changes in respiratory gas fractions and volumes. **Fig. 2** illustrates how the various components of the Fick equation, namely cardiac output and arteriovenous oxygen difference, respond during increasing levels of workload and oxygen extraction by the working muscle.

During submaximal exercise, an almost linear relationship exists between cardiac output and oxygen uptake as exercise progresses before volitional exhaustion. As exercise intensity increases, the muscles extract more oxygen and, therefore, the arteriovenous oxygen difference widens. Heart rate varies at rest depending on the participant's position, sitting versus standing. As the exercise workload increases, so does the heart rate and oxygen uptake in an almost linear relationship. Stroke volume at rest also depends on the participant's posture. Once oxygen uptake reaches about 40% of its maximal value, stroke volume increases to about 85% of its maximal value. As exercise intensity and oxygen uptake increase further, a continued increase in stroke volume occurs, at least in fit individuals.[3,8]

Maximal Oxygen Uptake

Maximal aerobic power, also called maximal $\dot{V}O_2$, is an important metric that defines the aerobic limits of the cardiopulmonary system. The term "peak $\dot{V}O_2$" is used generally when a graded exercise test is performed without documenting a plateau of $\dot{V}O_2$ with increasing work rate, and refers to the highest value obtained during the test averaged over at least 30 to 45 seconds. The $\dot{V}O_{2max}$ is governed by the Fick equation as mentioned, and has long been regarded as a valuable physiologic measure associated with performance in endurance sports.[3,9] Saltin and Astrand,[10] in one of the earliest studies supporting the link between $\dot{V}O_2$ max and athletic performance, measured the $\dot{V}O_2$ max of 95 males and 38 females representing the Swedish National Team in a variety of endurance sports. The mean $\dot{V}O_2$ max for the fittest 15 males was 5.8 L/min and was 3.6 L/min for the fittest 10 female athletes. Subsequent studies have confirmed consistently the association between athletic performance and $\dot{V}O_2$ max. For example, Foster and colleagues,[11] in a study involving 26 distance runners, measured the athletes' $\dot{V}O_2$ max and finish times in 1-, 2-, and 6-mile races. There was a strong correlation between running time and $\dot{V}O_2$ max, accounting for nearly 75% of the variation in completion times. However, when only groups of very high fitness are considered, the relationship between race performance and $\dot{V}O_{2max}$ may be less robust, because other factors influence the final time on the stop watch.

The $\dot{V}O_2$ max is expressed in either absolute or relative terms. Absolute $\dot{V}O_2$ max is measured in liters per minute (L.min^{-1}) or milliliters per minute (mL.min^{-1}). It is important to note that $\dot{V}O_2$ is directly related to body size with the assumption that larger individuals will have higher $\dot{V}O_2$ owing to increased muscle mass. Therefore, relative $\dot{V}O_2$ measured in mL.kg^{-1}.min^{-1} is usually reported to account for the differences in body weights between individuals. A conundrum exists, however, in the assessment of relative $\dot{V}O_2$ max in individuals who are obese and have larger body mass owing to an increase in fat mass, a less metabolically active tissue than muscle during exercise. In these individuals, $\dot{V}O_2$ scaled to lean body mass may be the better marker of aerobic fitness, because $\dot{V}O_2$ adjusted to total body mass likely underestimates their cardiorespiratory fitness.[12] In keeping with our car analogy at the beginning of this article, a perfectly strong and powerful Volkswagen engine will still have a hard time driving a large truck up a steep hill.

In addition to body weight, other factors that influence $\dot{V}O_2$ max are age and sex. With aging, $\dot{V}O_2$ max declines 5% per decade during early middle life (ages 30–64), but accelerates to 20% per decade after age 70.[13] The decrease in peak cardiac

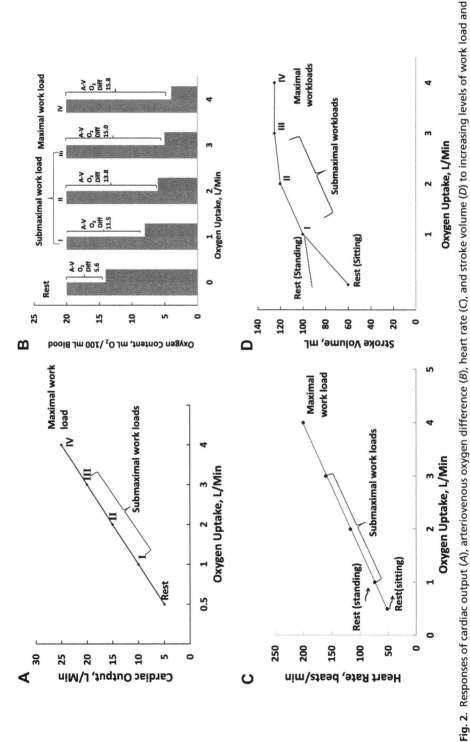

Fig. 2. Responses of cardiac output (*A*), arteriovenous oxygen difference (*B*), heart rate (*C*), and stroke volume (*D*) to increasing levels of work load and oxygen uptake. (*From* Mitchell JH, Blomqvist G. Maximal oxygen uptake. N Engl J Med 1971;284(18):1019; with permission from Massachusetts Medical Society.)

output is largely responsible for this decline in aerobic fitness, primarily owing to decreases in maximal achievable heart rate observed with aging.[14] However, the maintenance of lifelong active lifestyles with regular exercise can preserve $\dot{V}o_2$ to almost youthful levels. In Masters Athletes, defined as individuals older than 40 years who participate in competitive events, peak $\dot{V}o_2$ levels are often similar to much younger individuals.[15] Interestingly, even Masters Athletes are not immune from age-related declines and actually exhibit greater decrements in absolute $\dot{V}o_2$, although with similar relative declines, compared with sedentary, age-matched controls.[16,17]

In addition to age, sex is an important factor in aerobic performance and largely reflects differences in stroke volume between men and women, as well as differences in body composition. The larger body mass in men correlates with higher maximal cardiac output and, therefore, higher peak $\dot{V}o_2$. Even when adjusted for body surface area, men tend to have larger stroke volume indices at peak exercise.[18] The differences between sexes in relative maximal $\dot{V}o_2$ is attenuated (but not eliminated) if adjusted for fat-free mass, suggesting that some of the differences in aerobic fitness are a result of increased adiposity in women.

Thus, although $\dot{V}o_2$ max is a useful measure of overall fitness because it provides an integrated measure of cardiopulmonary and skeletal muscle function, certain caveats must be taken into account when assessing an individual's fitness and potential athletic performance. Peak $\dot{V}o_2$ must be understood within the context of age, sex, training status, and body fat content. Although it is difficult to ascribe "normal" values for peak $\dot{V}o_2$ and fitness for an individual, population-derived data established by the American College of Sports Medicine and Cooper Clinic can provide a helpful context for interpretation.[19]

The Athlete's Heart

Habitual exercise training leads to changes in cardiac structure and function. The most common observation in highly trained endurance sports participants is enlargement of all cardiac chambers and the presence of resting sinus bradycardia. Termed the "athlete's heart," the physiologic hypertrophy that occurs with repetitive bouts of sustained aerobic training reflects the cardiovascular system's adaptation to ensure adequate delivery of oxygen to exercising muscle in an efficient and effective manner. Described as early as the 19th century, advances in echocardiography, MRI, and understanding of molecular signaling pathways, have shed insight into the dramatic changes that progressively lead to cardiac enlargement.

The primary stimulus for cardiac chamber enlargement seems to be a repetitive volume challenge for the heart incurred during training. Although it is unclear what "dose," that is, frequency, duration, and intensity, of aerobic exercise is required to induce cardiac remodeling, at least 4 to 5 sessions per week of moderate aerobic activity is associated with increased cardiac chamber size[20] and can develop in as little as 1 year in young, but previously sedentary individuals. Given sufficient aerobic training impulse, changes in left and right ventricular morphology can be seen as early as 3 months, with the left ventricle displaying increases in mass (concentric hypertrophy) followed by enlargement (eccentric hypertrophy) with continued training.[21] Ventricular enlargement leads to a higher end-diastolic volume reserve, such that increasing stroke volume during exercise can be accomplished using the Starling mechanism, a process that is more energy efficient than increasing cardiac contractility.[22] The Starling mechanism describes the relationship between ventricular pressure and stroke volume. As ventricular filling pressure increases, the myofilaments within the myocyte are stretched, allowing for more actin–myosin cross-bridge formation and greater generation of contractile force.

The larger cardiac chambers are also associated with a more compliant or "flexible" ventricle. For any given filling pressure, the athlete's heart is much larger and distensible than the heart of a nonathlete.[23] The high compliance of the ventricular chamber really distinguishes the physiologic adaptation to chronic exercise training from pathologic conditions that can also be associated with cardiac hypertrophy, such as uncontrolled hypertension and systolic heart failure. The large flexible ventricle can easily adapt to increases in preload that occur with exercise and, in turn, can expel blood in an energy-efficient manner.

In addition to chamber enlargement, as noted, left ventricular mass and wall thickness also increases with training. The degree of thickening depends on gender and ethnicity. Athletes of African descent tend to have thicker ventricular walls than Caucasian athletes,[24] and women, even when adjusted for smaller body size, undergo less physiologic hypertrophy compared with men.[25]

Exercise Testing in Athletes

A graded exercise test (GXT) is a supervised and controlled exercise activity during which an individual exercises at gradually increasing workloads. Typically, treadmill walking or running, or stationery cycle ergometry are common modes of testing. The purpose of the GXT in athletes is 4-fold:

i. To evaluate baseline fitness and prescribe an exercise program or training thresholds;
ii. To evaluate continued progress after engaging in exercise training over a period of time;
iii. To diagnose cardiopulmonary conditions affecting exercise performance; and
iv. To provoke arrhythmias or evaluate hemodynamic response to exercise in an athlete with a known cardiovascular condition, and to determine whether it is safe to participate in competitive sports.

Thus, the key to evaluating athletes is to create a protocol that addresses the aforementioned questions and reproduces the demands of the sport. Relying on a standard Bruce protocol, common to many clinical exercise laboratories, may be an inadequate testing modality, particularly if the athlete is engaged in intermittent, explosive, and high-intensity bouts of exercise. If questions regarding sport-specific limitations are to be answered, recreating an athletic event's unique metabolic demand can provide more accurate insight into factors that limit performance.

Determinants of Performance Capacity

Exercise testing can provide a comprehensive evaluation of an athlete's performance capabilities. Measurement of (1) maximal oxygen uptake ($\dot{V}o_2$ max), (2) maximal steady state (MSS), (3) economy, and (4) anaerobic capacity describe an individual's exercise abilities under a variety of conditions. Maximal oxygen uptake has been described elsewhere in this article and, although it is a useful measure of maximal aerobic power, it does not characterize an athlete's performance at submaximal workloads, a level more commonly encountered during sports competition.

MSS is an important concept that describes an equilibrium point between the cardiac (supply) and skeletal muscle metabolic (demand) systems at which exercise intensity can be sustained for prolonged periods of time. MSS usually is between 50% and 70% of $\dot{V}o_2$ max, but in highly trained athletes, it can be as high as 95%. A high MSS allows an athlete to work near maximal aerobic power for very long periods of time, assuming adequate oxidative fuel (fatty acids, glycogen) stores and is the pace at which a good competitive marathon is run.

An individual's MSS can be identified by measuring ventilatory threshold or onset of blood lactate accumulation (OBLA). As aerobic work increases, the high glycolytic flux results not only in increased Kreb's cycle throughput, but also in increased pyruvate and lactate metabolism. At a certain point, lactate production exceeds the body's ability for clearance and lactate begins to accumulate. Commonly referred to as the "anaerobic threshold," this concept is better referred to as either the ventilatory or lactate threshold, depending on how it is actually measured. The concept of an anaerobic threshold implies a distinct onset of nonoxidative or glycolytic metabolism when in fact, glycolysis and substrate level phosphorylation occurs throughout exercise. OBLA more accurately describes the biochemical processes that occur at MSS, namely, the buildup of lactate owing to an imbalance between clearance and production.

Economy is also an important concept in exercise physiology, relating the work generated by exercising muscle to actual physical work accomplished. The slope of $\dot{V}o_2$ to physical work performed (commonly measured in Watts) is economy. The steeper the slope, that is, higher $\dot{V}o_2$ for the same work rate, the less economical an activity. Walking or cycling is very economical, whereas swimming is highly uneconomical with only 10% conversion of energy generated by the body into actual physical work.[26] Habitual exercise training can improve economy by improved neuromechanical coupling and coordination, changes in muscle fiber type, and ergonomic adaptations that lower $\dot{V}o_2$ requirements for similar work rates. Runners who have high economy (lower slope) are able to run at faster speeds for a similar $\dot{V}o_2$.

Last, anaerobic capacity is a measure of substrate-level phosphorylation capacity. For events that require short bouts of explosive activity (very rapid increase in work rate), high rates of substrate-level phosphorylation and regeneration are necessary to produce adenosine triphosphate in a short time frame before cardiac responses can adequately be ramped up to meet metabolic demand. This lag in cardiac response can be buffered by phosphocreatine or glycolytic stores that generate adenosine triphosphate essentially "anaerobically." The difference between the $\dot{V}o_2$ measured during "anaerobic work" and that measured if the work rate was increased gradually ("aerobically") represents the anaerobic capacity. Anaerobic capacity is an important parameter for short distance sprinters or athletes engaged in sudden bursts of high-intensity activity.

Contraindications to Exercise Testing

In athletes, who are presumably mostly healthy relative to the general population and therefore low risk with regard to the American College of Sports Medicine's risk classification, the overall risk for cardiac events during exercise testing may be low. However, adherence to the contraindications to exercise testing outlined by the American Heart Association/American College of Cardiology is of importance.[27]

Exercise Test Supervision

Major complications of exercise testing range from orthopedic injury, hemodynamic instability, cardiac arrhythmias, and myocardial infarction to death. When done under proper supervision, exercise stress testing entails a very small but finite risk with about 0 to 6 deaths or cardiac arrests per 10,000 tests and 2 to 10 myocardial infarctions per 10,000 tests. The American College of Cardiology/American Heart Association, in their clinical competency statement for exercise testing, recommend that testing should be performed under the supervision of a properly trained physician or individual incorporating appropriate technique and safety measures. The supervising physician or individual should be clear on the indications and contraindications of the test, know the normal endpoints and abnormal responses that call for test termination, and must be able to interpret the results (**Box 1**). Nonphysicians who supervise exercise tests must have sufficient knowledge of exercise physiology and the ability to recognize important changes in electrocardiographic rhythm and repolarization and other cognitive skills and competencies, as clearly outlined by the American College of Cardiology/American Heart Association.[28] A medical history, physical examination, and standard 12-lead electrocardiogram obtained before the graded exercise test can guide the determination of the level of supervision required for the test.[29]

VARIABLES MONITORED DURING EXERCISE TESTING AND THEIR PHYSIOLOGIC INTERPRETATION
Perceived Exertion

Perceived exertion is a subjective measure of the intensity of exertion as determined by the participant and it provides an indication of the relative fatigue. A rating of perceived exertion (RPE) scale used should be clearly explained to the participant before the test begins. Ratings of perceived exertion are obtained during the last 5 seconds of each exercise stage or every 2 minutes during ramp protocols. The 6 to 20 Borg scale is a commonly used RPE scale, with higher numbers indicating a higher level of fatigue. This scale was derived to represent the range of heart rate responses for a healthy young individual (possible range, 60–200).

Ventilatory Threshold

Immediately after beginning exercise, VE increases as a linear function of oxygen uptake until 45% to 65% of peak or $\dot{V}o_2$ max in healthy, untrained individuals and at a higher percentage in endurance trained individuals. The VT is the point at which

---

Box 1
General indications for stopping a graded exercise test in low-risk adults

- Onset of angina or angina-like symptoms
- A significant drop in systolic blood pressure (>10 mm Hg) from baseline blood pressure despite an increase in workload.
- Excessive increase in blood pressure (SBP >250 mm Hg or DBP >115 mm Hg).
- Dyspnea, wheezing, leg cramps, or claudication.
- Signs of poor perfusion such as dizziness, pallor, cyanosis, and ataxia.
- Failure of heart rate to increase with an increase in exercise intensity.
- A change in heart rhythm.
- Participant requests to stop the test.
- Severe fatigue; physical or verbal manifestation.
- Failure of testing equipment.

Abbreviations: DBP, diastolic blood pressure; SBP, systolic blood pressure.

Adapted from Gibbons RJ, Balady GJ, Bricker JT, et al. ACC/AHA 2002 guideline update for exercise testing: summary article. A report of the American College of Cardiology/American Heart Association Task Force on Practice Guidelines (committee to update the 1997 exercise testing guidelines). J Am Coll Cardiol 2002;40(8):1531–40.

the linear relationship changes as VE begins to increase exponentially relative to $\dot{V}O_2$ and corresponds with the onset of blood lactate accumulation.

Peak Respiratory Exchange Ratio

The respiratory exchange ratio (RER) is the ratio of carbon dioxide output (VCO_2) and $\dot{V}O_2$ obtained from the ventilatory expired gas analysis. During the exercise test, as the intensity of exercise is increased, lactate production increases and, as a result of lactate buffering, VCO_2 increases faster than $\dot{V}O_2$. This change in the $VCO_2/\dot{V}O_2$ ratio is consistent in all populations and makes the peak RER a reasonable gauge of a participant's effort. A peak RER of 1.10 or greater indicates a near maximal effort.

Minute Ventilation–Carbon Dioxide Output

The relationship between pulmonary VE and VCO_2 is a useful assessment of ventilatory efficiency. During exercise, VE is tightly coupled to VCO_2 because VE is driven by the amount of carbon dioxide produced. A VE/VCO_2 of less than 30 is considered normal for any age or gender. It is a highly reliable test that is not influenced by mode of exercise testing or type of protocol used.[2] VE/VCO_2 values of greater than 35 are associated with a variety of physiologic scenarios, including VE perfusion mismatch, decreased cardiac output, diminished heart rate variability, or an abnormal chemoreceptor sensitivity, which exaggerates the ventilatory response to exercise. It is important to evaluate the VE/VCO_2 relationship in the middle range of an exercise test and avoid low-intensity and high-intensity (above the ventilatory threshold) sections of the test.

Blood Pressure Response

During dynamic upright exercise, the expected blood pressure response is a progressive increase in systolic blood pressure, a slight decrease or no change in diastolic blood pressure, and a widening pulse pressure. An inadequate increase (<20–30 mm Hg) or a decrease of greater than 10 mm Hg from baseline is an abnormal response that may indicate myocardial ischemia, aortic outflow obstruction, severe left ventricular dysfunction, pulmonary hypertension, or antihypertensive therapy.

A systolic blood pressure of greater than 250 mm Hg or diastolic pressure of greater than 115 requires a termination of the test,[30] although it should be recognized that athletes often achieve blood pressures much greater than this during competition or intense training. Rowing and weight lifting[31,32] both can cause extreme hypertension. During postexercise recovery, systolic blood pressure declines progressively.

Heart Rate Response and Recovery

Heart rate responds to exercise with a progressively linear rise that is partly owing to a reduction in vagal tone, especially at the onset of exercise or at relatively low intensities, and then is sustained and enhanced by sympathetic activation and epinephrine release.

Recovery of the heart rate immediately after exercise is owing to reactivation of the vagal tone. A delayed decrease in heart rate after exercise is a powerful predictor of overall mortality independent of myocardial ischemia or changes in heart rate during exercise.[33] Despite the lack of standardized criteria, a decrease in the heart rate of less than 12 beats per minute 1 minute after stopping exercise is considered abnormal.[34]

SUMMARY

Exercise physiology has helped our understanding of the remarkable processes and adaptations that underlie human athletic performance. The cardiovascular system forms the core of this response allowing for the delivery of oxygen, removal of carbon dioxide, and dissipation of heat across a wide range of physical work rates. The plasticity of the cardiac system is well-reflected in the ability of the athlete to remodel his or her heart with habitual exercise training. There is a growing interest by athletes to maximize their exercise training and performance in competition. Exercise science has grown in leaps and bounds to provide a dynamic and comprehensive understanding of the cardiovascular system's adaptation to training for improved efficiency of oxygen delivery to the exercising muscles via cardiac remodeling. Athletes are increasingly aware of modern exercise science and frequently present to clinicians involved in sports medicine for exercise testing for the assessment of their fitness levels, modification of their training regimens, and for diagnostic purposes. Modern exercise science allows for sophisticated testing to meet these needs and it is important for clinicians involved in sports medicine to understand the unique attributes of an individual's competitive event and tailor testing to the athlete's needs.

REFERENCES

1. Eitzen DS. Fair and foul: beyond the myths and paradoxes of sport. Plymouth (United Kingdom): Rowman and Littlefield; 2012.
2. Balady GJ, Arena R, Sietsema K, et al. Clinician's guide to cardiopulmonary exercise testing in adults a scientific statement from the American heart association. Circulation 2010;122(2):191–225.
3. Mitchell JH, Blomqvist G. Maximal oxygen uptake. N Engl J Med 1971;284(18): 1018.
4. Bassett D, Howley ET. Limiting factors for maximum oxygen uptake and determinants of endurance performance. Med Sci Sports Exerc 2000;32(1):70–84.
5. Levine BD. VO2max: what do we know, and what do we still need to know? J Physiol 2008;586(1):25–34.
6. Levine BD, Stray-Gundersen J. "Living high-training low": effect of moderate-altitude acclimatization with low-altitude training on performance. J Appl Physiol (1985) 1997;83(1):102–12.
7. Coggan AR, Spina RJ, King DS, et al. Skeletal muscle adaptations to endurance training in 60- to 70-yr-old men and women. J Appl Physiol (1985) 1992;72(5): 1780–6.
8. Carrick-Ranson G, Hastings JL, Bhella PS, et al. The effect of lifelong exercise dose on cardiovascular function during exercise. J Appl Physiol (1985) 2014; 116(7):736–45.
9. Heyward VH, Gibson A. Advanced fitness assessment and exercise prescription. 7th edition. Champaign (IL): Human Kinetics; 2014.
10. Salting B, Astrand P-O. Maximal oxygen uptake in athletes. J Appl Physiol (1985) 1967;23(3):6.
11. Foster C, Costill D, Daniels J, et al. Skeletal muscle enzyme activity, fiber composition and VO2 max in relation to distance running performance. Eur J Appl Physiol 1978;39(2):73–80.
12. Goran M, Fields DA, Hunter GR, et al. Total body fat does not influence maximal aerobic capacity. Int J Obes Relat Metab Disord 2000;24(7):841–8.
13. Fleg JL, Morrell CH, Bos AG, et al. Accelerated longitudinal decline of aerobic capacity in healthy older adults. Circulation 2005;112(5):674–82.

14. Fleg JL, O'Connor F, Gerstenblith G, et al. Impact of age on the cardiovascular response to dynamic upright exercise in healthy men and women. J Appl Physiol (1985) 1995;78(3):890–900.
15. Stevenson ET, Davy KP, Seals DR. Maximal aerobic capacity and total blood volume in highly trained middle-aged and older female endurance athletes. J Appl Physiol (1985) 1994;77(4):1691–6.
16. Trappe SW, Costill DL, Vukovich MD, et al. Aging among elite distance runners: a 22-yr longitudinal study. J Appl Physiol (1985) 1996;80(1):285–90.
17. Tanaka H, Desouza CA, Jones PP, et al. Greater rate of decline in maximal aerobic capacity with age in physically active vs sedentary healthy women. J Appl Physiol (1985) 1997;83(6):1947–53.
18. Ogawa T, Spina RJ, Martin WH 3rd, et al. Effects of aging, sex, and physical training on cardiovascular responses to exercise. Circulation 1992;86(2): 494–503.
19. Amercian College of Sports Medicine. Guidelines for exercise testing and prescription. 6th edition. Baltimore (MD): Lippincot Williams & Wilkins; 2000.
20. Bhella PS, Hastings JL, Fujimoto N, et al. Impact of lifelong exercise "dose" on left ventricular compliance and distensibility. J Am Coll Cardiol 2014;64(12):1257–66.
21. Arbab-Zadeh A, Perhonen M, Howden E, et al. Cardiac remodeling in response to 1 year of intensive endurance training. Circulation 2014;130:2152–61.
22. Crawford MH, Petru MA, Rabinowitz C. Effect of isotonic exercise training on left ventricular volume during upright exercise. Circulation 1985;72(6):1237–43.
23. Levine BD, Lane LD, Buckey JC, et al. Left ventricular pressure-volume and Frank-Starling relations in endurance athletes. Implications for orthostatic tolerance and exercise performance. Circulation 1991;84(3):1016–23.
24. Basavarajaiah S, Boraita A, Whyte G, et al. Ethnic differences in left ventricular remodeling in highly-trained athletes relevance to differentiating physiologic left ventricular hypertrophy from hypertrophic cardiomyopathy. J Am Coll Cardiol 2008;51(23):2256–62.
25. Pelliccia A, Maron BJ, Culasso F, et al. Athlete's heart in women. Echocardiographic characterization of highly trained elite female athletes. JAMA 1996; 276(3):211–5.
26. Baudinette RV. The energetics and cardiorespiratory correlates of mammalian terrestrial locomotion. J Exp Biol 1991;160:209–31.
27. Gibbons RJ, Balady GJ, Bricker JT, et al. ACC/AHA 2002 guideline update for exercise testing: summary article. A report of the American College of Cardiology/American Heart Association Task Force on Practice Guidelines (committee to update the 1997 exercise testing guidelines). J Am Coll Cardiol 2002;40(8):1531–40.
28. Rodgers GP, Ayanian JZ, Balady G, et al. American College of Cardiology/American Heart Association Clinical Competence statement on stress testing: a report of the American College of Cardiology/American Heart Association/American College of Physicians–American Society of Internal Medicine Task Force on Clinical Competence. J Am Coll Cardiol 2000;36(4):1441–53.
29. Fletcher GF, Ades PA, Kligfield P, et al. Exercise standards for testing and training: a scientific statement from the American Heart Association. Circulation 2013;128(8):873–934.
30. American College of Sports Medicine (ACSM). ACSM's guidelines for exercise testing and prescription. Philadelphia: Lippincott Williams & Wilkins; 2013.
31. Clifford PS, Hanel B, Secher NH. Arterial blood pressure response to rowing. Med Sci Sports Exerc 1994;26(6):715–9.

32. MacDougall JD, Tuxen D, Sale DG, et al. Arterial blood pressure response to heavy resistance exercise. J Appl Physiol 1985;58(3):785–90.

33. Cole CR, Blackstone EH, Pashkow FJ, et al. Heart-rate recovery immediately after exercise as a predictor of mortality. N Engl J Med 1999;341(18):1351–7.

34. Lauer M, Froelicher ES, Williams M, et al. Exercise testing in asymptomatic adults a statement for professionals from the American Heart Association Council on Clinical Cardiology, subcommittee on exercise, cardiac rehabilitation, and prevention. Circulation 2005;112(5):771–6.

Cardiovascular Adaptation and Remodeling to Rigorous Athletic Training

 CrossMark

Rory B. Weiner, MD, Aaron L. Baggish, MD*

KEYWORDS

- Cardiac remodeling • Exercise • Sports • Endurance

KEY POINTS

- Exercise-induced cardiac remodeling is an adaptive process during which the cardinal hemodynamic stresses of pressure and volume lead to changes in cardiac structure and function.
- The morphology and magnitude of cardiac adaptation to sport are determined by numerous factors including age, gender, ethnicity, sporting discipline, and underlying genetics.
- Numerous unanswered clinical and scientific questions regarding exercise-induced cardiac remodeling remain and serve as a motivation for important future work.

INTRODUCTION

Adaptation is the process by which an organism changes structure, function, or behavior in response to an environmental condition in an effort to improve fitness or performance. Humans are remarkably adaptable and the numerous changes in cardiac structure and function that develop in response to repetitive bouts of vigorous physical exercise represent one of the most robust examples of our adaptive capability. During exercise, the cardiovascular system is exposed to variable and exercise discipline–specific amounts of hemodynamic stress in the forms of pressure and volume. If the exercise stimulus occurs with sufficient intensity, duration, and frequency, the cardiovascular system remodels in response to these cardinal forms of stress. In aggregate, specific changes in cardiac morphology and function that occur in response to exercise serve to minimize the energy cost of continued exercise exposure and simultaneously serve to enhance athletic performance.

Cardiovascular Performance Program, Massachusetts General Hospital, 55 Fruit Street, Boston, MA 02114, USA
* Corresponding author. Cardiovascular Performance Program, Massachusetts General Hospital, Yawkey Suite 5B, 55 Fruit Street, Boston, MA 02114.
E-mail address: abaggish@partners.org

Clin Sports Med 34 (2015) 405–418
http://dx.doi.org/10.1016/j.csm.2015.03.007
0278-5919/15/$ – see front matter © 2015 Elsevier Inc. All rights reserved.

Cardiac enlargement in athletes was first described by Henschen and Darling in 1899.[1,2] Using the rudimentary yet elegant physical examination techniques, these 2 pioneering investigators reported marked global cardiac enlargement among endurance-trained athletes. Over the ensuing century, much has been learned about the physiology of exercise-induced cardiac remodeling (EICR). Advances in our understanding of how the cardiovascular system responds to exercise have largely paralleled advances in diagnostic testing. The development of chest radiography and 12-lead electrocardiography set the stage for studies that confirmed Henschen's and Darling's original work and simultaneously shed novel insights on the electrical properties that accompany this phenomenon. Subsequently, noninvasive cardiac imaging, relying first exclusively on echocardiography and now including cardiac CT and MRI imaging, have further enhanced our quantitative understanding of how the heart responds to exercise. This article provides an overview of the relevant physiology, morphologic attributes, and principal determinants of EICR.

OVERVIEW OF RELEVANT EXERCISE PHYSIOLOGY

There is a direct relationship between exercise intensity (external work) and the body's demand for oxygen. Increasing oxygen demand is met by increasing pulmonary oxygen uptake (Vo_2). Peak oxygen consumption (peak Vo_2), a metric commonly measured in clinical practice, is defined as the amount of oxygen uptake/utilization that occurs at an individual athlete's peak level of exercise. The cardiovascular system is responsible for transporting oxygen-rich blood from the lungs to the skeletal muscles, a process that is quantified as cardiac output (liters per minute). The Fick equation [Vo_2 = cardiac output $\times$ (Δ arterial–venous O_2)] can be used to quantify the relationship between cardiac output and Vo_2. In the healthy human, there is a direct and inviolate relationship between Vo_2 and cardiac output.

Cardiac output, the product of stroke volume and heart rate, may increase 5- to 6-fold during maximal exercise effort. Coordinated autonomic nervous system function, characterized by rapid and sustained parasympathetic withdrawal coupled with sympathetic activation, is required for this to occur. Heart rates may range from fewer than 40 beats per minute at rest to greater than 200 beats per minute in a young, maximally exercising athlete. Heart rate increase is responsible for the majority of cardiac output augmentation during exercise. Maximal heart rate varies innately among individuals, decreases with age, and does not increase with exercise training.

In contrast, stroke volume both at rest and during exercise may increase significantly with prolonged exercise training. Stroke volume is defined as the quantity of blood ejected from the heart during each contraction. Cardiac chamber enlargement and the accompanying ability to generate a large stroke volume are direct results of exercise training and are the cardiovascular hallmarks of the endurance-trained athlete. Stroke volume increases during exercise as a result of increases in ventricular end-diastolic volume and, to a lesser degree, sympathetically mediated reduction in end-systolic volume.

Hemodynamic conditions, specifically changes in cardiac output and peripheral vascular resistance, vary widely across sporting disciplines. Although there is considerable overlap, exercise activity can be classified into 2 forms with defining hemodynamic differences. Isotonic exercise, or endurance exercise, involves sustained increases in cardiac output, with normal or reduced peripheral vascular resistance. Such activity represents a primary volume challenge for the heart that affects all 4 chambers. This form of exercise underlies activities such as long-distance running, cycling, rowing, and swimming. In contrast, isometric exercise, or strength training, involves activity characterized by increased peripheral vascular resistance and normal or only slightly increased cardiac output. This increase in peripheral vascular resistance causes transient but potentially marked increases in systolic blood pressure and left ventricular afterload. Strength training is the dominant form of exercise physiology in activities such as weightlifting, track and field throwing events, and American-style football. Many sports, including popular team-based activities, such as soccer, lacrosse, basketball, hockey, and field hockey, involve significant elements of both endurance and strength exercise.

STRUCTURAL AND FUNCTIONAL CARDIAC ADAPTATIONS
The Left Ventricle

The dilated left ventricle
Enlargement of the left ventricle (LV) is common among endurance trained athletes. This represents physiologic, eccentric LV hypertrophy (LVH) characterized by an increase in LV chamber size accompanied by proportionate increase in LV wall thickness. When distinguishing this from LV dilation seen in cardiomyopathic disease states (idiopathic dilated cardiomyopathy, toxin-mediated dilated cardiomyopathy, tachycardia mediated dilated cardiomyopathy, etc), it is important to recognize that pathologic dilation is typically accompanied by normal or reduced LV wall thickness. In general, "cutoff" values for LV end-diastolic diameter are not helpful to identify athletes' heart given overlap between EICR and cardiomyopathic states.

Pelliccia and colleagues[3] reported echocardiographic LV end-diastolic dimensions in a large group (n = 1309) of Italian elite athletes (73% men) representing 38 different sports. LV end-diastolic diameters varied widely from 38 to 66 mm in women (mean, 48 mm) and from 43 to 70 mm in men (mean, 55 mm). LV end-diastolic diameter was 54 mm or greater in 45% and greater than 60 mm in 14% of the cohort. Markedly dilated LV chambers (defined as >60 mm) were associated with increased body mass and were most common among those participating in endurance sports (cross-country skiing, cycling, etc). In clinical practice, 55 to 58 mm is commonly used to define the upper limits of normal for LV end-diastolic dimension,[4] meaning that approximately 40% of male athletes in this study were above the normal reference point. More recently, in a study of nearly 500 university athletes, approximately 25% exceeded the gender recommended limit for LV end-diastolic diameter.[5]

The function of the dilated LV in athletes has also been an area of active investigation. Several studies have examined resting LV systolic function in endurance athletes using cross-sectional, sedentary control study designs and found that LV ejection fraction is generally normal in athletes.[6–9] However, at least 1 study of 147 cyclists participating in the Tour de France found that 11% had an LV ejection fraction of 52% or less,[10] suggesting that healthy endurance athletes may demonstrate mildly reduced LV ejection fraction at rest. Exercise testing can be a very useful adjunct to confirm LV augmentation and to document greater than normal exercise capacity in the hearts of trained athletes.

Recent advances in functional myocardial imaging, including tissue Doppler and speckle tracking echocardiography, have also suggested that endurance exercise training may lead to changes in regional LV systolic function that are not detected by assessment of a global index, such as LV ejection fraction.[11,12] Cross-sectional studies have observed differences in LV rotation and twist when comparing cyclists[12] and soccer players with sedentary controls.[13] Furthermore, changes in LV apical rotation and twist have been identified in a longitudinal study of rowers participating in endurance exercise training.[14] The importance of these findings with respect to understanding functional aspects of EICR and for differentiating athletic from pathologic remodeling is an area of active investigation.

LV diastolic function has also been studied in endurance athletes with dilated LVs. Most studies have used pulsed Doppler (transmitral) and tissue Doppler echocardiography. Endurance exercise training leads to enhanced early diastolic LV filling as assessed by E-wave velocity and mitral annular/LV tissue velocities.[15–17] These changes are owing to a combination of enhanced intrinsic lusitropy and training-induced increases in LV preload. Speckle tracking echocardiography has provided further insight into diastolic function, with enhanced peak early diastolic untwisting rate observed in rowers after 90 days of endurance exercise training.[14] This ability of the LV to relax briskly during early diastole is an essential mechanism of stroke volume preservation during exercise at high heart rates.

The thick left ventricle

Thickening of the LV, without associated LV chamber dilation, occurs infrequently in trained athletes. When LV wall thickening (ie, exercise-induced concentric LVH) occurs, it is most likely in strength (isometric) trained athletes.[18] This often presents a diagnostic challenge given the potential for overlap with mild forms of hypertrophic cardiomyopathy (HCM). Wall thickness "cutoff" values may be helpful, because a LV wall thickness of greater than 15 mm should be considered pathologic until proven otherwise. Additionally, the pattern of LVH may be useful. LVH in strength-trained athletes is typically symmetric, and the presence of asymmetry typically suggests HCM, although this notion has been questioned in a recent study of healthy young athletic men.[19]

Pelliccia and colleagues[20] reported echocardiographic measurements of LV wall thicknesses among 947 elite Italian athletes. Within this exclusively white cohort, a small but significant percentage of athletes (1.7%) had LV wall thicknesses of 13 mm or greater, and all of these individuals had concomitant LV cavity dilation. Sharma and colleagues[21] also reported a low incidence (0.4%) of LV wall thickness greater than 12 mm in 720 elite junior athletes and confirmed that increased LV wall thickness is associated with increased chamber size in young athletes. Furthermore, in a more recent study of nearly 500 collegiate athletes, not a single healthy university athlete had LV wall thickness of greater than 14 mm.[5] In summary, LV wall thickness in excess of 13 mm is a rare finding in healthy athletes, although it can be seen in a small number of healthy, highly trained individuals. This finding is more common in athletes with relatively large body size and those of Afro-Caribbean descent.[22]

Diastolic function evaluation of the thick LV in athlete's heart has been investigated to determine functional correlates and in an effort to differentiate from HCM. Athletes with increased LV wall thickness have shown normal LV diastolic filling by transmitral velocities,[23] whereas most patients with HCM show abnormal Doppler diastolic indices of LV filling.[24] However, use of the transmitral filling pattern as an assessment of diastolic function can be limited, given the load dependency. More recent studies have, therefore, focused on tissue Doppler echocardiography because it is less load dependent.[25] A longitudinal study of male American-style football players with concentric exercise-induced LVH showed relative impairment of LV early diastolic relaxation (E′) velocity by tissue Doppler,[26] and this finding may be explained by resting hypertension in these athletes (Weiner RB, Wang F, Isaacs S, et al: The impact of American style football participation on the development of hypertension and left ventricular hypertrophy. Circulation. 2013. Submitted for publication). The study of diastolic function in strength-trained athletes requires further investigation, although recent evidence does suggest that athletes with thick LV walls have higher E' velocity by tissue Doppler imaging compared with patients with HCM.[27] Furthermore, study of myocardial mechanics and deformation parameters may be a useful adjunct in the assessment of exercise-induced concentric LVH. Specifically, delayed diastolic untwisting in HCM patients may account for increased LV filling pressures and reduced exercise capacity,[28] and analysis of diastolic untwisting in strength athletes is an area of active investigation. Better understanding of strain and twist parameters in strength athletes has the potential to define more clearly this phenotypic form of athletes' heart.

The Right Ventricle

EICR is not confined to the LV. Endurance exercise training requires both the LV and right ventricle (RV) to accept and eject relatively large quantities of blood. Therefore, the cardiovascular response to repetitive endurance training includes biventricular remodeling. For the thin-walled RV, this remodeling typically takes the form of mild to moderate RV dilation without significant concomitant hypertrophy. Importantly, RV dilation in the endurance-trained athlete is associated with LV remodeling (eccentric LVH) and the finding of isolated RV enlargement should raise suspicion of a pathologic process. Furthermore, RV dilation in endurance athletes tends to be a global process, without sacculation, aneurysmal dilation, or segmental dysfunction. Similar to LV dilation, in general strict "cutoff" values for RV end-diastolic diameter are not helpful in distinguishing exercise-related adaptation and pathologic cardiomyopathy.

Biventricular remodeling was documented in an early M-mode echocardiographic study, which demonstrated symmetric RV and LV enlargement in a small cohort of highly trained endurance athletes.[29] In a larger M-mode and 2-dimensional echocardiography study of 127 male elite endurance athletes, the athletes demonstrated significantly larger RV cavities and a trend toward thicker RV free walls compared with historical control subjects.[30] More recently, in an echocardiographic study of 102 endurance athletes, RV chamber dimensions were larger than "normal" values in more than one-half of the athletes and 28% of the athletes had RV outflow tract values greater than the proposed major criteria for arrhythmogenic RV cardiomyopathy.[31] Cardiac MRI studies have also shown that RV enlargement is common among endurance athletes.[32,33] Differentiating exercise-induced RV changes from the diagnosis of arrhythmogenic RV cardiomyopathy is among the most important clinical challenges that can arise, and awareness of the diagnostic criteria for arrhythmogenic RV cardiomyopathy that integrate family history, electrocardiography, and cardiac imaging is essential.[34]

The impact of strength training on the RV has not been as well-studied. A recent echocardiographic study of endurance and strength athletes found that endurance athletes had greater internal RV dimensions, although RV function (systolic strain and diastolic function) were similar between the 2 groups.[35] A longitudinal study of RV structure in collegiate athletes before and after 90 days of team-based exercise training showed significant RV dilation in endurance athletes, but no changes in RV architecture in strength athletes.[26] Further characterization of how the RV responds to different forms of exercise and its contribution to exercise capacity is an important area for future investigation.

In terms of global RV systolic function, a mild reduction in RV function can be considered a physiologic phenomenon because stroke volume at higher end-diastolic volumes will consequently be achieved at a lower ejection fraction. A cardiac MRI study of more than 300 subjects showed that RV ejection fraction was lower compared with nonathletic controls.[36] However, in a recent 3-dimensional echocardiography study, RV systolic indices were comparable between athletes and controls.[37] Therefore, preserved or mildly reduced RV systolic function can be expected in endurance athletes, although severe reductions in global function should be considered abnormal in any athlete. Regional function of the RV has also been assessed in athletes. In endurance athletes, both tissue Doppler and 2-dimensional strain studies have shown reduced systolic deformation in athletes compared with controls.[38,39] However, segments with reduced regional function showed complete normalization at peak exercise, indicating normal contractile reserve.[39]

Atria

An early echocardiographic study showed that endurance athletes have larger left atria (LA) than sedentary controls,[29] and that older individuals with a significant history of exercise training had LA enlargement.[40] Pelliccia and colleagues[41] studied a large number of athletes (n = 1777) and demonstrated that LA enlargement ($\geq$40 mm anterior–posterior dimension by echocardiography) was present in 20% of athletes. Interestingly, atrial fibrillation and other supraventricular tachyarrhythmias proved to be uncommon (prevalence of <1%) and similar to that in the general population, despite the frequency of LA enlargement. More recently, in a study of more than 600 athletes, the LA volume index determined by echocardiography confirmed a high prevalence of LA enlargement in trained athletes, particularly endurance athletes.[42] Recent studies have also begun to examine the right atrium in athletes and have documented an increase in right atrium size in endurance athletes.[35,43]

Atrial function in athletes, assessed with speckle tracking echocardiography, has become an area of active investigation. A longitudinal study of elite female athletes before and after 16 weeks of training showed that LA global peak longitudinal strain and peak atrial contraction strain significantly decreased after training in athletes.[44] In contrast, other studies have not shown differences in atrial strain when comparing athletes and sedentary controls.[35,45] More studies in various groups of athletes are needed before conclusions can be drawn regarding atrial function in the athlete's heart. This information is needed to help determine whether there is a mechanistic relationship between atrial size/function and the potential for increased incidence of atrial arrhythmias in certain athletic populations.[46]

Aorta

The aorta experiences a significant hemodynamic load during exercise and the nature of this load depends on sport type. It has been hypothesized that the pressure overload during strength training may lead to aortic remodeling and a study comparing elite strength-trained athletes and matched controls showed significantly larger aortic dimensions (annulus, sinuses of Valsalva, and proximal ascending aorta) in athletes.[47] Another study compared strength and endurance trained athletes and found that the aortic root diameter was significantly larger in among strength-trained athletes.[48] However, in contrast, in a large study of more than 2000 Italian athletes, the largest aortic root dimensions were observed in endurance-trained athletes, specifically swimmers and cyclists.[49] To help resolve these conflicting data regarding aortic size in athletes, a recent metaanalysis was conducted to determine whether endurance or strength training is associated with increased aortic dimensions. This analysis found that the weighted mean aortic root diameter measured at the sinuses of Valsalva was 3.2 mm larger in athletes compared with nonathletic controls, whereas aortic root size at the aortic valve annulus was 1.6 mm greater in athletes than in controls.[50] Therefore, the present data indicate that athletes have a small and likely clinically insignificant increase in aortic root diameter, and clinicians evaluating athletes should be aware that marked aortic root dilatation likely represents a pathologic process and not physiologic adaptation to exercise.

DETERMINANTS OF ADAPTATION

Cardiovascular adaptations to exercise vary considerably across individual athletes. Explanatory factors including gender, ethnicity, sporting discipline, underlying genetics, and duration of prior exercise exposure explain most but not all of this variability. Available data indicate that female athletes exhibit quantitatively less physiologic remodeling than their male counterparts. In an important early study, Pelliccia and colleagues[51] presented cross-sectional echocardiographic data on 600 elite female Italian athletes and small group of sedentary controls. Athletes in this study demonstrated larger left ventricular end-diastolic cavity dimension (49 ± 4 mm) and greater maximal wall thickness (8.2 ± 0.9 mm) than controls (46 ± 3 mm and 7.2 ± 0.6 mm, respectively; $P<.001$). Compared with data from previously studied male athletes (n = 738), female athletes showed significantly smaller left ventricular cavity dimension (11% less; $P<.001$) and wall thickness (23% less; $P<.001$) and were far less likely to have absolute measurements that exceeded normal cutpoints. Similar findings have been reproduced by numerous investigators.[42,52–56] Although there are conflicting data in the literature, not all of the difference in absolute cardiac dimensions between men and women is eliminated when cardiac dimensions are corrected for the typically smaller female body size. Definitive mechanistic explanation for the gender-specific magnitude of EICR remains elusive.

Ethnicity is also an important determinant of EICR. Most notably, athletes of Afro-Caribbean descent, often termed black athletes, tend to have thicker LV walls than Caucasian athletes. Basavarajaiah and colleagues[57] studied a group of Caucasian and black male athletes using echocardiographic imaging and found that nearly 20% of the black athletes were found to have LV wall thickness of at least 12 mm as compared with 4% of white athletes. Importantly, 3% of black athletes in this cohort were found to have wall thickness of greater than 15 mm. Similarly, Rawlins and colleagues[22] studied ethnicity/race-related differences in a group of 440 black and white female athletes using echocardiography. Black female athletes demonstrated significantly higher left ventricular wall thickness and mass compared with the white women (LV wall thickness = 9.2 ± 1.2 mm, LV mass = 187.2 ± 42 g in the black athletes vs LV wall thickness = 8.6 ± 1.2 mm, LV mass = 172.3 ± 42 g in the white athletes). At present, there are many ethnic populations that participate in athletics that have not been studied.

As discussed in detail, exercise physiology differs markedly across sporting disciplines. In a landmark early paper, Morganroth and colleagues[18] presented cross-sectional echocardiographic data that demonstrated strong associations between sport type and left ventricular morphology. Specifically, athletes participating in sports with predominantly isotonic physiology—swimmers and runners—were found to have larger left ventricular chamber diameters than athletes practicing wrestling, a sport with largely isometric physiology. Although the notion that cardiac dimensions vary as a function of sporting physiology has been challenged,[58] findings similar to those presented by Morganroth and colleagues[18] have been reproduced by other investigators.[26,59,60] It must be emphasized that physiologic dichotomization of sporting disciplines into isometric and isotonic activities is a very simplistic and inherently limited way of defining the cardiac stressors of exercise. Contemporary descriptions of exercise physiology acknowledge the fact that all athletic disciplines involve some element of each form stress.[61] This is best illustrated by considering the broad category of endurance sport that all share in common substantial amounts of isotonic stress but that involve variable amounts of concomitant isometric stress. To what degree cardiac adaptations differ across the specific endurance disciplines has been largely unexplored and represents and an area of important future work.

The genetics of exercise adaptation are an area of active investigation. Initial insights were gained from studies examining polymorphisms within genes coding for proteins of the renin–angiotensin–aldosterone axis. Among military recruits, the angiotensin-converting enzyme DD polymorphism was associated with more LVH than the II polymorphism during 10 weeks of exercise training.[62] Specific polymorphisms of the angiotensinogen gene have been similarly associated with LV remodeling.[63] Further work is required to examine alternative gene candidates in a similar fashion. We previously demonstrated that familial hypertension, as defined by an individual with 1 or both parents with hypertension, is associated with both the magnitude and geometry of LV EICR.[64] Further work is required to determine the genetic and hemodynamic mechanisms underlying this observation. Most recently, animal models of exercise have begun to clarify the molecular pathways that are responsible for cardiac adaptations to exercise. Several molecular mechanisms including the CCAAT/enhancer-binding protein β (C/EBPβ)/CITED4 [CBP/p300-interacting transactivators with E (glutamic acid)/D (aspartic acid)-rich-arboxylterminal domain] pathway and the IGF-1/neuregulin-1 (NRG-1) activated PI3K-AKT1 signaling pathway seems to be central to the process of exercise-induced cardiac remodeling.[65–68] Translational work documenting the role of such pathways in the human response to exercise is required.

Finally, the influence of exercise exposure duration has recently been shown to play a role in the process of cardiac adaptation. Arbab-Zadeh and colleagues[69] used a progressive exercise protocol to prepare 12 sedentary subjects (men, n = 7; age = 29 ± 6 years) for a marathon run (42 km) in which participants advanced through an incremental training protocol that began with light aerobic work characteristic of a clinical cardiac rehab program (1.5–3 h/wk) and progressed to a more intense, recreational endurance athlete regimen (7–9 h/wk).[69] In this setting, the authors observed a biphasic increase in LV mass with initial hypertrophy caused by LV wall thickening (0–6 months) and subsequent hypertrophy attributable to LV dilation (6–12 months). Our group recently completed an observation study in which elite male rowers were followed with serial echocardiography over a 39-month period of high-intensity, team-based training. In this study, we observed a phasic remodeling response with distinct acute adaptations, including increases in LV chamber size, early diastolic function, and systolic twist followed by a chronic phase of adaptation characterized by increasing wall thickness and regression in LV twist. Although many questions about the role of exercise dose remain unanswered, it is increasingly clear that training duration is an important determinant of myocardial structure and function in athletes.

UNCERTAINTIES AND AREAS FOR FUTURE WORK

Although the last century of scientific investigation has led to numerous advances in our understanding of how the heart and vascular system responds to exercise, key areas of uncertainty persist. The dose–response relationship between exercise and cardiac adaptation represents one such area. Although it is well-established that routine, moderate intensity exercise promotes optimal cardiovascular health, several recent studies suggest that increasing "doses" of exercise may come with diminishing returns.[70,71] Although this remains a controversial topic and is not the focus of this paper, it serves to emphasize that we know relatively little about how varying levels of exercise volume and intensity dictate cardiac adaptation. There are several lines of evidence that suggest at least some association between the amount of exercise and the degree of cardiac remodeling. Large, descriptive studies of elite athletes routinely report indices of cardiac chamber volume and mass that exceed those seen in less competitive athlete cohorts. One prior study by our group addressed this question directly by comparing cardiac parameters in international caliber rowers (22 ± 6 hours of weekly training) with those in sub-elite rowers (11 ± 4 hours of weekly training; $P<.001$).[15] In this study, the metrics of both left and right ventricular size were significantly larger in the international-caliber athletes. Although some of the observed differences were accounted for by the significantly larger body sizes of the elite competitors, left ventricular volume, right ventricular volume, and left ventricular mass remained significantly greater after body size correction among the international-level competitors. Owing to the cross-sectional nature of the study design, this effort does not establish a cause and effect link between exercise dose and cardiac size, but serves as a hypothesis generating impetus for more definitive longitudinal studies.

The majority of data describing cardiac adaptation to sport have been derived from studies such as the one noted that examine high-level competitors, leaving questions about whether remodeling occurs in athletes of lower caliber who perform less exercise. Zilinski and colleagues[72] recently conducted a prospective study in which approximately 50 recreational runners were studied with echocardiography before and after an 18-week marathon training plan that consisted of a relatively modest exercise dose of approximately 25 miles per week. Interestingly, many of the adaptations that have been well-described among high-level competitive athletes, including mild eccentric left ventricular hypertrophy, left atrial dilation, and improvements in left ventricular diastolic function, were observed. Although more work is required to characterize the myocardial response to moderate levels of exercise, it does seem that the process of EICR is relevant to more than just elite athletes.

A final point about the exercise dose and cardiac remodeling relationship deserves mention. There are 2 principal components that define the magnitude of exercise the exercise exposure: dose and intensity. The relative contribution of these 2 distinct factors to the process of cardiac remodeling remains completely unknown. The vast majority of studies examining EICR provide quantitation of the exercise exposure as a sole function of duration, usually measured as hours per unit time. This fact is largely one of convenience, because exercise duration is far simpler to measure and report with accuracy than exercise intensity. As such, we know very little about the role of exercise intensity as a determinant of the remodeling process. Although methods that integrate both duration and intensity have been developed and applied in a limited capacity, we are unaware of any studies that have been completed with a primary goal of addressing this important issue. Although speculative, we suspect that both components of the exercise stimulus have independent and perhaps mechanistically discrete effects on cardiac remodeling.

Cardiac remodeling in response to exercise has been viewed traditionally as a benign and even health-promoting phenomenon. However, recent preliminary data suggest that the most extreme degrees of remodeling may be accompanied by some maladaptive attributes. Two complementary studies of high-level master's athletes, men and women with decades of intense, high-volume exercise exposure, have documented the presence of patchy myocardial fibrosis and associated ventricular arrhythmias.[73,74] When considered in tandem, these provocative cross-sectional studies raise the possibility that extreme amounts of exercise may lead to an ultimately maladaptive form of cardiac remodeling with potential adverse clinical implication. At present, we view these data as hypothesis generating and as compelling grounds for longitudinal work in extreme performers with careful control for other factors that may cause cardiac muscle damage such as occult myocardial infection. While we await such work, it remains uncertain whether high levels of exercise should be discouraged but it must be emphasized that moderate exercise exposure remains a key element of clinical disease prevention and should be encouraged in all patient populations.

Finally, to what degree EICR is reversible with detraining in the contexts of both short- and long-term exercise abstinence remains uncertain. As described, concentric LVH (LV wall thickening without chamber dilation) may develop in response to strength training. This form of athlete's heart may pose the greatest challenge when a clinician is asked to distinguish physiologic adaptation (EICR) from pathology (HCM). At present, there is no single diagnostic test with adequate accuracy for making this distinction. Consequently, an integrated approach with consideration of personal and family history, 12-lead electrocardiography, imaging (echocardiography and/or cardiac MRI) and exercise testing is recommended.[75] Despite use of a systematic approach, situations of "gray-zone" hypertrophy (13–15 mm) may remain ambiguous and prescribed detraining and follow-up cardiac imaging to assess for LVH regression may be required.

Despite the theoretic role of prescribed detraining, the time course and degree of expected LVH regression has not been well-described. Most prior studies examining the LV response to exercise cessation have focused on eccentric LVH and have not standardized the duration of detraining. Maron and colleagues[76] documented regression of eccentric LVH among Olympic athletes over 6 to 34 weeks (mean, 13 weeks). The largest detraining report to date included 40 elite Italian male athletes with eccentric LVH (LV dimension = 61.2 ± 2.9 mm; LV wall thickness = 12.0 ± 1.3 mm).[77] These athletes demonstrated complete normalization of wall thickness and significant but incomplete reduction in cavity dilation after 5.8 ± 3.6 years of detraining. The response of concentric LVH in strength athletes, the true mimicker of HCM, to prescribed detraining has not been well-studied. A recent small study of 5 strength-trained athletes with concentric LVH showed significant regression of LV mass and LV wall thickness during detraining.[78] However, despite the improvement in LV structural parameters, there was persistent impairment of diastolic function as measured by lateral E' velocity. Further investigation is needed to address this important area of uncertainty and delineate the expected structural and functional changes in athletes with concentric LVH undergoing a period of exercise cessation (prescribed detraining).

SUMMARY

EICR is a complex process by which the cardinal hemodynamic stresses of pressure and volume lead to a host of structural or functional adaptations. In aggregate, the constellation of changes that accompany this process serve to facilitate athletic performance by minimizing the cardiac work inherent in athletic activity. Although several key determinants of athletic cardiac adaptation have been described, observed variability across athlete cohorts remains incompletely understood area. Ongoing and future work are required to further understand this process and ultimately to determine where the boundary lies between adaptive physiology and maladaptive disease.

REFERENCES

1. Henschen S. Skidlauf und Skidwettlauf. Eine medizinische Sportstudie. Mitt Med Klin Upsala; 1899. p. 2.

2. Darling EA. The effects of training. A study of the Harvard University Crews. Boston Med Surg J 1899;CXLI:229–33.
3. Pelliccia A, Culasso F, Di Paolo FM, et al. Physiologic left ventricular cavity dilatation in elite athletes. Ann Intern Med 1999;130:23–31.
4. Lang RM, Badano LP, Mor-Avi V, et al. Recommendations for cardiac chamber quantification by echocardiography in adults: an update from the American Society of Echocardiography and the European Association of Cardiovascular Imaging. Eur Heart J Cardiovasc Imaging 2015;16:233–71.
5. Weiner RB, Wang F, Hutter AM Jr, et al. The feasibility, diagnostic yield, and learning curve of portable echocardiography for out-of-hospital cardiovascular disease screening. J Am Soc Echocardiogr 2012;25:568–75.
6. Fagard R, Aubert A, Staessen J, et al. Cardiac structure and function in cyclists and runners. Comparative echocardiographic study. Br Heart J 1984; 52:124–9.
7. Bar-Shlomo BZ, Druck MN, Morch JE, et al. Left ventricular function in trained and untrained healthy subjects. Circulation 1982;65:484–8.
8. Bekaert I, Pannier JL, Van de Weghe C, et al. Non-invasive evaluation of cardiac function in professional cyclists. Br Heart J 1981;45:213–8.
9. Douglas PS, O'Toole ML, Hiller WD, et al. Left ventricular structure and function by echocardiography in ultraendurance athletes. Am J Cardiol 1986;58:805–9.
10. Abergel E, Chatellier G, Hagege AA, et al. Serial left ventricular adaptations in world-class professional cyclists: implications for disease screening and follow-up. J Am Coll Cardiol 2004;44:144–9.
11. Baggish AL, Yared K, Wang F, et al. The impact of endurance exercise training on left ventricular systolic mechanics. Am J Physiol Heart Circ Physiol 2008;295: H1109–16.
12. Nottin S, Doucende G, Schuster-Beck I, et al. Alteration in left ventricular normal and shear strains evaluated by 2D-strain echocardiography in the athlete's heart. J Physiol 2008;586:4721–33.
13. Zocalo Y, Bia D, Armentano RL, et al. Assessment of training-dependent changes in the left ventricle torsion dynamics of professional soccer players using speckle-tracking echocardiography. Conf Proc IEEE Eng Med Biol Soc 2007; 2007:2709–12.
14. Weiner RB, Hutter AM Jr, Wang F, et al. The impact of endurance exercise training on left ventricular torsion. JACC Cardiovasc Imaging 2010;3:1001–9.
15. Baggish AL, Yared K, Weiner RB, et al. Differences in cardiac parameters among elite rowers and subelite rowers. Med Sci Sports Exerc 2010;42:1215–20.
16. D'Andrea A, Cocchia R, Riegler L, et al. Left ventricular myocardial velocities and deformation indexes in top-level athletes. J Am Soc Echocardiogr 2010;23: 1281–8.
17. Caso P, D'Andrea A, Galderisi M, et al. Pulsed Doppler tissue imaging in endurance athletes: relation between left ventricular preload and myocardial regional diastolic function. Am J Cardiol 2000;85:1131–6.
18. Morganroth J, Maron BJ, Henry WL, et al. Comparative left ventricular dimensions in trained athletes. Ann Intern Med 1975;82:521–4.
19. Lee PT, Dweck MR, Prasher S, et al. Left ventricular wall thickness and the presence of asymmetric hypertrophy in healthy young army recruits: data from the LARGE heart study. Circ Cardiovasc Imaging 2013;6:262–7.
20. Pelliccia A, Maron BJ, Spataro A, et al. The upper limit of physiologic cardiac hypertrophy in highly trained elite athletes. N Engl J Med 1991;324: 295–301.

21. Sharma S, Maron BJ, Whyte G, et al. Physiologic limits of left ventricular hypertrophy in elite junior athletes: relevance to differential diagnosis of athlete's heart and hypertrophic cardiomyopathy. J Am Coll Cardiol 2002;40:1431–6.

22. Rawlins J, Carre F, Kervio G, et al. Ethnic differences in physiological cardiac adaptation to intense physical exercise in highly trained female athletes. Circulation 2010;121:1078–85.

23. Lewis JF, Spirito P, Pelliccia A, et al. Usefulness of Doppler echocardiographic assessment of diastolic filling in distinguishing "athlete's heart" from hypertrophic cardiomyopathy. Br Heart J 1992;68:296–300.

24. Maron BJ, Spirito P, Green KJ, et al. Noninvasive assessment of left ventricular diastolic function by pulsed Doppler echocardiography in patients with hypertrophic cardiomyopathy. J Am Coll Cardiol 1987;10:733–42.

25. Vinereanu D, Florescu N, Sculthorpe N, et al. Differentiation between pathologic and physiologic left ventricular hypertrophy by tissue Doppler assessment of long-axis function in patients with hypertrophic cardiomyopathy or systemic hypertension and in athletes. Am J Cardiol 2001;88:53–8.

26. Baggish AL, Wang F, Weiner RB, et al. Training-specific changes in cardiac structure and function: a prospective and longitudinal assessment of competitive athletes. J Appl Physiol (1985) 2008;104:1121–8.

27. Caselli S, Maron MS, Urbano-Moral JA, et al. Differentiating left ventricular hypertrophy in athletes from that in patients with hypertrophic cardiomyopathy. Am J Cardiol 2014;114:1383–9.

28. Wang J, Buergler JM, Veerasamy K, et al. Delayed untwisting: the mechanistic link between dynamic obstruction and exercise tolerance in patients with hypertrophic obstructive cardiomyopathy. J Am Coll Cardiol 2009;54:1326–34.

29. Hauser AM, Dressendorfer RH, Vos M, et al. Symmetric cardiac enlargement in highly trained endurance athletes: a two-dimensional echocardiographic study. Am Heart J 1985;109:1038–44.

30. Henriksen E, Landelius J, Wesslen L, et al. Echocardiographic right and left ventricular measurements in male elite endurance athletes. Eur Heart J 1996;17:1121–8.

31. Oxborough D, Sharma S, Shave R, et al. The right ventricle of the endurance athlete: the relationship between morphology and deformation. J Am Soc Echocardiogr 2012;25:263–71.

32. Scharhag J, Schneider G, Urhausen A, et al. Athlete's heart: right and left ventricular mass and function in male endurance athletes and untrained individuals determined by magnetic resonance imaging. J Am Coll Cardiol 2002;40:1856–63.

33. Scharf M, Brem MH, Wilhelm M, et al. Cardiac magnetic resonance assessment of left and right ventricular morphologic and functional adaptations in professional soccer players. Am Heart J 2010;159:911–8.

34. Marcus FI, McKenna WJ, Sherrill D, et al. Diagnosis of arrhythmogenic right ventricular cardiomyopathy/dysplasia: proposed modification of the Task Force Criteria. Eur Heart J 2010;31:806–14.

35. Pagourelias ED, Kouidi E, Efthimiadis GK, et al. Right atrial and ventricular adaptations to training in male Caucasian athletes: an echocardiographic study. J Am Soc Echocardiogr 2013;26:1344–52.

36. Prakken NH, Velthuis BK, Teske AJ, et al. Cardiac MRI reference values for athletes and nonathletes corrected for body surface area, training hours/week and sex. Eur J Cardiovasc Prev Rehabil 2010;17:198–203.

37. D'Andrea A, Riegler L, Morra S, et al. Right ventricular morphology and function in top-level athletes: a three-dimensional echocardiographic study. J Am Soc Echocardiogr 2012;25:1268–76.

38. Teske AJ, Prakken NH, De Boeck BW, et al. Effect of long term and intensive endurance training in athletes on the age related decline in left and right ventricular diastolic function as assessed by Doppler echocardiography. Am J Cardiol 2009;104:1145–51.
39. La Gerche A, Burns AT, D'Hooge J, et al. Exercise strain rate imaging demonstrates normal right ventricular contractile reserve and clarifies ambiguous resting measures in endurance athletes. J Am Soc Echocardiogr 2012;25:253–62.e1.
40. Hoglund C. Enlarged left atrial dimension in former endurance athletes: an echocardiographic study. Int J Sports Med 1986;7:133–6.
41. Pelliccia A, Maron BJ, Di Paolo FM, et al. Prevalence and clinical significance of left atrial remodeling in competitive athletes. J Am Coll Cardiol 2005;46:690–6.
42. D'Andrea A, Riegler L, Cocchia R, et al. Left atrial volume index in highly trained athletes. Am Heart J 2010;159:1155–61.
43. Grunig E, Henn P, D'Andrea A, et al. Reference values for and determinants of right atrial area in healthy adults by 2-dimensional echocardiography. Circ Cardiovasc Imaging 2013;6:117–24.
44. D'Ascenzi F, Pelliccia A, Natali BM, et al. Morphological and functional adaptation of left and right atria induced by training in highly trained female athletes. Circ Cardiovasc Imaging 2014;7:222–9.
45. McClean G, George K, Lord R, et al. Chronic adaptation of atrial structure and function in elite male athletes. Eur Heart J Cardiovasc Imaging 2015;16(4):417–22.
46. Andersen K, Farahmand B, Ahlbom A, et al. Risk of arrhythmias in 52 755 long-distance cross-country skiers: a cohort study. Eur Heart J 2013;34:3624–31.
47. Babaee Bigi MA, Aslani A. Aortic root size and prevalence of aortic regurgitation in elite strength trained athletes. Am J Cardiol 2007;100:528–30.
48. D'Andrea A, Cocchia R, Riegler L, et al. Aortic root dimensions in elite athletes. Am J Cardiol 2010;105:1629–34.
49. Pelliccia A, Di Paolo FM, De Blasiis E, et al. Prevalence and clinical significance of aortic root dilation in highly trained competitive athletes. Circulation 2010;122:698–706.
50. Iskandar A, Thompson PD. A meta-analysis of aortic root size in elite athletes. Circulation 2013;127:791–8.
51. Pelliccia A, Maron BJ, Culasso F, et al. Athlete's heart in women. Echocardiographic characterization of highly trained elite female athletes. JAMA 1996;276:211–5.
52. George KP, Wolfe LA, Burggraf GW, et al. Electrocardiographic and echocardiographic characteristics of female athletes. Med Sci Sports Exerc 1995;27:1362–70.
53. Sun B, Ma JZ, Yong YH, et al. The upper limit of physiological cardiac hypertrophy in elite male and female athletes in China. Eur J Appl Physiol 2007;101:457–63.
54. Whyte GP, George K, Nevill A, et al. Left ventricular morphology and function in female athletes: a meta-analysis. Int J Sports Med 2004;25:380–3.
55. Haykowsky M, Chan S, Bhambhani Y, et al. Effects of combined endurance and strength training on left ventricular morphology in male and female rowers. Can J Cardiol 1998;14:387–91.
56. Rowland T, Roti M. Influence of sex on the "Athlete's Heart" in trained cyclists. J Sci Med Sport 2010;13:475–8.
57. Basavarajaiah S, Boraita A, Whyte G, et al. Ethnic differences in left ventricular remodeling in highly-trained athletes relevance to differentiating physiologic left ventricular hypertrophy from hypertrophic cardiomyopathy. J Am Coll Cardiol 2008;51:2256–62.
58. Naylor LH, George K, O'Driscoll G, et al. The athlete's heart: a contemporary appraisal of the 'Morganroth hypothesis'. Sports Med 2008;38:69–90.

59. D'Andrea A, Riegler L, Golia E, et al. Range of right heart measurements in top-level athletes: the training impact. Int J Cardiol 2013;164:48–57.
60. D'Andrea A, Limongelli G, Caso P, et al. Association between left ventricular structure and cardiac performance during effort in two morphological forms of athlete's heart. Int J Cardiol 2002;86:177–84.
61. Mitchell JH, Haskell W, Snell P, et al. Task Force 8: classification of sports. J Am Coll Cardiol 2005;45:1364–7.
62. Montgomery HE, Clarkson P, Dollery CM, et al. Association of angiotensin-converting enzyme gene I/D polymorphism with change in left ventricular mass in response to physical training. Circulation 1997;96:741–7.
63. Karjalainen J, Kujala UM, Stolt A, et al. Angiotensinogen gene M235T polymorphism predicts left ventricular hypertrophy in endurance athletes. J Am Coll Cardiol 1999;34:494–9.
64. Baggish AL, Weiner RB, Yared K, et al. Impact of family hypertension history on exercise-induced cardiac remodeling. Am J Cardiol 2009;104:101–6.
65. Buerke M, Murohara T, Skurk C, et al. Cardioprotective effect of insulin-like growth factor I in myocardial ischemia followed by reperfusion. Proc Natl Acad Sci U S A 1995;92:8031–5.
66. McMullen JR, Shioi T, Zhang L, et al. Phosphoinositide 3-kinase(p110alpha) plays a critical role for the induction of physiological, but not pathological, cardiac hypertrophy. Proc Natl Acad Sci U S A 2003;100:12355–60.
67. DeBosch B, Treskov I, Lupu TS, et al. Akt1 is required for physiological cardiac growth. Circulation 2006;113:2097–104.
68. Bostrom P, Mann N, Wu J, et al. C/EBPbeta controls exercise-induced cardiac growth and protects against pathological cardiac remodeling. Cell 2010;143:1072–83.
69. Arbab-Zadeh A, Perhonen M, Howden E, et al. Cardiac remodeling in response to 1 year of intensive endurance training. Circulation 2014;130:2152–61.
70. Lee DC, Pate RR, Lavie CJ, et al. Leisure-time running reduces all-cause and cardiovascular mortality risk. J Am Coll Cardiol 2014;64:472–81.
71. Schnohr P, O'Keefe JH, Marott JL, et al. Dose of jogging and long-term mortality: the Copenhagen City Heart Study. J Am Coll Cardiol 2015;65:411–9.
72. Zilinski JL, Contursi ME, Isaacs SK, et al. Myocardial adaptations to recreational marathon training among middle-aged men. Circ Cardiovasc Imaging 2015;8:e002487.
73. Wilson M, O'Hanlon R, Prasad S, et al. Diverse patterns of myocardial fibrosis in lifelong, veteran endurance athletes. J Appl Physiol (1985) 2011;110:1622–6.
74. La Gerche A, Burns AT, Mooney DJ, et al. Exercise-induced right ventricular dysfunction and structural remodelling in endurance athletes. Eur Heart J 2012;33:998–1006.
75. Maron BJ. Distinguishing hypertrophic cardiomyopathy from athlete's heart physiological remodelling: clinical significance, diagnostic strategies and implications for preparticipation screening. Br J Sports Med 2009;43:649–56.
76. Maron BJ, Pelliccia A, Spataro A, et al. Reduction in left ventricular wall thickness after deconditioning in highly trained Olympic athletes. Br Heart J 1993;69:125–8.
77. Pelliccia A, Maron BJ, De Luca R, et al. Remodeling of left ventricular hypertrophy in elite athletes after long-term deconditioning. Circulation 2002;105:944–9.
78. Weiner RB, Wang F, Berkstresser B, et al. Regression of "gray zone" exercise-induced concentric left ventricular hypertrophy during prescribed detraining. J Am Coll Cardiol 2012;59:1992–4.

The Electrocardiogram in Highly Trained Athletes

Keerthi Prakash, MBChB, MRCP, Sanjay Sharma, MD, FRCP, FESC*

KEYWORDS

- Electrocardiography • Athlete's heart • 2010 ESC criteria • Refined criteria
- Ethnicity • Cardiomyopathy • Primary electrical disease

KEY POINTS

- The normal electrical manifestations of athletic training reflect an increase in vagal tone and in cardiac chamber size and/or wall thickness. Certain repolarization changes observed in athletes overlap with diseases implicated in sudden cardiac death.
- Electrocardiogram (ECG) interpretation must account for the age, sex, and ethnicity of the athlete as well as the type of sports and level of participation.
- The ECG is just one diagnostic tool for differentiating between physiological adaptation and potentially serious cardiac disorders and should be used in conjunction with a clinical history and physical examination, with further investigations as deemed necessary.
- This article provides a review of the normal ECG patterns associated with athletic training to facilitate the differentiation from electrical patterns suggestive of cardiac diseases implicated in exercise-related sudden cardiac death.

INTRODUCTION

Participation in regular intensive physical exercise is associated with a constellation of structural and functional changes within the heart that promote increases in cardiac output and/or blood pressure for both burst activities and for prolonged periods. These changes are referred to as the athlete's heart. These physiological changes are commonly manifested on the surface electrocardiogram (ECG). Over the past 3 decades, several studies in large athlete populations have revealed a spectrum of ECG patterns that are considered benign and can be divided broadly into those that reflect autonomic changes (increased vagal tone) and those that reflect an increase in cardiac chamber size and ventricular wall thickness. The magnitude with which these electrical patterns manifest is determined by several demographic factors and the intensity of exercise.

Disclosure: The authors have nothing to disclose.
Department of Cardiovascular Sciences, St. George's University of London, Cranmer Terrace, London, SW17 ORE, UK
* Corresponding author.
E-mail address: sasharma@sgul.ac.uk

In some instances, the repolarization changes that occur partly as a result of increased vagal tone may overlap with morphologically mild or incomplete phenotypic expressions of both the cardiomyopathies and ion channel diseases. Marked repolarization changes overlapping with disease processes are usually observed in male endurance athletes and athletes of African/Afro-Caribbean origin. The differentiation of benign physiological adaptation from electrical harbingers of diseases implicated in exercise-related sudden cardiac death is crucial because an erroneous diagnosis either way has potentially serious consequences.

The steady trickle of deaths among athletes and the high visibility of these catastrophes have led several sporting bodies, including the International Olympic Committee, the National Basketball Association, and the Union of European Football Associations, to advocate cardiac screening for their athletes. This practice frequently incorporates a 12-lead ECG hence the interpretation of the ECG is pivotal for the assessment of individuals engaged in competitive sport or high-level routine recreational exercise.

In 2010, the European Society of Cardiology (ESC) published consensus guidelines.[1] ECG changes were divided into 2 groups (**Box 1**) based on findings in more than 33,000 nonselect Italian athletes. Group 1 contains ECG changes that occurred in up to 80% of athletes and were deemed to be normal physiological variants. Anomalies occurring in less than 5% of athletes were categorized as group 2 changes and were considered to warrant further investigation to exclude cardiac disease; specifically cardiomyopathy or ion channel disorders.[1]

Since the publication of the ESC guidelines, several other publications have improved the understanding of the ECGs of athletes and stimulated further modifications of these recommendations. This article provides a critical appraisal of the ECGs of athletes using the ESC 2010 guidelines as the current gold standard.

GROUP 1 EUROPEAN SOCIETY OF CARDIOLOGY CRITERIA

Group 1 changes include sinus bradycardia, sinus arrhythmia, first degree atrioventricular (AV) block, and early repolarization consisting of J-point elevation, ST segment elevation, and tall T waves. Most group 1 changes are attributable to increased vagal tone. Sinus bradycardia (heart rate <60 beats per minute [bpm]) is common and observed in more than 80% of athletes. Less than 5% have a heart rate less than

---

Box 1
ESC 2010 criteria for interpretation of an athlete's ECG

Group 1	Group 2
Sinus bradycardia	T-wave inversion
First-degree atrioventricular block	ST depression
Early repolarization	Pathologic Q waves
Isolated QRS voltage criteria for left ventricular hypertrophy	Left atrial enlargement
Incomplete right bundle branch block	Left axis deviation/left anterior hemiblock
—	Right axis deviation/left posterior hemiblock
—	Right ventricular hypertrophy
—	Complete left bundle branch block/right bundle branch block
—	Long or short QT interval
—	Brugada-like early repolarization
—	Ventricular pre-excitation

40 bpm and a resting pulse of less than 35 bpm is exceptionally rare. Sinus arrhythmia is common, particularly in young athletes. First-degree AV block is detected in 5% of athletes, whereas Mobitz type 1 AV block, sinus pauses, and junctional rhythms may be observed at rest or during sleep in a smaller proportion of athletes. These group 1 changes are more common in endurance athletes[2] and resolve with exercise once sympathetic tone overrides vagal tone.

An ectopic atrial rhythm is suggested by p waves of differing morphology to sinus p waves. The detection of more than 2 types of p-wave morphology on an ECG is described as a wandering atrial pacemaker, which is also recognized in athletes and a result of increased vagal tone. In contrast, Mobitz type 2 or third-degree AV block are extremely rare and are more suggestive of cardiac conduction tissue disease, particularly in the presence of symptoms such as dizziness or syncope.

Repolarization Changes

Repolarization changes involving the J point, ST segment, and T wave are present in more than 60% of athletes.[3–5] J-point elevation in most leads associated with concave ST segments is a common finding in slim men. Such repolarization changes are seen particularly in people of African/Afro-Caribbean origin. In the latter group, the ST segments in leads V1 to V4 may be convex and associated with biphasic T waves or asymmetrical and occasionally deep T-wave inversion (TWI) (**Fig. 1**). This pattern has been shown in up to 13% of African/Afro-Caribbean athletes, including women and adolescent athletes of both sexes.

Early Repolarization Pattern

J-point elevation has always been considered a normal variant in athletes; however, there have been associations between certain early repolarization patterns in the

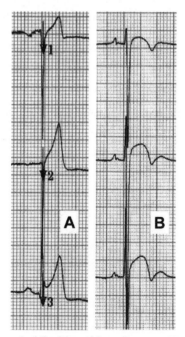

Fig. 1. Repolarization changes in (*A*) white athletes (concave ST elevation [STE]) and peaked upright T waves; (*B*) African/Afro-Caribbean athletes (convex STE with TWI).

inferior and lateral leads with idiopathic ventricular fibrillation (VF). Specifically, the presence of notched J waves (after the S wave) or terminal slurring of the S wave (J wave embedded in the S wave) are considered harbingers for fatal arrhythmias in some individuals (**Fig. 2**). In our experience these changes are present in 20% of white and 40% of African/Afro-Caribbean athletes and are likely to be vagally mediated because they resolve with exercise and are most profound in athletes with the slowest heart rates.[6] Consistent with the ESC recommendations we think that the early repolarization pattern changes discussed earlier are normal variants in athletes and do not warrant investigation in the absence of symptoms.

Incomplete Right Bundle Branch Block

Incomplete right bundle branch block (RBBB) (rSR′ in V1, QRS <120 milliseconds) may be seen in almost one-third of athletes and is regarded as a normal finding.[3,5,7] This pattern is thought to result from right ventricular (RV) dilatation and remodeling, resulting in increased conduction time rather than disease of the His-Purkinje fibers. In the absence of precordial TWI, symptoms, or a cardiac murmur suggestive of an intracardiac shunt, no further investigation is required.

Voltage Criteria for Left Ventricular Hypertrophy

Isolated voltage criteria for left ventricular hypertrophy (LVH) is common in athletes and present in around 70% of male athletes because of chamber enlargement and left ventricular (LV) mass. There are numerous definitions for voltage criteria for ventricular hypertrophy, but the most commonly used are the Sokolow-Lyon criteria (S wave V1 + largest R wave V5/V6 ≥35 mV or R wave AVL ≥11 mV). Voltage criteria for LVH are more common in adolescent athletes (possibly because of their thin chest walls) and African/Afro-Caribbean male athletes (probably because of an increased LV mass). Increased QRS voltage in isolation does not warrant investigation. The coexistence with ST depression, TWI, and pathologic Q waves is highly suggestive of pathologic LVH.[8]

An example of the plethora of electrical patterns observed in highly trained athletes is shown in **Fig. 3**.

GROUP 2 EUROPEAN SOCIETY OF CARDIOLOGY CRITERIA

Of the group 2 changes, TWI and ST segment depression are most likely to be associated with a structural cardiac abnormality such as a cardiomyopathy. ST segment

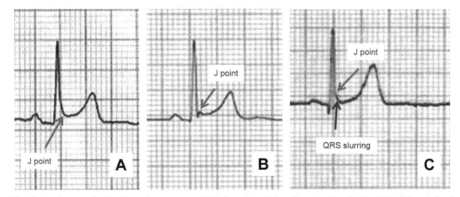

Fig. 2. Early repolarization changes on ECG showing (*A*) a discrete J point in STE; (*B*) notched J point after S wave; (*C*) terminal slurring of S wave with J point embedded in the S wave.

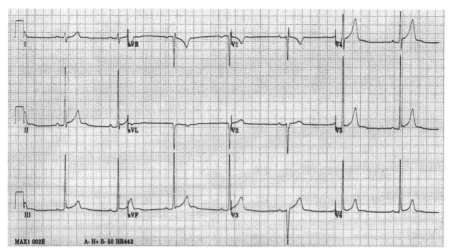

Fig. 3. An athlete's ECG showing sinus bradycardia, right axis deviation, voltage criteria for LVH, partial RBBB and early repolarization.

depression is always considered abnormal irrespective of the athlete's demographics or the lack of symptoms.

T-wave Inversion

T-wave inversion (TWI) is present in 3% to 4% of adolescent (14–18 years old) and adult white athletes; in adolescent athletes the juvenile ECG pattern comprising TWI in V1 to V3 is observed in 9% of athletes less than 14 years of age. After the age of 16 years, TWI beyond V2 is rare. Occasionally endurance athletes show biphasic T waves or inverted T waves in V3,[3,7,9] which do not warrant investigation in asymptomatic athletes if preceded by ST elevation.

TWI in the lateral leads (I, AVL, V5, V6) has been associated with hypertrophic cardiomyopathy (HCM) and always warrants investigation (**Fig. 4**).[8,9] The significance of TWI in contiguous inferior leads is uncertain but our practice is to investigate such athletes.

The situation is different in African/Afro-Caribbean athletes in whom TWI is common (23% of African/Afro-Caribbean athletes) (**Fig. 5**).[3,4,7] TWI confined to the anterior leads (V1–V4) preceded by convex ST elevation is considered a normal ethnic variant[4,10] and does not warrant investigation in asymptomatic athletes. TWI in the inferior and lateral leads occurs in 1.5% to 1.8% of white adult athletes but is seen in 10% of African/Afro-Caribbean adult athletes (6% with inferior and 4% with lateral TWI).[11]

TWI in the absence of overt cardiomyopathy outside the context of the circumstances mentioned earlier is an indication for ongoing surveillance; in 2 studies, TWI heralded the onset of cardiomyopathy in the ensuing years.[12,13]

Pathologic Q Waves

Pathologic Q waves are a recognized manifestation of cardiomyopathies. The prevalence of pathologic Q waves depends on the precise definition. Our practice is to consider a Q wave as pathologic when the Q/R ratio is greater than 0.25 or when the Q wave duration is greater than 40 milliseconds. Definitions based purely on the

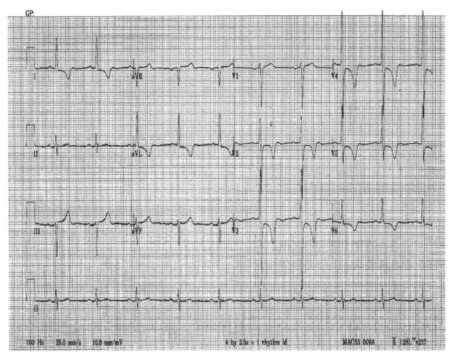

Fig. 4. ECG from a patient with HCM showing ST segment depression, TWI V2 to V6, I and AVL and voltage criteria for LVH.

depth of the Q wave (>0.3 mV) lack specificity, especially in adolescent athletes, who frequently show large QRS complexes involving deep Q waves.[14]

Bundle Branch Block

Complete RBBB is seen in only 1% of athletes. Studies suggest that RBBB correlates with RV size and may be part of the normal spectrum of physiological adaptation.[15]

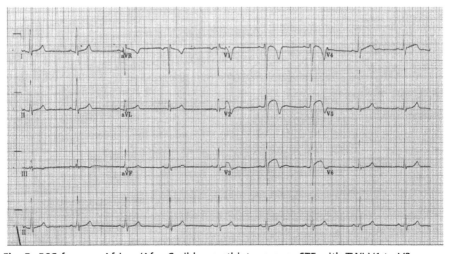

Fig. 5. ECG from an African/Afro-Caribbean athlete: convex STE with TWI V1 to V3.

Given its rarity, it is our practice to perform an echocardiogram to exclude an intracardiac shunt or RV disorder in athletes with RBBB. Left bundle branch block (LBBB) is not a marker of athlete's heart and always requires further investigation.

Voltage Criteria for Right Ventricular Hypertrophy, Atrial Enlargement, and Axis Deviation

The ESC recommendations consider voltage criteria for right ventricular hypertrophy (RVH), atrial enlargement, and axis deviation as abnormal findings; however, our experience suggests that voltage criteria for RVH, and atrial enlargement are significantly common in highly trained athletes versus sedentary individuals and echocardiography in athletes with these findings in isolation or along with other changes is not associated with structural heart disease.[12]

RVH by the Sokolow-Lyon criteria (R wave V1 + S wave V5/V6 >10.5 mm) is present in almost 12% of athletes and does not require investigation in the absence of symptoms.[16]

Voltage criteria for atrial enlargement in athletes vary with age and are more common in adolescent athletes compared with adult athletes (14%–16% vs 4%–5% respectively).[7,17]

We consider right axis deviation to be a normal variant in athletes. Isolated left axis deviation is a nonspecific anomaly with a poor diagnostic yield and does not warrant further investigation in asymptomatic athletes with a normal cardiac examination.

Long QT Interval

A prolonged QT interval raises concerns about congenital long QT syndromes (LQTS), which are genetic ion channel diseases that have a propensity to degenerate to polymorphic ventricular tachycardia and sudden cardiac death. Athletes have a slightly longer QT interval compared with nonathletes.

Measurement of the QT interval in athletes may be difficult, particularly in the presence of sinus arrhythmia, U waves, or indistinct termination of the T wave. The QT interval should be corrected for heart rate and the most commonly used formula for this purpose is the Bazett formula ($QTc = QT/\sqrt{RR}$ interval). The most accurate method to identify the end of the QT interval is to identify the intercept of the tangent of the downslope of the T wave (**Fig. 6**), which is often best seen in lead II or V5. In the setting of sinus arrhythmia, an average RR and QT interval should be used.

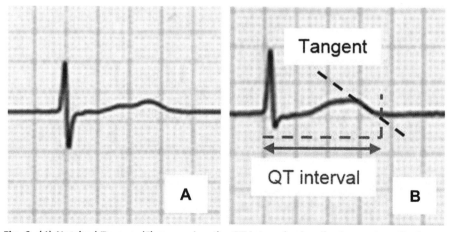

Fig. 6. (*A*) Notched T wave; (*B*) measuring the QT interval using the tangent method.

The recommended upper limit for the QT interval is the same as with nonathletes according to the ESC recommendations (440 milliseconds for men; 460 milliseconds for women). Based on several reports, approximately 6% of athletes have a QT interval longer than these upper limits. The American Heart Association recommends a corrected QTc greater than 470 milliseconds in men and greater than 480 milliseconds in women. These values have a positive predictive accuracy of just 7% in isolation. Our own experience suggests that a QT greater than 500 milliseconds is usually associated with other phenotypic features of LQTS, such as paradoxic QT prolongation with exercise, identification of another family member with a long QT interval, or a positive genotype.[18] In athletes with a long QT interval, notched or bifid T waves may also be suggestive of a genuine ion channel disorder.

Brugada Electrocardiogram Pattern

Brugada syndrome (BrS) is a hereditary cardiac sodium channel disorder associated with fatal ventricular arrhythmias during resting conditions when the heart rate is slow. Theoretically, deaths from BrS should not occur during intense exercise; however, vagotonia may promote arrhythmia at rest. The diagnostic type 1 pattern comprises a high takeoff and downsloping ST segment with J-point elevation ($\geq$2 mm) before TWI in the right precordial leads (V1–V3) (**Fig. 7**). Another nondiagnostic pattern (type 2 pattern) is described as a saddleback ST elevation (>1 mm) with J-point elevation ($\geq$2 mm) and either a biphasic or positive T wave, which may convert to a type 1 pattern using high-lead ECGs or the use of a sodium channel blocker agent such as ajmaline.

The type 1 pattern may resemble repolarization changes in African/Afro-Caribbean athletes. The key difference being that in African/Afro-Caribbean athletes, there is more of a domed ST elevation. Another method to differentiate between BrS and

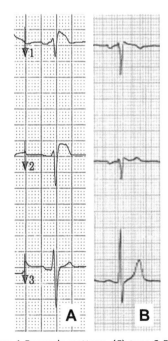

Fig. 7. ECGs showing (*A*) type 1 Brugada pattern, (*B*) type 2 Brugada pattern.

repolarization changes is to measure the ST segment elevation at the J point (STJ) and also 80 milliseconds after the J point (ST80). In BrS, the ratio of STJ/ST80 is greater than 1, whereas with repolarization the ratio is less than 1 (**Fig. 8**). Brugada can often mimic incomplete RBBB; however, a differentiating feature is J-point elevation confined to V1 to V2 without reciprocal S waves in I and V6.

Wolff-Parkinson-White Electrocardiogram Pattern

The presence of an accessory pathway allowing excitation of the ventricles bypassing the AV node results in ventricular preexcitation and hence is seen on the ECG as a short PR (<120 milliseconds), a slurred upstroke of the QRS (delta wave), and a prolonged QRS (>120 milliseconds): this is known as Wolff-Parkinson-White (WPW) (**Fig. 9**). The prevalence is similar to that in the normal population: 0.1% to 0.3%. Rapid conduction of atrial fibrillation can result in VF and hence sudden cardiac death.

Refined Criteria

The ESC 2010 criteria were an excellent starting point for interpretation of the ECGs of athletes; however, with evidence suggesting that isolated axis deviation, atrial enlargement, and RVH were poor indicators of cardiac disease in athletes, and taking into account normal variants between different ethnic groups, we recently proposed the refined criteria to help improve the specificity of the ECG without compromising sensitivity. These criteria categorize ECG findings into normal, borderline, and training-unrelated variants (**Fig. 10**). Further investigations to exclude cardiomyopathy or primary ion channel disorders are suggested with borderline anomalies in the presence of symptoms, family history, or abnormal examination, or in the presence of more than 1 borderline ECG pattern. Tested retrospectively in a cohort of 5550 athletes, the refined criteria were associated with improved specificity of the ECG, particularly in African/Afro-Caribbean athletes, from 40.3% to 84.2%, whereas sensitivity remained similar between the 3 criteria (70% for African/Afro-Caribbean athletes, 60% for white athletes).[12]

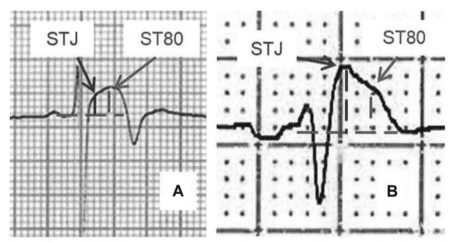

Fig. 8. Measuring the ST segment elevation at the J point (STJ) and at 80 milliseconds after the J point (ST80) in (A) an athlete (STJ/ST80 ratio <1); (B) Brugada pattern (STJ/ST80 ratio >1).

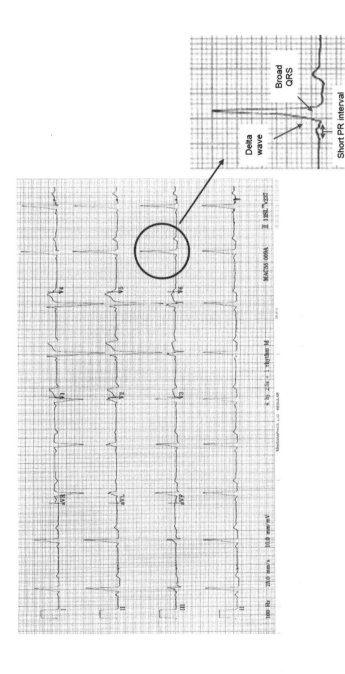

Fig. 9. ECG from a patient with WPW: short PR interval, delta wave, and broad QRS.

Normal ECG changes

- Sinus bradycardia
- First-degree AV block
- Incomplete RBBB
- Early repolarisation
- Isolated QRS voltage criteria for LVH

Training unrelated ECG changes

- ST depression
- Pathological Q waves
- Ventricular pre-excitation
- TWI beyond V1 in Caucasians
- TWI beyond V4 in African/Afro-Caribbeans
- LBBB/RBBB
- QTc ≥470msec (males)
- QTc ≥480msec (females)
- Brugada-like ER
- Atrial/ventricular arrhythmia
- ≥2PVCs per 10sec

- Left/right atrial enlargement
- Left/right axis deviation
- Right ventricular hypertrophy
- TWI preceeded by convex ST segment elevation upto V4 in African/Afro-Caribbeans

Borderline ECG changes

Fig. 10. Data from the refined criteria. AV, atrio-ventricular; ER, early repolarization; LBBB, left bundle branch block; LVH, left ventricular hypertrophy; PVCs, premature ventricular complexes; QTc, corrected QT interval; RBBB, right bundle branch block; TWI, T-wave inversion. (*Data from* Sheikh N, Papadakis M, Ghani S, et al. Comparison of electrocardiographic criteria for the detection of cardiac abnormalities in elite black and white athletes. Circulation 2014;129(16):1637–49.)

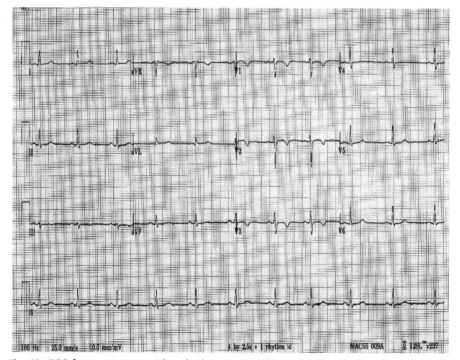

Fig. 11. ECG from a patient with arrhythmogenic right ventricular cardiomyopathy.

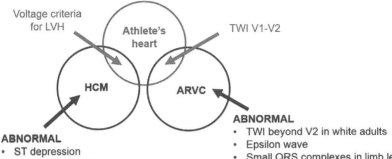

Voltage criteria for LVH

Athlete's heart

TWI V1-V2

HCM

ARVC

ABNORMAL
- ST depression
- Infero-lateral TWI
- LBBB
- Pathological Q waves

ABNORMAL
- TWI beyond V2 in white adults
- Epsilon wave
- Small QRS complexes in limb leads
- Terminal S wave duration >55msec
- Ventricular ectopics of LBBB morphology

Fig. 12. Summary of ECG changes in an athlete's heart and the overlap between cardiomyopathy.

SUMMARY

Athletic training induces a plethora of electrical changes on the surface ECG that are usually benign but may mimic those observed in cardiomyopathy or ion channel disease. Voltage criteria for LVH are common in athletes but accompanying ST depression, TWI, and Q waves should raise the suspicion of HCM. TWI in V1 to V3/V4 are normal in all adolescents (<16 years) and adult Afro-Caribbean athletes. TWI beyond V2 in white athletes may be suggestive of arrhythmogenic RV cardiomyopathy **(Fig. 11)**, particularly in the presence of epsilon waves. LBBB, WPW ECG pattern, Br ECG pattern, and QTc greater than 500 milliseconds are always abnormal **(Fig. 12)**.

REFERENCES

1. Corrado D, Pelliccia A, Heidbuchel H, et al. Recommendations for interpretation of 12-lead electrocardiogram in the athlete. Eur Heart J 2010;31(2):243–59.
2. Brosnan M, La Gerche A, Kalman J, et al. Comparison of frequency of significant electrocardiographic abnormalities in endurance versus nonendurance athletes. Am J Cardiol 2014;113(9):1567–73.
3. Papadakis M, Basavarajaiah S, Rawlins J, et al. Prevalence and significance of T-wave inversions in predominantly Caucasian adolescent athletes. Eur Heart J 2009;30(14):1728–35.
4. Papadakis M, Carre F, Kervio G, et al. The prevalence, distribution, and clinical outcomes of electrocardiographic repolarization patterns in male athletes of African/Afro-Caribbean origin. Eur Heart J 2011;32(18):2304–13.
5. Di Paolo FM, Schmied C, Zerguini YA, et al. The athlete's heart in adolescent Africans: an electrocardiographic and echocardiographic study. J Am Coll Cardiol 2012;59(11):1029–36.
6. Noseworthy PA, Weiner R, Kim J, et al. Early repolarization pattern in competitive athletes: clinical correlates and the effects of exercise training. Circ Arrhythm Electrophysiol 2011;4(4):432–40.
7. Sharma S, Whyte G, Elliott P, et al. Electrocardiographic changes in 1000 highly trained junior elite athletes. Br J Sports Med 1999;33(5):319–24.
8. Schnell F, Riding N, O'Hanlon R, et al. The recognition and significance of pathological T-wave inversions in athletes. Circulation 2015;131(2):165–73.

9. Calò L, Sperandii F, Martino A, et al. Echocardiographic findings in 2261 peri-pubertal athletes with or without inverted T waves at electrocardiogram. Heart 2015;101(3):193–200.
10. Sheikh N, Papadakis M, Carre F, et al. Cardiac adaptation to exercise in adolescent athletes of African ethnicity: an emergent elite athletic population. Br J Sports Med 2013;47(9):585–92.
11. Wilson MG, Sharma S, Carré F, et al. Significance of deep T-wave inversions in asymptomatic athletes with normal cardiovascular examinations: practical solutions for managing the diagnostic conundrum. Br J Sports Med 2012;46(Suppl 1):151–8.
12. Sheikh N, Papadakis M, Ghani S, et al. Comparison of electrocardiographic criteria for the detection of cardiac abnormalities in elite black and white athletes. Circulation 2014;129(16):1637–49.
13. Pelliccia A, Di Paolo FM, Quattrini FM, et al. Outcomes in athletes with marked ECG repolarization abnormalities. N Engl J Med 2008;358(2):152–61.
14. Konno T, Shimizu M, Ino H, et al. Diagnostic value of abnormal Q waves for identification of preclinical carriers of hypertrophic cardiomyopathy based on a molecular genetic diagnosis. Eur Heart J 2004;25(3):246–51.
15. Kim JH, Noseworthy PA, McCarty D, et al. Significance of electrocardiographic right bundle branch block In trained athletes. Am J Cardiol 2011;107(7):1083–9.
16. Zaidi A, Ghani S, Sheikh N, et al. Clinical significance of electrocardiographic right ventricular hypertrophy in athletes: comparison with arrhythmogenic right ventricular cardiomyopathy and pulmonary hypertension. Eur Heart J 2013; 34(47):3649–56.
17. Gati S, Sheikh N, Ghani S, et al. Should axis deviation or atrial enlargement be categorised as abnormal in young athletes? The athlete's electrocardiogram: time for re-appraisal of markers of pathology. Eur Heart J 2013;34(47):3641–8.
18. Basavarajaiah S, Wilson M, Whyte G, et al. Prevalence and significance of an isolated long QT interval in elite athletes. Eur Heart J 2007;28(23):2944–9.

Advanced Imaging of Athletes

Added Value of Coronary Computed Tomography and Cardiac Magnetic Resonance Imaging

Matthew W. Martinez, MD

KEYWORDS

- Cardiac MRI • Cardiac CT • Athletes • Sports
- Hypertrophic cardiomyopathy (HCM)
- Arrhythmogenic right ventricular cardiomyopathy (ARVC) • Dilated cardiomyopathy

KEY POINTS

- Advanced imaging is complementary with the best option being based on the clinical question.
- Cardiac computed tomography (CCT) is a robust method for the assessment of anatomic structures of athletes, while cardiac magnetic resonance imaging (CMR) is a robust method for the assessment of athlete volumes and function.
- CMR for evaluation of scar/fibrosis is a powerful risk predictor for myocardial disease.
- CCT with and without contrast is a robust tool for the coronary arteries.

Videos of a steady state free precession (SSFP – white blood) cine image of hypertrophic cardiomyopathy with an apical aneurysm and a contrast enhanced gated computed tomography image illustrating a bicuspid aortic valve in short axis accompany this article at http://www.sportsmed.theclinics.com/

INTRODUCTION

Adaptations of the athlete, often termed as the athlete's heart, refers to the pattern of morphologic, functional, and electrical changes that result from intensive training. Assessment of athletes has led to the discovery of reversible training-related electrocardiographic (ECG) changes, diastolic parameters, atrial and ventricular dimensions, and more recently the possibility of intramyocardial fibrotic changes associated with exercise. When evaluating athletes each of these is encountered, some more often

Disclosures/Supporting Grants: None.
Division of Cardiology, Lehigh Valley Health Network, 1250 South Cedar Crest Boulevard, Suite 300, Allentown, PA 18103, USA
E-mail address: matthew_w.martinez@lvhn.org

than the others. The distinction between physiologic adaptation of the athlete's heart and sinister disease is problematic because of the substantial overlap between normal and pathologic changes. This controversial area referred to as the gray zone first emerged as a description of overlap for left ventricular (LV) wall thickness.[1,2] However, physiologic adaptations related to training are not limited to LV wall thickness but include enlargement of both the LV and the right ventricle (RV).[3–6] Most agree that exercise testing and echocardiography are the initial diagnostic steps for evaluating athletes when cardiac abnormalities are suspected. In the recent decades there has been rapid growth and use of advanced imaging modalities such as CMR and CCT. These modalities are now integral tools for most practices to assess cardiovascular disease and are now increasingly used for the evaluation of athletes with suspected cardiac disease. Causes of sudden cardiac arrest (SCA) differ by age with a larger proportion of those younger than 30 years having hypertrophic cardiomyopathy (HCM) and those older than 30 years having coronary artery disease.[7] This article provides a practical guide for CMR and CCT assessment of young and adult athletes.

IMAGING BACKGROUND

Both CMR and CCT provide highly reproducible and accurate assessments of cardiovascular structures. CCT is faster and less operator dependent than CMR. In some instances they are complementary, but for patient evaluations, the best choice depends on the clinical question (**Fig. 1**).

Cardiac Magnetic Resonance Imaging

CMR provides superior image quality with accuracy and reproducibility that exceeds those of most other techniques without requiring contrast media administration or ionizing radiation. CMR measures cardiac volumes including atrial volumes, ventricular volumes, and mass by acquiring a 3-dimensional stack of contiguous short-axis images. LV as well as RV volume and mass are determined by planimetry for each slice and summed for the entire ventricle. The accuracy of the volume assessments allows normalization of the measurements to body size, gender, and age to provide a confident diagnosis of both normal adaptations and abnormal conditions. Contrast-enhanced CMR is widely used for MRI of the vessels with near-instantaneous imaging after contrast injection. However, the myocardium can be assessed for abnormal myocardial interstitium using contrast-enhanced CMR to identify late gadolinium enhancement (LGE) (**Fig. 2**).[8,9] Gadolinium bound to diethylenetriamine pentaacetic acid localizes to the interstitial space in areas where there is cell membrane disruption resulting in increased concentrations of gadolinium in areas of myocardial scar or fibrosis (LGE), which is distinctly different from the normal myocardium.[10–12] LGE, as its name implies, occurs late and requires the contrast to wash in and out of myocardium before myocardial imaging is done. LGE has emerged as a newer technique for cardiovascular assessment and has the unique ability to illustrate both ischemic scar tissue and nonischemic fibrosis.[10,13–16]

Cardiovascular Computed Tomography

Initially, CCT emerged as a rudimentary tool with limited image quality primarily because of the small caliber and near-continuous motion of the coronary vessels during the cardiac cycle. Rapid evolution in CT technology has led to modern CT scanners with improved spatial and temporal resolution allowing cardiovascular details well beyond the initial images. In the current era, 64-slice or more multidetector CT is used to provide noninvasive coronary artery visualization, which in many instances

Athlete

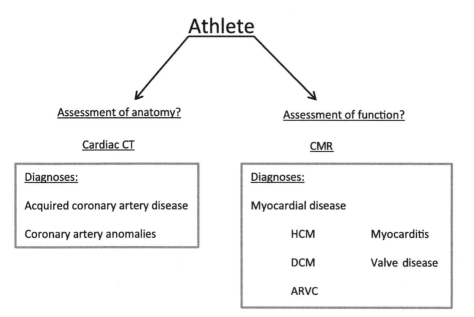

Assessment of anatomy?

Cardiac CT

Diagnoses:

Acquired coronary artery disease

Coronary artery anomalies

Assessment of function?

CMR

Diagnoses:

Myocardial disease

HCM   Myocarditis

DCM   Valve disease

ARVC

CAVEATS:

Under age 30 with suspected coronary artery anomalies -> consider CMR.

Suspected ARVC with a device → cardiac CT

Fig. 1. Algorithm for imaging choice based on clinical question of anatomic or functional assessment. DCM, dilated cardiomyopathy.

is well beyond that provided by other noninvasive methods and approaches that provided by conventional coronary angiography.[17] CCT can be either non–contrast enhanced or contrast enhanced with each requiring some measure of radiation exposure. CCT has been criticized for its previously described high radiation exposure and

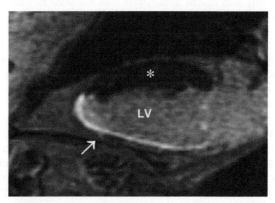

Fig. 2. LGE imaging illustrating normal myocardium (*asterisk*) as well as a transmural infarction (*arrow*). LV, left ventricular.

requirement of iodinated contrast agent. However, if assessment of function is not required, prospectively gated CCT using very low radiation dose (3–5 mSv) can replace the retrospectively gated CCT using relatively high dose (10–15 mSv).[18,19] Despite significant radiation reductions in recent years and exposure that is often less than that of other imaging modalities, radiation exposure should be taken into consideration when choosing this modality.

CARDIOMYOPATHIES
Hypertrophic Cardiomyopathy

A classic description of criteria for HCM includes LV wall thickness greater than 12 mm combined with a relatively nondilated LV in association with impaired diastolic function.[2,20] HCM is a frequent cause of SCA in young people, and in well-trained athletes, the disease is most often associated with the controversial discussion of how to evaluate the gray zone.[1,21] Physiologic hypertrophy associated with athletic physiologic adaptations, up to 15 mm, can overlap with the pathologic increases that represent HCM. This overlap represents the so-called gray zone between the physiologic adaptation of the athlete and pathologic expression of HCM. In a previous landmark study, athletic hypertrophy has been described as occurring in approximately 2% of athletes.[22] However, these data may be incomplete and may not represent all modern athletes. Athletic adaptations are affected by various factors including gender, race, genetics, and type of sport and perhaps the presence of confounding factors such as weight, body mass index, hypertension, and obstructive sleep apnea. A recent description of American football players indicates that hypertrophy in this group of athletes exceeds 13 mm nearly 10% of the time.[1] The degree of hypertrophy is paramount to make the diagnosis of HCM and is primarily made by echocardiographic assessment. However, it is well known that echocardiography has poor acoustic windows, provides incomplete visualization of the entire LV wall, and can miss HCM particularly when the hypertrophy is localized and regional.[23,24]

   CMR is able to overcome these limitations to more accurately identify and more precisely measure wall thickness or distribution of hypertrophy.[8,23,24] This fact was demonstrated by Rickers and colleagues[8] who found that CMR was better able to identify hypertrophy, especially in the LV anterolateral free wall. In the same study, echocardiography was found to underestimate the degree of hypertrophy in the basal anterolateral free wall. It was also found that the diagnostic capability of CMR in HCM for apical hypertrophy and apical aneurysms was superior to that of 2-dimensional echocardiography (Video 1).[25,26] Myocardial scarring identified by LGE has been found to be a common feature in HCM and a robust predictor of arrhythmias and subsequent risk of SCA.[2,16,27] LGE has been found to occur in a patchy multifocal distribution located in the midventricular wall confined to areas of cardiac hypertrophy and is rarely present, if ever, in athletic hearts. For assessment of the athlete, the presence of LGE with borderline LV wall thickness would strongly suggest pathologic hypertrophy rather than physiologic adaptation.[28,29]

   CCT is not often used for the assessment of patients with HCM with a few exceptions. In patients with questionable wall thickness measurements by echocardiography and who are unable to tolerate a CMR, CCT could be considered. This technique would allow for an equally accurate measurement of wall thickness; however, no LGE images would be obtained.

   Before surgical myectomy, assessment of the coronary arteries is common and recommended.[20,30] CCT offers an opportunity to exclude coronary artery disease without the need for an invasive catheterization.

Arrhythmogenic Right Ventricular Cardiomyopathy

Arrhythmogenic right ventricular cardiomyopathy (ARVC) is a common cause of SCA in athletes because of exercise-induced ventricular arrhythmias, especially in the Italian athletes.[31–33] ARVC is characterized by structural and functional abnormalities of the RV as a result of fatty and fibrous tissue replacement in the myocardium.[34] Although the gray zone assessment of athletes is classically discussed in the context of LV changes; the RV is now a focus of athletic changes that mimic pathologic processes. In this manner, it fits into the so-called gray zone assessment of athletes in a similar way that the hypertrophied ventricle does. Both physiologic athletic changes of the RV and pathologic features of patients with ARVC result in increased RV dilatation/volumes compared with LV volumes.[29,34] Echocardiographic measurements of the RV using standard published criteria place many athletes in the abnormal category.[35,36] CMR provides noninvasive evaluation of the RV with more accurate volumetric and functional measurements to differentiate pathologic from physiologic changes of the athlete.[31,37–39]

CMR findings associated with ARVC include (**Box 1**)[34,37]:

- RV dilatation with associated systolic impairment
- Segmental or localized dilatation
- Regional wall motion abnormalities
- RV aneurysms
- RV LGE

Calkins[34] described the accordion sign of the RV for patients identified to have ARVC, which was present in 60% of those with genetic mutations for ARVC and in 0% of noncarriers. The accordion sign refers to the crinkling of the RV outflow tract and below the tricuspid valve of the RV free wall during systole.[40,41] Further study is needed to investigate its clinical usefulness and observer variability.

CCT can provide reliable diagnostic information in patients in whom CMR is not possible.[42,43] Quantitative RV volume and function are measured in the same way as they are for CMR. A retrospective gated CCT is used to assess RV volumes, function, and characteristic wall motion abnormalities, similar to the features found on CMR.[44,45]

Left Ventricular Abnormalities

The athletic heart is highly efficient and able to maintain stroke volumes that exceed typical age- and gender-matched groups.[46] LV volumes that significantly exceed published normal values for age- and gender-matched nonathletes are common among

---

Box 1
Imaging criteria for the diagnosis of ARVD/ARVC

Major

     Severe dilatation and reduction of RV ejection fraction with no (or only mild) LV impairment

     Localized RV aneurysms (akinetic or dyskinetic areas with diastolic bulging)

     Severe segmental dilatation of the RV

Minor

     Regional RV akinesia or dyskinesia or dyssynchronous RV contraction, and 1 of the following:

     Ratio of RV end diastolic volume to BSA $\geq$110 mL/m^2 (male) or $\geq$100 mL/m^2 (female)

     RV ejection fraction $\leq$40%

Abbreviations: ARVD, arrhythmogenic right ventricular dysplasia; BSA, body surface area.

endurance athletes. In the same way, athletic LV wall thickness exceeds accepted normal values, LV dimensions and volumes do as well.[1–3] Echocardiographic criteria for dilated cardiomyopathy include an LV diameter greater than 60 mm, which is found in as much as 15% of elite athletes.[33,47] The precision and reproducibility of volumetric measurements of CMR make it most useful for definitive measurements of athletic ventricles. As a general rule, true LV dysfunction is an uncommon finding in athletes with current publications indicating that athletic ejection fractions are normal with increased stroke volume and LV volumes.[46] Dilated cardiomyopathy is characterized by ventricular dilatation and dysfunction and often biventricular dilation (**Fig. 3**) with other supporting features that suggest pathology rather than physiologic chamber adaptations.[48] The cause of dilated cardiomyopathies is often idiopathic but may be a genetic condition such as LV noncompaction cardiomyopathy (LVNC) or secondary to acute or chronic myocarditis.[49] Myocarditis is an inflammatory illness resulting in acute necrosis of myocytes with subsequent acute LV dysfunction.[50–53] Myocarditis is most frequently caused by a viral infection, but it can also be caused by drugs and toxic agents with most patients recovering function.[51,53] CMR has become the noninvasive standard for investigation of myocarditis with sensitivity and specificity of 100% and 90%, respectively, and a diagnostic accuracy of approximately 80%.[54,55] Different CMR sequences have the ability to uncover the pathophysiology of myocarditis by illustrating the increased capillary permeability, myocyte necrosis, and increased extracellular space.[16,48] CMR offers a unique opportunity for assessment of LV dysfunction with LGE. Unique to CMR, LGE is able to differentiate ischemic (including subendocardial to transmural enhancement) from nonischemic (none, midwall, or epicardial enhancement) causes of dilated cardiomyopathy.[10] Patterns of myocarditis include a diffuse or patchy distribution involving the epicardial surface of the lateral wall or midwall and have been found to be a better predictor of cardiac events, including arrhythmias and death, than LV function.[55] For athletes, this pattern of distribution would help differentiate physiologic dilation from an underlying pathologic process.

LVNC is characterized by a prominent trabecular network most often at the apex but may involve any part of the LV.[56] Accepted diagnostic criteria, with limited supportive

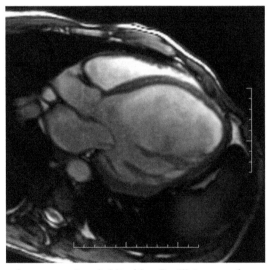

Fig. 3. Steady-state free precession (white blood) still image of a severely dilated left ventricle consistent with a dilated cardiomyopathy.

data, include a noncompact to compact myocardium ratio greater than 2.3 in end diastole by CMR and a ratio greater than 2.0 in end systole by echocardiography.[56] However, a high proportion of young athletes exhibit conventional criteria for LVNC highlighting the nonspecific nature of current diagnostic criteria if applied to elite athletic populations[57]; its high prevalence among otherwise healthy athletes suggests that it is more of a physiologic than a pathologic finding. Therefore, identification of a trabeculated apex without the presence of LV dysfunction or LGE most likely represents normal athletic features.

ARTERIAL DISEASE
Anomalous Coronary Artery

Anomalous coronary arteries (ACAs) are uncommon yet can represent a high risk for SCA in the young.[58,59] Most consider CCT to be the optimal way to identify the presence, course, and significance of ACAs as well as assist with surgical planning.[60] There are many types of ACAs with variable importance with regard to patient outcomes (**Box 2**).[61,62]

Coronary arteries with a posterior course between the aorta and low-pressure atrium have little clinical importance, but an anomalous right coronary artery arising from the left sinus with a course between the great vessels has variable outcomes and a controversial association with SCA.[63,64]

The most common coronary arterial anomaly associated with SCA of the young originates from the opposite sinus of Valsalva or opposite coronary artery, with an interarterial course between the aortic root and pulmonary artery.[59,61,62,65] It has been postulated that the coronary artery may be compressed between the aorta and pulmonary artery, which leads to acute ischemia or arrhythmia (**Fig. 4**). However, some investigators have described the ACA as having an acute angle (less than 45°) at its takeoff and have implicated this feature along with others as features that lead to SCA.[66] When an anomalous left main coronary artery arises from the right sinus of Valsalva, an interarterial course at or above the level of the pulmonary valve with narrowing of the orifice in a slitlike manner are features associated with risk of SCA. In a large retrospective study of 6.3 million military recruits, of the 64 patients who

---

Box 2
Description of different types of ACAs divided into those with high-risk features and those without

ACAs

Potential for symptoms and ischemia: coronary artery that arises from the opposite sinus of Valsalva

    Intramural: slitlike coronary artery orifice

    Interarterial: passes between the aorta and pulmonary artery at the pulmonary valve level.

Typically benign ACA: opposite coronary artery that takes a

    Retroaortic course

    Prepulmonic course

    Intramural course

    Transseptal course

    High takeoff point from the aorta or coronary artery duplication

    Coronary artery fistulas

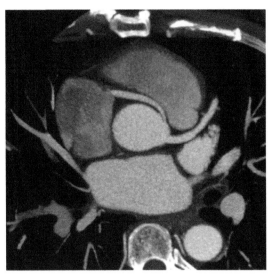

Fig. 4. Maximum intensity projection contrast-enhanced CT image of the coronary arteries illustrating an ACA.

died of a cardiac cause, 54% had a left main coronary artery arising from the right sinus of Valsalva and these features.[59] A benign subtype of the anomalous left coronary artery has a subpulmonic course through the ventricular septum and may give rise to a septal perforator before exiting the epicardial surface.

The most serious and rarest coronary artery anomalies are a right or left coronary artery arising from the pulmonary artery trunk. These are typically highly symptomatic early in life and usually require surgical intervention to relieve symptoms.[67]

Coronary artery ostia including the course of the anomalous vessel can be visualized using either CMR or CCT, with consistent results and generally without requiring rate-reducing medication as a result of the athlete's low resting heart rate. CMR is preferred below 35 years of age because it requires no radiation or intravenous contrast agent, but it is usually unable to visualize the entire vessel.

Cardiac magnetic resonance imaging

Three-dimensional coronary magnetic resonance angiography (CMRA) can be included to screen for coronary artery anomalies in asymptomatic athletes.[68,69] Whole-heart MRA allows 3-dimensional volumetric assessment of the coronary vasculature. In addition, steady-state free precession (SSFP, white blood) sequences allow free breathing and improved anatomic sharpness, signal-to-noise ratio, and contrast-to-noise ratio when compared with older CMR sequences. However, motion-free visualization of coronary vasculature using CMR remains the exception because of motion artifact and spatial resolution limitations.[70]

Cardiovascular computed tomography

CCT is able to demonstrate ACAs in all patients with superior image quality compared with other imaging techniques. Several studies have demonstrated the accuracy of ACA identification and vessel course even in patients who could not be correctly classified at angiography.[61,62]

Prospective gating and low-voltage CCT techniques that routinely have radiation doses of less than 4 mSv are allowing for more widespread use of CCT. The newest generations of CCT systems now produce radiation exposure of less than 1 mSv in many cases. Various imaging planes and reconstructions should be used to visualize the coronary artery segment as it courses in the aortic wall, which may be compressed throughout the cardiac cycle, especially during systole.[65] Narrowing of an intramural segment within the aortic wall can be initially seen on axial views with optimal identification of the slitlike orifice and lateral compression best visualized on orthogonal short-axis cross-sectional views. When the vessel is outside the aortic wall, the artery has a round appearance distally. The acute angle takeoff can be best seen on axial and oblique maximum intensity projection images.

Coronary Artery Bridging and Aneurysm

Myocardial bridging or coronary artery tunneling into the myocardium, usually the left anterior descending artery, can easily be identified by CCT or CMR and may be associated with systolic compression. Myocardial bridging is a commonly encountered variant on coronary CT and is rarely associated with symptoms.[71]

Coronary artery aneurysms can be identified by CMR or CCT with or without associated symptoms. CMRA has limited data that suggest excellent agreement with invasive coronary angiography for detection of coronary artery aneurysms as well as measurement of aneurysm length and diameter.[72,73] Magnetic resonance angiography is often used to monitor aneurysm diameter progression, an essential part of patient follow-up because the risk of thrombosis is correlated to aneurysm size.[72]

Coronary Artery Disease

The role of CMR in identifying coronary artery anatomic stenosis is limited because image quality is hampered by relatively low contrast-to-noise-ratios and relatively poor spatial resolution compared with CCT. At the expense of radiation exposure, CCT is superior to CMR for visualizing the coronary arteries and coronary artery disease.

Coronary artery calcium (CAC) scoring with CCT is a noncontrast rapidly acquired study with radiation exposures of approximately 1 to 2 mSv. CAC scoring with CCT may be used to assess the risk of exercise-related coronary events in athletes.[74] A paucity of data exists in competitive athletes identifying the presence and severity of coronary artery disease related to athletic participation.[74,75] Associations of CAC and athletes have been described, but further investigation reveals that these studies show that prior traditional risk factors, tobacco abuse, hypertension, and hyperlipidemia are not erased when one decides to increase aerobic interests.

The identification of the presence of coronary artery stenosis using stress MRI has been found to be effective for excluding significant stenosis with high negative predictive value.[76,77] Importantly, the patients in this study were those with a higher pretest probability of disease than would be expected in many athletes. Further investigation is required to identify what role, if any, there is for asymptomatic athletes.

Valve disease

Most valve diseases are evaluated using echocardiography, considered the test of choice.[30] The aortic valve is normally composed of 3 leaflets; young athletes with aortic stenosis typically have unicuspid or bicuspid aortic valves. Bicuspid aortic valve is the most common congenital cardiac disorder in the general population and has a prevalence between 0.5% and 2.0%, with a 3:1 male predominance.[78,79]

SCA secondary to aortic stenosis is rare and most often occurs during physical exertion.[64] In cases in which the valve morphology is uncertain, transesophageal echocardiography is used, but CMR and CCT are good alternatives to assess morphology and the severity of the valve. Calcification of aortic valve leaflet the aortic annulus is well visualized by CCT (Video 2). CMR with SSFP has been found to be superior to echocardiography for diagnosis of bicuspid aortic valve with sensitivity of 100% and specificity of 95%.[80] CCT has produced equal precision as CMR for diagnosis along with identification of important related conditions such as aortic root diameter.[81]

Mitral Valve Prolapse

The prevalence of mitral valve prolapse has been described as high as 2.5% and is commonly caused by myxomatous valve leaflets.[82] Echocardiographic diagnosis requires valve prolapse of 2 mm or more beyond the mitral annulus in the long-axis parasternal view. The addition of leaflet thickening of more than 5 mm is associated with a greater risk of sudden death.[30,83] Contemporary studies have evaluated CMR compared with echocardiography for detection of leaflet prolapse and found a sensitivity and specificity of 100% along with accurate identification of leaflet thickness.[84]

AORTIC ROOT DILATION

Aortic root dilation among athletes, especially basketball and volleyball players, is reported as having a prevalence of 1.3% in male athletes and 0.9% in female athletes.[85,86] Causes may be related to valve disease or an inherited condition. Marfan syndrome is a common inherited disease that is transmitted in an autosomal dominant manner with a prevalence of 1 in 5000.[87] Individuals with Marfan syndrome have multi–organ system involvement with cardiovascular manifestations that are associated with risk of SCA. The cardiovascular manifestations of Marfan syndrome are numerous; they include aortic root disease including aneurysm formation, dissection, and mitral valve disease.[88,89]

As much as 60% of those with Marfan syndrome have aortic root dilation, with a 2:1 male predominance.[88,89] Aortic dissection is the most feared complication of Marfan syndrome, resulting from an intimal tear involving the proximal ascending aorta, sino-tubular junction, and aortic sinuses.[90,91]

Contrast-enhanced CCT and CMR (gated chest MRI) are considered optimal for precise aortic root measurements of diameter when suspected aortic pathology is present.[92] CMR offers the advantage of no ionizing radiation exposure compared with CT.[58,93] Therefore, in the author's practice, CMR is the imaging modality of choice for aortic root evaluations.

SUMMARY

The imaging approach to the athlete should be comprehensive. Any one single modality is rarely the only test needed for all patients. Decisions regarding which imaging study to use should be dictated by the clinical question at hand. The types of cardiovascular pathology described in this article are commonly encountered by those who regularly evaluate athletes. The advanced imaging techniques discussed in this article may each be the best option depending on the clinical scenario of the athlete. Unclear or borderline findings may require discussion or consultation with other experts in the field.

SUPPLEMENTARY DATA

Supplementary data related to this article can be found online at http://dx.doi.org/10.1016/j.csm.2015.02.005.

REFERENCES

1. Martinez MW, Nair S. The athlete grey zone: distinguishing pathologic from physiologic left ventricular hypertrophy. 2014. Available at: http://www.cardiosource. org/Science-And-Quality/Hot-Topics/2014/09/The-Athlete-Grey-Zone.aspx. Accessed November 2014.
2. Maron BJ, Ommen SR, Semsarian C, et al. Hypertrophic cardiomyopathy: present and future, with translation into contemporary cardiovascular medicine. J Am Coll Cardiol 2014;64(1):83–99.
3. Maron BJ. Distinguishing hypertrophic cardiomyopathy from athlete's heart physiological remodelling: clinical significance, diagnostic strategies and implications for preparticipation screening. Br J Sports Med 2009;43(9):649–56.
4. Lauschke J, Maisch B. Athlete's heart or hypertrophic cardiomyopathy? Clin Res Cardiol 2009;98(2):80–8.
5. Lai EJ, Rakowski H. Physiologic or pathologic hypertrophy: how can we know? Expert Rev Cardiovasc Ther 2014;12(8):919–22.
6. Baggish AL, Wang F, Weiner RB, et al. Training-specific changes in cardiac structure and function: a prospective and longitudinal assessment of competitive athletes. J Appl Physiol 2008;104(4):1121–8.
7. Corrado D, Schmied C, Basso C, et al. Risk of sports: do we need a preparticipation screening for competitive and leisure athletes? Eur Heart J 2011; 32(8):934–44.
8. Rickers C, Wilke NM, Jerosch-Herold M, et al. Utility of cardiac magnetic resonance imaging in the diagnosis of hypertrophic cardiomyopathy. Circulation 2005;112(6):855–61.
9. Petersen SE, Selvanayagam JB, Francis JM, et al. Differentiation of athlete's heart from pathological forms of cardiac hypertrophy by means of geometric indices derived from cardiovascular magnetic resonance. J Cardiovasc Magn Reson 2005;7(3):551–8.
10. Kuruvilla S, Adenaw N, Katwal AB, et al. Late gadolinium enhancement on cardiac magnetic resonance predicts adverse cardiovascular outcomes in nonischemic cardiomyopathy: a systematic review and meta-analysis. Circ Cardiovasc Imaging 2014;7(2):250–8.
11. El Aidi H, Adenaw N, Katwal AB, et al. Cardiac magnetic resonance imaging findings and the risk of cardiovascular events in patients with recent myocardial infarction or suspected or known coronary artery disease: a systematic review of prognostic studies. J Am Coll Cardiol 2014;63(11):1031–45.
12. Pennell DJ. Cardiovascular magnetic resonance. Circulation 2010;121(5):692–705.
13. Wu E, Judd RM, Vargas JD, et al. Visualisation of presence, location, and transmural extent of healed Q-wave and non-Q-wave myocardial infarction. Lancet 2001;357(9249):21–8.
14. Mahrholdt H, Wagner A, Judd RM, et al. Delayed enhancement cardiovascular magnetic resonance assessment of non-ischaemic cardiomyopathies. Eur Heart J 2005;26(15):1461–74.
15. Deshpande A, Pakkal M, Agrawal B, et al. Cardiac magnetic resonance imaging of non-ischaemic cardiomyopathy. Postgrad Med J 2012;88(1035):38–48.
16. Hoey ET, Teoh JK, Das I, et al. The emerging role of cardiovascular MRI for risk stratification in hypertrophic cardiomyopathy. Clin Radiol 2014;69(3):221–30.
17. Vanhoenacker PK, Heijenbrok-Kal MH, Van Heste R, et al. Diagnostic performance of multidetector CT angiography for assessment of coronary artery disease: meta-analysis. Radiology 2007;244(2):419–28.

18. Rubin GD, Leipsic J, Joseph Schoepf U, et al. CT angiography after 20 years: a transformation in cardiovascular disease characterization continues to advance. Radiology 2014;271(3):633–52.
19. Brix G, Lechel U, Nekolla E, et al. Radiation protection issues in dynamic contrast-enhanced (perfusion) computed tomography. Eur J Radiol 2014. pii: S0720-048X(14)00518. [Epub ahead of print].
20. Gersh BJ, Maron BJ, Bonow RO, et al. 2011 ACCF/AHA guideline for the diagnosis and treatment of hypertrophic cardiomyopathy: a report of the American College of Cardiology Foundation/American Heart Association Task Force on Practice Guidelines. J Thorac Cardiovasc Surg 2011;142(6):e153–203.
21. Baggish A, Thompson PD. Thick hearts, high stakes, great uncertainties: screening athletes for hypertrophic cardiomyopathy. Heart 2009;95(5):345–7.
22. Pelliccia A, Maron BJ, Spataro A, et al. The upper limit of physiologic cardiac hypertrophy in highly trained elite athletes. N Engl J Med 1991;324(5):295–301.
23. Posma JL, Blanksma PK, van der Wall EE, et al. Assessment of quantitative hypertrophy scores in hypertrophic cardiomyopathy: magnetic resonance imaging versus echocardiography. Am Heart J 1996;132(5):1020–7.
24. Allison JD, Flickinger FW, Wright JC, et al. Measurement of left ventricular mass in hypertrophic cardiomyopathy using MRI: comparison with echocardiography. Magn Reson Imaging 1993;11(3):329–34.
25. Moon JC, McKenna WJ. The emerging role of cardiovascular magnetic resonance in refining the diagnosis of hypertrophic cardiomyopathy. Nat Clin Pract Cardiovasc Med 2009;6(3):166–7.
26. Morita Y, Kato T, Okano M, et al. A rare case of hypertrophic cardiomyopathy with subendocardial late gadolinium enhancement in an apical aneurysm with thrombus. Case Rep Radiol 2014;2014:780840.
27. Wong TC. Cardiovascular magnetic resonance imaging of myocardial interstitial expansion in hypertrophic cardiomyopathy. Curr Cardiovasc Imaging Rep 2014; 7:9267.
28. Franzen E, Mangold S, Erz G, et al. Comparison of morphological and functional adaptations of the heart in highly trained triathletes and long-distance runners using cardiac magnetic resonance imaging. Heart Vessels 2013; 28(5):626–31.
29. Camm CF, Tichnell C, James CA, et al. Premature ventricular contraction variability in arrhythmogenic right ventricular dysplasia/cardiomyopathy. J Cardiovasc Electrophysiol 2015;26(1):53–7.
30. Nishimura RA, Otto CM, Bonow RO, et al. 2014 AHA/ACC guideline for the management of patients with valvular heart disease: a report of the American College of Cardiology/American Heart Association Task Force on Practice Guidelines. J Thorac Cardiovasc Surg 2014;148(1):e1–132.
31. Luijkx T, Velthuis BK, Prakken NH, et al. Impact of revised Task Force Criteria: distinguishing the athlete's heart from ARVC/D using cardiac magnetic resonance imaging. Eur J Prev Cardiol 2012;19(4):885–91.
32. Maron BJ. Sudden death in young athletes. N Engl J Med 2003;349(11):1064–75.
33. Maron BJ, Douglas PS, Graham TP, et al. Task Force 1: preparticipation screening and diagnosis of cardiovascular disease in athletes. J Am Coll Cardiol 2005;45(8): 1322–6.
34. Calkins H. Arrhythmogenic right ventricular dysplasia. Curr Probl Cardiol 2013; 38(3):103–23.
35. Oxborough D, Shave R, Warburton D, et al. Dilatation and dysfunction of the right ventricle immediately after ultraendurance exercise: exploratory insights from

conventional two-dimensional and speckle tracking echocardiography. Circ Cardiovasc Imaging 2011;4(3):253–63.

36. Oxborough D, Sharma S, Shave R, et al. The right ventricle of the endurance athlete: the relationship between morphology and deformation. J Am Soc Echocardiogr 2012;25(3):263–71.

37. Zaidi A, Ghani S, Sheikh N, et al. Clinical significance of electrocardiographic right ventricular hypertrophy in athletes: comparison with arrhythmogenic right ventricular cardiomyopathy and pulmonary hypertension. Eur Heart J 2013; 34(47):3649–56.

38. Scott JM, Esch BT, Haykowsky MJ, et al. Effects of high intensity exercise on biventricular function assessed by cardiac magnetic resonance imaging in endurance trained and normally active individuals. Am J Cardiol 2010; 106(2):278–83.

39. Claessen G, Claus P, Ghysels S, et al. Right ventricular fatigue developing during endurance exercise: an exercise cardiac magnetic resonance study. Med Sci Sports Exerc 2014;46(9):1717–26.

40. Calkins H. Arrhythmogenic right ventricular dysplasia. Trans Am Clin Climatol Assoc 2008;119:273–86 [discussion: 287–8].

41. James CA, Calkins H. Update on arrhythmogenic right ventricular dysplasia/cardiomyopathy (ARVD/C). Curr Treat Options Cardiovasc Med 2013;15(4):476–87.

42. Omichi C, Sugiyabu Y, Kakizawa Y, et al. Three-dimensional image of arrhythmogenic right ventricular dysplasia/cardiomyopathy reconstructed with 64-multislice computed tomography. Heart Rhythm 2008;5(11):1631–2.

43. Kantarci M, Bayraktutan U, Sevimli S, et al. Multidetector computed tomography findings of arrhythmogenic right ventricular dysplasia: a case report. Heart Surg Forum 2008;11(1):E56–8.

44. Valsangiacomo Buechel ER, Mertens LL. Imaging the right heart: the use of integrated multimodality imaging. Eur Heart J 2012;33(8):949–60.

45. Nakajima T, Kimura F, Kajimoto K, et al. Utility of ECG-gated MDCT to differentiate patients with ARVC/D from patients with ventricular tachyarrhythmias. J Cardiovasc Comput Tomogr 2013;7(4):223–33.

46. Scharhag J, Schneider G, Urhausen A, et al. Athlete's heart: right and left ventricular mass and function in male endurance athletes and untrained individuals determined by magnetic resonance imaging. J Am Coll Cardiol 2002;40(10): 1856–63.

47. Maron BJ. Distinguishing hypertrophic cardiomyopathy from athlete's heart: a clinical problem of increasing magnitude and significance. Heart 2005;91(11): 1380–2.

48. Nishimura RA, Chareonthaitawee P, Martinez MW. Noninvasive imaging: echocardiography, nuclear cardiology, and MRI/CT imaging. In: Fauci AS, Longo DL, Kasper DL, et al, editors. Harrison's principles of internal medicine. New York: McGraw-Hill; 2012.

49. Koikkalainen JR, Antila M, Lötjönen JM, et al. Early familial dilated cardiomyopathy: identification with determination of disease state parameter from cine MR image data. Radiology 2008;249(1):88–96.

50. Tandri H, Saranathan M, Rodriguez ER, et al. Noninvasive detection of myocardial fibrosis in arrhythmogenic right ventricular cardiomyopathy using delayed-enhancement magnetic resonance imaging. J Am Coll Cardiol 2005;45(1):98–103.

51. Bowles NE, Ni J, Kearney DL, et al. Detection of viruses in myocardial tissues by polymerase chain reaction. evidence of adenovirus as a common cause of myocarditis in children and adults. J Am Coll Cardiol 2003;42(3):466–72.

52. Radunski UK, Lund GK, Stehning C, et al. CMR in patients with severe myocarditis: diagnostic value of quantitative tissue markers including extracellular volume imaging. JACC Cardiovasc Imaging 2014;7(7):667–75.

53. Luetkens JA, Doerner J, Thomas DK, et al. Acute myocarditis: multiparametric cardiac MR imaging. Radiology 2014;273(2):383–92.

54. Friedrich MG, Sechtem U, Schulz-Menger J, et al. Cardiovascular magnetic resonance in myocarditis: A JACC white paper. J Am Coll Cardiol 2009;53(17): 1475–87.

55. Schumm J, Greulich S, Wagner A, et al. Cardiovascular magnetic resonance risk stratification in patients with clinically suspected myocarditis. J Cardiovasc Magn Reson 2014;16(1):14.

56. Bellavia D, Michelena HI, Martinez M, et al. Speckle myocardial imaging modalities for early detection of myocardial impairment in isolated left ventricular non-compaction. Heart 2010;96(6):440–7.

57. Gati S, Chandra N, Bennett RL, et al. Increased left ventricular trabeculation in highly trained athletes: do we need more stringent criteria for the diagnosis of left ventricular non-compaction in athletes? Heart 2013;99(6):401–8.

58. Yim ES. Aortic root disease in athletes: aortic root dilation, anomalous coronary artery, bicuspid aortic valve, and Marfan's syndrome. Sports Med 2013;43(8): 721–32.

59. Lee HJ, Hong YJ, Kim HY, et al. Anomalous origin of the right coronary artery from the left coronary sinus with an interarterial course: subtypes and clinical importance. Radiology 2012;262(1):101–8.

60. Datta J, White CS, Gilkeson RC, et al. Anomalous coronary arteries in adults: depiction at multi-detector row CT angiography. Radiology 2005;235(3):812–8.

61. Angelini P. Novel imaging of coronary artery anomalies to assess their prevalence, the causes of clinical symptoms, and the risk of sudden cardiac death. Circ Cardiovasc Imaging 2014;7(4):747–54.

62. Yildiz A, Okcun B, Peker T, et al. Prevalence of coronary artery anomalies in 12,457 adult patients who underwent coronary angiography. Clin Cardiol 2010; 33(12):E60–4.

63. Angelini P. Coronary artery anomalies: an entity in search of an identity. Circulation 2007;115(10):1296–305.

64. Graham TP Jr, Driscoll DJ, Gersony WM, et al. Task Force 2: congenital heart disease. J Am Coll Cardiol 2005;45(8):1326–33.

65. Angelini P. Coronary artery anomalies–current clinical issues: definitions, classification, incidence, clinical relevance, and treatment guidelines. Tex Heart Inst J 2002;29(4):271–8.

66. Iskandar EG, Thompson PD. Exercise-related sudden death due to an unusual coronary artery anomaly. Med Sci Sports Exerc 2004;36(2):180–2.

67. Pena E, Nguyen ET, Merchant N, et al. ALCAPA syndrome: not just a pediatric disease. Radiographics 2009;29(2):553–65.

68. Jahnke C, Paetsch I, Nagel E. 3D MR coronary angiography: optimization of the technique and preliminary results. Int J Cardiovasc Imaging 2006;22(3–4): 489–91.

69. Prakken NH, Vonken EJ, Velthuis BK, et al. 3D MR coronary angiography: optimization of the technique and preliminary results. Int J Cardiovasc Imaging 2006; 22(3–4):477–87.

70. Bluemke DA, Achenbach S, Budoff M, et al. Noninvasive coronary artery imaging: magnetic resonance angiography and multidetector computed tomography angiography: a scientific statement from the American Heart Association Committee

on Cardiovascular Imaging and Intervention of the Council on Cardiovascular Radiology and Intervention, and the Councils on Clinical Cardiology and Cardiovascular Disease in the Young. Circulation 2008;118(5):586–606.

71. Jodocy D, Aglan I, Friedrich G, et al. Left anterior descending coronary artery myocardial bridging by multislice computed tomography: correlation with clinical findings. Eur J Radiol 2010;73(1):89–95.

72. Mavrogeni S, Papadopoulos G, Douskou M, et al. Magnetic resonance angiography is equivalent to X-ray coronary angiography for the evaluation of coronary arteries in Kawasaki disease. J Am Coll Cardiol 2004;43(4):649–52.

73. Greil GF, Stuber M, Botnar RM, et al. Coronary magnetic resonance angiography in adolescents and young adults with Kawasaki disease. Circulation 2002;105(8): 908–11.

74. Sanchez LD, Pereira J, Berkoff DJ. The evaluation of cardiac complaints in marathon runners. J Emerg Med 2009;36(4):369–76.

75. Kim JH, Malhotra R, Chiampas G, et al. Cardiac arrest during long-distance running races. N Engl J Med 2012;366(2):130–40.

76. Palios J, Karangelis D, Roubelakis A, et al. The prominent role of cardiac magnetic resonance imaging in coronary artery disease. Expert Rev Cardiovasc Ther 2014;12(2):167–74.

77. Heydari B, Kwong RY. Cardiac magnetic resonance imaging for ischemic heart disease: update on diagnosis and prognosis. Top Magn Reson Imaging 2014; 23(1):21–31.

78. Basso C, Boschello M, Perrone C, et al. An echocardiographic survey of primary school children for bicuspid aortic valve. Am J Cardiol 2004;93(5):661–3.

79. Clementi M, Notari L, Borghi A, et al. Familial congenital bicuspid aortic valve: a disorder of uncertain inheritance. Am J Med Genet 1996;62(4):336–8.

80. Gleeson TG, Mwangi I, Horgan SJ, et al. Steady-state free-precession (SSFP) cine MRI in distinguishing normal and bicuspid aortic valves. J Magn Reson Imaging 2008;28(4):873–8.

81. Manghat NE, Rachapalli V, Van Lingen R, et al. Imaging the heart valves using ECG-gated 64-detector row cardiac CT. Br J Radiol 2008;81(964):275–90.

82. Freed LA, Levy D, Levine RA, et al. Prevalence and clinical outcome of mitral-valve prolapse. N Engl J Med 1999;341(1):1–7.

83. Hayek E, Gring CN, Griffin BP. Mitral valve prolapse. Lancet 2005;365(9458): 507–18.

84. Han Y, Peters DC, Salton CJ, et al. Cardiovascular magnetic resonance characterization of mitral valve prolapse. JACC Cardiovasc Imaging 2008;1(3):294–303.

85. Pelliccia A, Di Paolo FM, De Blasiis E, et al. Prevalence and clinical significance of aortic root dilation in highly trained competitive athletes. Circulation 2010; 122(7):698–706, 3 p following 706.

86. Kinoshita N, Mimura J, Obayashi C, et al. Aortic root dilatation among young competitive athletes: echocardiographic screening of 1929 athletes between 15 and 34 years of age. Am Heart J 2000;139(4):723–8.

87. von Kodolitsch Y, Blankart CR, Vogler M, et al. Genetics and prevention of genetic aortic syndromes (GAS) and of the Marfan syndrome. Bundesgesundheitsblatt Gesundheitsforschung Gesundheitsschutz 2015;58(2):146–53 [in German].

88. Radke RM, Baumgartner H. Diagnosis and treatment of Marfan syndrome: an update. Heart 2014;100(17):1382–91.

89. Paterick TE, Humphries JA, Ammar KA, et al. Aortopathies: etiologies, genetics, differential diagnosis, prognosis and management. Am J Med 2013;126(8): 670–8.

90. Treasure T, Takkenberg JJ, Pepper J. Surgical management of aortic root disease in Marfan syndrome and other congenital disorders associated with aortic root aneurysms. Heart 2014;100(20):1571–6.
91. Chu LC, Johnson PT, Dietz HC, et al. CT angiographic evaluation of genetic vascular disease: role in detection, staging, and management of complex vascular pathologic conditions. AJR Am J Roentgenol 2014;202(5):1120–9.
92. Tsai SF, Trivedi M, Daniels CJ. Comparing imaging modalities for screening aortic complications in patients with bicuspid aortic valve. Congenit Heart Dis 2012; 7(4):372–7.
93. Dormand H, Mohiaddin RH. Cardiovascular magnetic resonance in Marfan syndrome. J Cardiovasc Magn Reson 2013;15:33.

Cardiovascular Concerns in Water Sports

Alfred A. Bove, MD, PhD

KEYWORDS

- Diving • Triathlon • Immersion • Swimming-induced pulmonary edema
- Immersion pulmonary edema • Decompression sickness • Arterial gas embolism

KEY POINTS

- Excess dyspnea and cough during the swimming phase of a triathlon is likely caused by swimming-induced pulmonary edema.
- Divers who develop extensive pulmonary barotrauma on ascent from depth may develop shock and pulseless electrical activity of the heart because of obstruction of the central circulation with air.
- Adults with congenital, valvular, and acquired heart disease may require special training to avoid adverse hemodynamic effects of water immersion and underwater exercise.
- Divers and swimmers with a long QT syndrome may develop ventricular tachycardia when swimming or diving.

Although there are a variety of water sports that have effects on the cardiovascular system, this article is confined to the sports that are affected by two important factors involved with water exposure. These include the physiologic effects of immersion on the cardiovascular system and the effects of exposure to increased pressure that include the physical effects of pressure based on the principles of Boyle's law (direct pressure effects[1,2]), and the effects of increased pressure on kinetics of gases in tissues and organs based on Henry's law (indirect pressure effects[3]). In some exposures all three effects may combine to cause abnormal stresses on the circulatory and the respiratory systems. To understand these various physiologic effects, it is necessary to provide a brief review of the physics of immersion and diving.

DEPTH AND PRESSURE

Pressure, defined as force/unit area, is related to the weight of a fluid column by the formula: pressure = height·density. Thus, pressure in water is directly related to depth below the surface. **Table 1** shows the relation between depth in seawater and

Cardiology Section, Temple University School of Medicine, 3501 N. Broad Street, Philadelphia, PA 19140, USA
E-mail address: Alfred.bove@tuhs.temple.edu

Clin Sports Med 34 (2015) 449–460
http://dx.doi.org/10.1016/j.csm.2015.02.003
0278-5919/15/$ – see front matter © 2015 Elsevier Inc. All rights reserved.

Table 1				
Relationship between depth in seawater and ambient pressure				
	feet	atm	mm Hg	psi
Sea level	0	1	760	14.7
	33	2	1520	29.4
Depth in seawater	66	3	2280	44.1
	99	4	3040	58.8
	132	5	3800	73.5
	165	6	4560	88.2

pressure. In seawater, an increase in pressure of 1 atm (14.7 psi; 100 kPa) occurs for each 33 feet of seawater (FSW). Because of the slightly lower density of freshwater, the depth to achieve 1 atm pressure is 34 feet. Because of the fixed relationship between height and pressure, pressure is often expressed in units of length (millimeters of mercury, FSW, and so forth).

BOYLE'S LAW

For a fixed mass of an ideal gas, Boyle's law states that the product of pressure and volume ($P \cdot V$) is constant.[1] Thus a volume of gas at the surface of seawater at a pressure of 1 atm absolute pressure (ATA) is reduced to one-half of the original volume at 33 FSW (2 ATA). Conversely, a volume of gas at 33 FSW doubles as it rises from 33 FSW to the surface. This relationship has important implications related to lung volumes during excursions underwater.

HENRY'S LAW

This law states that the volume of dissolved gas in a liquid is proportional to the partial pressure of the gas.[3] Gas partial pressure is determined by the product of the ambient pressure and the proportion of the gas in the gas mixture. In air (79% nitrogen) at 33 FSW for example, partial pressure of nitrogen is $0.79 \cdot 2$ ATA $= 1.58$ ATA. This relationship is particularly applicable to decompression sickness (DCS) that results from supersaturation of inert gas in tissues and water with the risk of formation of a gas phase (bubbles) and tissue injury.

IMMERSION

When an individual is immersed in water, the vertical fluid column produces a pressure that counters the intravascular pressures that result from the height of the blood column below the heart. This effect results in an estimated 600 to 700 mL of blood to shift from the veins into the central circulation.[4] This volume is accommodated by expansion of the pulmonary vasculature, and by increased stroke volume based on the Starling relationship.[4,5] In individuals with reduced systolic or diastolic ventricular function, this shift can result in an increase in left ventricular end diastolic pressure with subsequent pulmonary venous congestion and pulmonary edema. Stickland and colleagues[6] demonstrated that exercise-trained individuals show a lower pulmonary capillary wedge pressure at high exercise loads compared with untrained individuals. Their data suggest that dyspnea related to extreme exercise is related to increased pulmonary capillary pressure and interstitial lung edema that impairs gas exchange. The work of West and colleagues[7,8] in race horses performing extreme exercise supports this hypothesis. He studied several horses that developed exercise-induced pulmonary hemorrhage when racing at maximum performance (**Fig. 1**). When added to

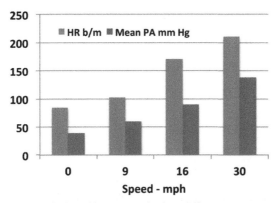

Fig. 1. Pulmonary pressure (PA) and heart rate (HR) at different running speeds in miles per hour (mph) in a race horse that demonstrated exercise-induced pulmonary hemorrhage. (*Data from* West JB, Mathieu-Costello O, Jones JH, et al. Stress failure of pulmonary capillaries in racehorses with exercise-induced pulmonary hemorrhage. J Appl Physiol 1993;75:1097–109.)

the increased pulmonary vascular volume associated with immersion, there is an increased likelihood that exercising in water would result in lung congestion, dyspnea, and pulmonary edema. Abnormal left ventricular diastolic function with impaired relaxation[9] would further aggravate this situation.

In-water exercise occurs in triathletes, divers, and other water sport athletes. In addition, military tactical divers are trained to work in water at high exercise loads. Swimming-induced pulmonary edema (SIPE) has been reported from several military training programs where swimming for long distances at high aerobic load has resulted in pulmonary edema in well-conditioned, trained swimmers with no evidence of cardiac or pulmonary disorders.[10–12] Similar reports described triathletes who developed pulmonary edema during the swimming phase of the event.[13,14] In most cases detailed cardiac evaluation found no evidence of cardiac pathology.

Wilmshurst and colleagues[15] studied a group of divers who developed pulmonary edema while diving (immersion pulmonary edema [IPE]). In these subjects, they demonstrated a hyperreactivity to immersion, cold, and increased oxygen partial pressure.[15] **Fig. 2** shows results from their report. Increased blood pressure and peripheral vasoconstriction with high vascular resistance were characteristic of the divers who developed IPE. Subsequent studies, however, suggested that IPE can occur in individuals who do not have evidence of abnormal vascular reactivity.[16,17]

Immersion effects on cardiac and pulmonary function are well understood. Studies over several decades have elucidated the physiologic effects of head-out immersion.[18,19] Swimmers, divers, and others who are immersed in water to the neck undergo these fluid shift effects caused by the physical effects of water pressure countering usual gravitational pooling of blood in the venous circulation when in the upright position. The work of West and colleagues[7,8] suggests that there may be an intrinsic susceptibility to capillary leakage and pulmonary edema. The effects of exercise on lung capillary pressure under circumstances of increased lung capillary volume, abnormal left ventricular relaxation that results in increased pulmonary venous pressure, and increased pulmonary arterial pressure that results from extreme exercise[20–22] may combine to cause IPE.

Prevention of IPE or SIPE can be based on the known physiology of the disorder.[18–22] Avoiding overhydration to minimize fluid load on the heart and lungs is

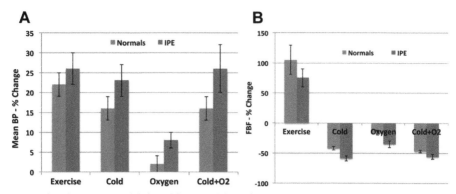

Fig. 2. Blood pressure (BP) (*A*) and forearm blood flow (FBF) (*B*) response to cold and oxygen exposure in normal subjects and subjects who demonstrated immersion pulmonary edema (IPE) while diving or swimming. (*Data from* Wilmshurst PT, Nuri M, Crowther A, et al. Cold-induced pulmonary oedema in scuba divers and swimmers and subsequent development of hypertension. Lancet 1989;1(8629):62–5.)

essential. In some cases of SIPE during competitive swimming, the participant's fluid loaded before entering the water to swim at a high intensity.[10] For triathletes, entering the water before starting the swim is helpful but some events do not allow prerace entry into the water. Starting the swim with a less than maximum effort minimizes diastolic pressure increases and avoids elevated pulmonary venous pressure. Diuretics have been proposed to lower fluid volume, but in competitive endurance races where loss of fluid is a concern, diuretics should not be recommended.

DIVING
Barotrauma

Diving injuries related to direct effects of pressure are caused by changing gas volumes in body spaces according to Boyle's law. Air spaces in the middle ear and paranasal sinuses are highly susceptible to volume changes during descent. Middle ear barotrauma is the most common diving-related injury.[23] Sinus barotrauma is also common.[24,25] Other injuries related to descent include lung injury caused by barotrauma at extreme depths in competitive breathhold diving (discussed later).

Increasing pressure can also affect implanted pacemakers and defibrillators; however, most pacemakers and defibrillators are designed to withstand pressures to about 100 FSW (4 ATA).[26] Manufacturers should be consulted to obtain pressure specifications for each model of device. Divers can safely dive with a pacemaker in the absence of significant cardiac abnormalities that would impair normal exercise capacity.

Although middle ear barotrauma of descent is the most common diving-related injury, lung barotrauma of ascent is the most lethal.[27–30] Recreational scuba divers breathe compressed air at depth to maintain normal tidal volume for usual oxygen and carbon dioxide exchange. Air pressure regulators provide breathing gas at the ambient pressure so no pressure gradient exists between the air supply and the lungs.[31] During ascent the compressed gas in the lungs must be ventilated because it expands according to Boyle's law. If proper ventilation is not maintained or there is a local airway obstruction, expanding gas distends the lungs, ultimately disrupting lung tissue.[27] Air can dissect into the pleural space or the mediastinum, and enters the torn pulmonary capillaries and veins to produce arterial gas embolism (AGE). The common presentation is sudden unconsciousness on reaching the surface with evidence of cerebral injury.[32,33] In extreme cases enough air enters the circulation that it obstructs the left ventricle and results in an air lock that blocks forward blood flow through the heart.[34] Fatal air embolism has been reported from central circulatory obstruction with air.[35] Pulmonary barotrauma has been reported from depths of 4 FSW,[36] and use of scuba equipment in a swimming pool is known to result in pulmonary barotrauma. Prevention is essential to avoid this disorder. Scuba training programs emphasize the need to properly ventilate when ascending to avoid lung overpressure. Several studies have demonstrated that risk for pulmonary barotrauma is increased in the presence of lung abnormalities.[37] Treatment of cerebral and circulatory abnormalities related to AGE requires recompression in a hyperbaric chamber.[38,39] The increased pressure reduces the volume of intravascular gas and improves perfusion. With added oxygen in the breathing gas, nitrogen in the air bubbles can be replaced by oxygen, which is metabolized to more rapidly reduce the volume of intravascular gas.[40–42]

Decompression Sickness

The content of inert gas dissolved in tissue is related to the partial pressure of the gas as described by Henry's law.[3] When air is breathed at increased pressure during diving, nitrogen content of tissues is increased. The equilibrium concentration of nitrogen described by Henry's law, however, is not achieved instantaneously; different tissues and organs take up nitrogen at different rates, and nitrogen concentration changes as an exponential function of time.[43] The work of Boycott and coworkers[44] demonstrated that different tissue compartments in the body take up and wash out nitrogen at different rates. Because of the finite time needed to remove nitrogen from tissue, nitrogen becomes supersaturated in tissues on ascent. Haldane and Colleagues[44] developed a method of avoiding excess supersaturation of nitrogen by incorporating periodic stops during ascent to minimize nitrogen supersaturation. **Fig. 3** demonstrates the uptake and washout of nitrogen from five tissue compartments. By stopping during ascent, the nitrogen concentration of supersaturated tissues can be lowered to avoid conversion to a gas phase in tissue, thereby avoiding

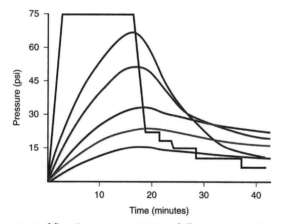

Fig. 3. Nitrogen content of five tissue compartments following exposure to air at 75 psi (168 FSW), and decompression. Blue line represents exposure profile, curved lines demonstrate nitrogen content of five tissue compartments. (*Adapted from* Boycott AE, Damant GC, Haldane J. The prevention of compressed air illness. J Hyg (Lond) 1908;8:363.)

DCS. Numerous observations[45,46] subsequent to the work of Haldane and colleagues in 1908[44] demonstrated that venous gas emboli (VGE) appear before symptoms of overt DCS are evident. Doppler ultrasound surveillance of the pulmonary vein after a diving exposure has demonstrated asymptomatic bubbles transported from the peripheral veins to the central circulation to be trapped by the lung.[45] Of interest is the role of intracardiac shunts in allowing VGE to enter the arterial circulation to become AGE. Based on this concern, individuals with evident right to left shunts have been discouraged from diving to avoid the risk of cerebral injury from AGE. Recent interest has focused on the role of a patent foramen ovale (PFO) on risk for DCS.[47–50] Presence of a PFO has been demonstrated to increase risk for DCS[48]; however, absolute risk is low and a PFO, estimated to be present in 25% to 30% of the population,[50] is not a contraindication to diving. Recent studies of divers exposed to high-stress dives that are known to produce VGE demonstrated an increased incidence of AGE in divers with a large PFO, and a trend toward increased clinical DCS.[50] Although a PFO is likely to increase risk for DCS under certain extreme exposures, closing a PFO in divers is not recommended.[51]

Breathhold Diving

Diving beneath the surface while apneic with a single breath has been described for more than 2000 years.[18,40,52] Besides the recreational aspects of breathhold diving to observe the undersea environment, commercial breathhold divers have been active in the Pacific for more than five centuries. The Ama of Japan[53,54] perform underwater harvesting of food by repetitive breathhold dives. More recent efforts at competitive breathhold diving events have included spear fishing contests and attempts to set depth records on a single breath. Based on Boyle's law, with a residual lung volume of 20% of maximum lung volume, the residual volume would be attained at 5 ATA (132 FSW) depth. Diving below that level would theoretically result in rib cage compression and injury. However, the record for a single breathhold dive exceeds 500 FSW and the deep breathhold divers do not seem to sustain overt lung injury from these deep exposures. Dahlback and colleagues[55] demonstrated that the shrinking lung volume with increasing depth is accommodated by blood shifts into the lung vasculature to fill the diminishing air space resulting from increased pressure. As gas volume diminishes, more blood fills the lung vasculature, and the diaphragms are displaced upward. At a depth of 500 FSW (16 ATA), an initial lung volume of 6 L is reduced to 375 mL (Fig. 4). Several reports of pulmonary congestion following deep breathhold dives[56,57] suggest that progressive distention of lung capillaries with blood to accommodate the shrinking air space results in lung injury.

Diving Effects on Heart Rhythm

Diving mammals (dolphin, seal, whale) exhibit a profound bradycardia when diving (diving reflex[58]). The reduced heart rate and vasoconstriction of muscle vasculature preserves blood flow to the brain and heart and allows those animals to spend substantial time underwater.[58,59] Whales are thought to dive for up to 2 hours on a single breath, and seals have demonstrated dives more than 30 minutes on a single breath.[60] The bradycardia is mediated by an increase in parasympathetic activity.[61] A less profound diving reflex can be found in humans who may exhibit a reduction in heart rate from 70 to 50 during diving.[62,63]

Ackerman and colleagues[64] found a high incidence of the inherited long QT syndrome in victims of drowning. The long QT1 variant seems to be sensitive to swimming or immersion, and can result in sudden death while swimming caused by ventricular fibrillation.[65] Divers with paroxysmal atrial flutter or fibrillation may experience the

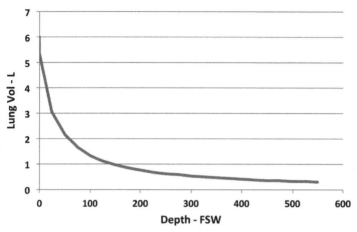

Fig. 4. Change in lung volume versus depth in a diver with a 6-L total lung capacity.

arrhythmia while diving, likely caused by atrial distention resulting from the central fluid shift associated with immersion.

Fitness for Diving

Usual forms of recreational diving do not require high levels of exercise. Most diving requires 3 to 4 metabolic equivalents (Mets) of exercise activity.[66] However to manage adverse conditions, a steady state capacity of 6 to 7 Mets is recommended. To sustain a steady state 6- to 7-Met activity, peak capacity should be about 12 to 13 Mets.[67] Divers with less than 13 Mets peak capacity should be cautioned to avoid diving that might require high levels of physical activity.

Coronary Disease

Because certification for sport diving is lifelong after one training encounter, many certified divers seek to return to diving after developing coronary artery disease and undergoing therapy many years after their initial certification. Divers with evidence of ischemia at low workloads are at risk for coronary events during diving.[68] Those with a history of coronary artery disease should have exercise tests performed to assess physical capacity with the understanding that 6 to 7 Mets of capacity should be tolerated without evidence of ischemia. Individuals can return to diving after percutaneous coronary intervention or coronary artery bypass graft if there is no evidence of ischemia at moderate workloads and there are no serious arrhythmias.

Valvular Disease

Mild or moderate valvular disease that does not impair exercise capacity is not a contraindication to diving. Significant aortic stenosis impairs exercise capacity and is a contraindication, whereas mild or moderate stenosis that allows normal exercise tolerance to 6 to 7 mets is not a contraindication. Regurgitant lesions result in left ventricular failure when severe, and the combined fluid shift centrally and exercise demands can result in acute onset of heart failure while diving.

Heart Rhythm Disorders and Pacemakers

Divers with chronic atrial fibrillation on anticoagulant therapy seem to have low risk for significant cardiac events when diving. Barotrauma to sinuses or middle ear often is accompanied by hemorrhage and anticoagulant therapy causes significant bleeding into middle ear or sinuses if a diver sustains barotrauma. Appropriate caution regarding ability to equalize ears and sinuses prevents severe bleeding related to barotrauma.

Divers with serious ventricular arrhythmias should be evaluated for etiology before being cleared for diving. Long QT syndrome can result in immersion- or swimming-induced ventricular fibrillation (discussed previously). Divers with evidence of this disorder should be cautioned about diving. Pacemakers and implantable cardioverter-defibrillators are discussed previously.

Congenital Heart Disease

Most patient with cyanotic congenital heart disease have reduced exercise capacity, and often right to left shunts that limit diving ability and increase risk for DCS.[69] Divers with a PFO are discussed previously. Divers with the restrictive ventricular septal defect with normal right-sided pressures can dive safely because the shunt is left to right, unless significant pulmonary hypertension develops and an Eisenmenger syndrome results in right to left shunting. An atrial septal defect is considered a contraindication to diving because of the potential for VGE to cross into the arterial circulation. Patients with corrected tetralogy of Fallot are known to dive safely,[70] whereas patients with a Fontan conduit and absence of right ventricular function are susceptible to hemodynamic aberrations related to central fluid shift, exercise and fluid volume changes, and may have left residual right to left shunting.[71]

Heart Failure and Cardiomyopathy

Patients with clinical evidence of heart failure should not dive because the fluid shift from immersion coupled with need for exercise often results in acute decompensation. Patients with left ventricular dysfunction should be tested for exercise capacity, particularly with swimming to evaluate capacity for exercise while immersed.

Aortic Disease

Patients with a significant thoracic aortic aneurysm may be at risk for aortic rupture related to blood surges into the aorta following a Valsalva maneuver commonly used to equalize the middle ear during descent.[72]

SUMMARY

Aquatic sports have increased in popularity with the increasing numbers of participants in triathlon events and long distance swimming competition. In addition, recreational sport diving with a single breath and with a portable air supply (scuba) has increased in popularity. Competitive breathhold diving to extreme depths is also now a recognized sport that brings a new form of pressure exposure and barotrauma risk to the diver. These exposures are accompanied by unique physiologic changes in the heart and circulation, and in addition demand an understanding of the environment to provide informed advice regarding safety for participation for athletes of all ages, and for those with documented heart disease. Knowledge of the aquatic environment and its effects on swimmers and divers is an important component of the knowledge base for the cardiologist interested in sports medicine.

REFERENCES

1. Boyle R. Defence of the doctrine touching the spring and the weight of the air. In: New experiments physico-mechanical. Touching the air. Oxford University Press; 1662.
2. Navy Department. U.S. Navy diving manual, rev 6, vol. 5: diagnosis and treatment of decompression sickness and arterial gas embolism (publication no. NAVSEA 0910-LP-106–0957). Washington, DC: U.S. Navy Department; 2008. p. 2–17. Available at: http://www.supsalv.org/00c3_publications.asp.
3. Henry W. Experiments on the quantity of gases absorbed by water, at different temperatures, and under different pressures. Phil Trans Roy Soc Lond 1803;93: 29–274.
4. Ferrigno M. Breath hold diving. In: Bove AA, editor. Bove and Davis' diving medicine. Philadelphia: Elsevier; 2004. p. 77–94.
5. Katz AM. Ernest Henry Starling, his predecessors, and the "Law of the Heart". Circulation 2002;106:2986–92.
6. Stickland MK, Welsh RC, Petersen SR, et al. Does fitness level modulate the cardiovascular hemodynamic response to exercise? J Appl Physiol 2006;100: 1895–901.
7. West JB, Mathieu-Costello O, Jones JH, et al. Stress failure of pulmonary capillaries in racehorses with exercise-induced pulmonary hemorrhage. J Appl Physiol 1993;75:1097–109.
8. West JB. Invited review: pulmonary capillary stress failure. J Appl Physiol 2000; 89:2483–9.
9. Rigolli M, Whalley GA. Heart failure with preserved ejection fraction. J Geriatr Cardiol 2013;10:369–76.
10. Adir Y, Shupak A, Gil A, et al. Swimming-induced pulmonary edema: clinical presentation and serial lung function. Chest 2004;126:394–9.
11. Lund KL, Mahon RT, Tanen DA, et al. Swimming-induced pulmonary edema. Ann Emerg Med 2003;41:251–6.
12. Mahon RT, Kerr S, Amundson D, et al. Immersion pulmonary edema in special forces combat swimmers. Chest 2002;122:383–4.
13. Boggio-Alarco JL, Jaume-Anselmi F, Ramirez-Rivera J. Acute pulmonary edema during a triathlon occurrence in a trained athlete. Bol Asoc Med P R 2006;98:110–3.
14. Stefanko G, Lancashire B, Coombes JS, et al. Pulmonary oedema and hyponatraemia after an ironman triathlon. BMJ Case Rep 17 Aug 2009 [pii:bcr04.2009.1764].
15. Wilmshurst PT, Nuri M, Crowther A, et al. Cold-induced pulmonary oedema in scuba divers and swimmers and subsequent development of hypertension. Lancet 1989;1(8629):62–5.
16. Koehle MS, Lepawsky M, McKenzie DC. Pulmonary oedema of immersion. Sports Med 2005;35:183–90.
17. Pons M, Blickenstorfer D, Oechslin E, et al. Pulmonary oedema in healthy persons during scuba-diving and swimming. Eur Respir J 1995;8:762–7.
18. Hong SK, Cerretelli P, Cruz JC, et al. Mechanics of respiration during submersion in water. J Appl Physiol 1969;27:537–8.
19. Craig AB Jr, Ware DE. Effect of immersion in water on vital capacity and residual volume of the lungs. J Appl Physiol 1967;23:423–5.
20. Zavorsky GS, Anholm JD. Mild interstitial pulmonary edema occurs during sea level strenuous exercise. J Appl Physiol 2010;109:1276 [discussion: 1281–2].
21. Hopkins SR. Point: pulmonary edema does occur in human athletes performing heavy sea-level exercise. J Appl Physiol 2010;109:1270–2.

22. Ma JL, Dutch MJ. Extreme sports: extreme physiology. Exercise-induced pulmonary oedema. Emerg Med Australas 2013;25:368–71.
23. Hunter SE, Farmer JC. Ear and sinus problems in diving. In: Bove AA, editor. Bove and Davis' diving medicine. 4th edition. Philadelphia: WB Saunders; 2004. p. 431–60.
24. Butler F. Orbital hemorrhage following facemask barotrauma. Undersea Hyperb Med 2001;28:31–4.
25. Uzun C. Paranasal sinus barotrauma in sports self-contained underwater breathing apparatus divers. J Laryngol Otol 2009;123:80–4.
26. Lafay V, Trigano JA, Gardette B, et al. Effects of hyperbaric exposures on cardiac pacemakers. Br J Sports Med 2008;42:212–6.
27. Schaefer KE, Nulty WP, Carey C, et al. Mechanisms in development of interstitial emphysema and air embolism on decompression from depth. J Appl Physiol 1958;13:15–29.
28. Behnke AR. Analysis of accidents occurring in training with the submarine "lung". US Naval Med Bull 1932;30:177–84. Available at: http://catalog.hathitrust.org/Record/005637982.
29. Polak B, Adams H. Traumatic air embolism in submarine escape training. US Naval Med Bull 1932;30:165–77. Available at: http://catalog.hathitrust.org/Record/005637982.
30. Tetzlaff K, Reuter M, Leplow B, et al. Risk factors for pulmonary barotrauma in divers. Chest 1997;112:654–9.
31. Egstrom GH. Diving equipment. In: Bove AA, editor. Bove and Davis diving medicine. Philadelphia: Elsevier; 2003. p. 41–3.
32. Muth CM, Shank ES. Gas embolism. N Engl J Med 2000;342:476–82.
33. Leitch DR, Green RD. Pulmonary barotrauma in divers and the treatment of cerebral arterial gas embolism. Aviat Space Environ Med 1986;57:931.
34. Harker CP, Neuman TS, Olson LK, et al. The roentgenographic findings associated with air embolism in sport scuba divers. J Emerg Med 1993;11:443–9.
35. Neuman TS, Jacoby J, Bove AA. Fatal pulmonary barotrauma due to obstruction of the central circulation with air. J Emerg Med 1998;16:413–7.
36. Benton PJ, Woodfine JD, Westwood PR. Arterial gas embolism following a 1 metre ascent during helicopter escape training: a case report. Aviat Space Environ Med 1996;67:63–4.
37. Reuter M, Tetzlaff K, Warninghoff V, et al. Computed tomography of the chest in diving-related pulmonary barotrauma. Br J Radiol 1997;70:440–5.
38. Kizer KW. Dysbaric cerebral air embolism in Hawaii. Ann Emerg Med 1987;16:535–41.
39. Hawes J, Massey EW. Neurologic injuries from scuba diving. Neurol Clin 2008;26:297–308, xii.
40. Bove AA, Clark JM, Simon AJ, et al. Successful therapy of cerebral air embolism with hyperbaric oxygen at 2.8 ATA. Undersea Biomed Res 1982;9:76–80.
41. Moon RE. Treatment of decompression illness. In: Bove AA, editor. Bove and Davis' diving medicine. 4th edition. Philadelphia: Elsevier; 2004. p. 195–224.
42. Bennett MH, Lehm JP, Mitchell SJ, et al. Recompression and adjunctive therapy for decompression illness. Cochrane Database Syst Rev 2012;(5):CD005277.
43. Vann RD. Mechanisms and risk of decompression sickness. In: Bove AA, editor. Bove and Davis' diving medicine. Philadelphia: Elsevier; 2004. p. 127–64.
44. Boycott AE, Damant GC, Haldane J. The prevention of compressed air illness. J Hyg (Lond) 1908;8:342–443.

45. Conkin J, Waligora JM, Foster PP, et al. Information about venous gas emboli improves prediction of hypobaric decompression sickness. Aviat Space Environ Med 1998;69:8–16.
46. Eftedal OS, Lydersen S, Brubakk AO. The relationship between venous gas bubbles and adverse effects of decompression after air dives. Undersea Hyperb Med 2007;34:99–105.
47. Torti SR, Billinger M, Schwerzmann M, et al. Risk of decompression illness among 230 divers in relation to the presence and size of patent foramen ovale. Eur Heart J 2004;25:1014–20.
48. Bove AA. Risk of decompression sickness with patent foramen ovale. Undersea Hyperb Med 1998;25:175–8.
49. Germonpré P, Dendale P, Unger P, et al. Patent foramen ovale and decompression sickness in sports divers. J Appl Physiol 1998;84:1622–6.
50. Honek J, Sramek M, Sefc L, et al. Effect of catheter-based patent foramen ovale closure on the occurrence of arterial bubbles in scuba divers. J Am Coll Cardiol Intv 2014;7:403–8.
51. Moon RE, Bove AA. Transcatheter occlusion of patent foramen ovale: a prevention for decompression illness? Undersea Hyperb Med 2004;31:271–4.
52. Landsberg PG. Hyperventilation: an unpredictable danger to the sports diver. In: Lundgren CE, Ferrigno M, editors. The physiology of breath-hold diving. Bethesda (MD): Undersea and Hyperbaric Medical Society; 1987. p. 256–67.
53. Schagatay E, Lodin-Sundström A, Abrahamsson E. Underwater working times in two groups of traditional apnea divers in Asia: the Ama and the Bajau. Diving Hyperb Med 2011;41:27–30.
54. Nukada M. Historical development of the Ama's diving activities. In: Rahn H, Yokoyama T, editors. physiology of breath-hold diving and the Ama of Japan. Washington, DC: National Academy of Sciences; National Research Council; 1965. p. 25–40.
55. Dahlbäck GO, Jönsson E, Linér MH. Influence of hydrostatic compression of the chest and intrathoracic blood pooling on static lung mechanics during head-out immersion. Undersea Biomed Res 1978;5(1):71–85.
56. Muth CM, Radermacher P, Pittner A, et al. Arterial blood gases during diving in elite apnea divers. Int J Sports Med 2003;24:104–7.
57. Lindholm P, Lundgren CE. Alveolar gas composition before and after maximal breath-holds in competitive divers. Undersea Hyperb Med 2006;33:463–7.
58. Elsner RW, Franklin DL, Vancitters RL. Cardiac output during diving in an unrestrained sea lion. Nature 1964;202:809–10.
59. Scholander PF. Experimental investigations on the respiratory function in diving animals and birds, vol. 22. Oslo (Norway): Hvalrådets Skrifter; Norske Videnskaps-Akad; 1940. p. 1–131.
60. Tyack PL, Johnson M, Soto NA, et al. Extreme diving of beaked whales. J Exp Biol 2006;209:4238–53.
61. Kawakami Y, Natelson BH, DuBois AB. Cardiovascular effects of face immersion and factors affecting diving reflex in man. J Appl Physiol 1967;23:964–70.
62. Bove AA, Lynch PR, Connell JV, et al. Diving reflex after physical training. J Appl Physiol 1968;25:70–2.
63. Foster GE, Sheel AW. The human dive response, its function, and its control. Scand J Med Sci Sports 2005;15:3–12.
64. Ackerman MJ, Tester DJ, Porter CJ. Swimming, a gene-specific arrhythmogenic trigger for inherited long QT syndrome. Mayo Clin Proc 1999;74:1088–94.

65. Bradley T, Dixon J, Easthope R. Unexplained fainting, near drowning, and unusual seizures in childhood: screening for long QT syndrome in New Zealand families. N Z Med J 1999;112:299–302.

66. Pendergast DR, Tedesco M, Nawrocki DM, et al. Energetics of underwater swimming with SCUBA. Med Sci Sports Exerc 1996;28:573–80.

67. Levine BD. Exercise physiology for the clinician. In: Thompson PD, editor. Exercise and sports cardiology. New York: McGraw Hill; 2001. p. 6–868.

68. Åkesson A, Larsson SC, Discacciati A, et al. Low-risk diet and lifestyle habits in the primary prevention of myocardial infarction in men. A population-based prospective cohort study. J Am Coll Cardiol 2014;64:1299–306.

69. Bove AA. The cardiovascular system and diving risk. Undersea Hyperb Med 2011;38:261–9.

70. Takagi J. A new "complex exercise test" for children with cardiac diseases. Kurume Med J 1994;41:97–107.

71. Goldberg DJ, Avitabile CM, McBride MG, et al. Exercise capacity in the Fontan circulation. Cardiol Young 2013;23:824–30.

72. Hiratzka LF, Bakris GL, Beckman JA, et al. ACCF/AHA/AATS/ACR/ASA/SCA/SCAI/SIR/STS/SVM guidelines for the diagnosis and management of patients with thoracic aortic disease. J Am Coll Cardiol 2010;55(14):1509–44.

Diseases of the Aorta in Elite Athletes

Aline Iskandar, MD[a], Paul D. Thompson, MD[b],*

KEYWORDS

- Aortic dilation • Bicuspid aortic valve • Acute aortic syndromes
- Sudden cardiac death in athletes

KEY POINTS

- Sudden cardiovascular deaths in athletes are rare and only a fraction are due to aortic events.
- There has been concern that the hemodynamic load during exercise, specifically pressure overload during strength training, may also lead to aortic dilation, but the aortic dimensions in endurance and strength-trained athletes are only slightly larger than those in sedentary comparison subjects.
- Consequently, routine echocardiography for aortic size assessment in athletes is not recommended and athletes with moderate aortic dilation can continue sports participation with monitoring.
- The presence of a bicuspid aortic valve without significant valvular dysfunction and normal aortic dimensions should not influence eligibility to practice sport.
- Patients with genetic syndromes associated with aortopathy, such as Marfan, Loeys-Dietz, and Ehlers-Danlos vascular-type syndromes, generally should be restricted from vigorous sports participation.

INTRODUCTION

Aortic disease accounts for approximately 1.6% of sudden cardiac death in young athletes.[1] The importance of aortic disease in athletes was highlighted when Flo Hyman, a member of the US volleyball team that won an Olympic silver medal in 1984, collapsed

Disclosures: A. Iskandar: None; P.D. Thompson has received research support from the NHLBI, NIAMS, NCCAM, Genomas, RocheSanofi, Regeneron, Esperion, Amarin and Pfizer. He has served as a consultant for Amgen, AstraZeneca, Regeneron, Merck, Genomas, Runners World, Sanofi, Esperion, and Amarin. He has received speaker honoraria from Merck, AstraZeneca, and Kowa. He owns stock in AbbVie, Abbott Labs, J&J; General Electric, and JA Wiley.
a Division of Cardiovascular Medicine, UMass Memorial Medical Center, 55 North Lake Avenue, Worcester, MA 01655, USA; b Division of Cardiology, Hartford Hospital, 80 Seymour Street, Hartford, CT 06102, USA
* Corresponding author.
E-mail address: paul.thompson@hhchealth.org

and died during a match in 1986 from aortic rupture associated with Marfan syndrome (MFS). The threat of aortic disease in athletes has attracted additional attention with the increased awareness of the association of bicuspid aortic valve and aortic abnormalities, including aortic dilation, coarctation, acute dissection, and rupture. This article reviews the diagnosis and management of diseases of the aorta in athletes.

Pathophysiology

Acute aortic syndromes refer to a spectrum of aortic emergencies that include aortic dissection, intramural hematoma (IMH), and symptomatic aortic ulcer.

Aortic Dissection

Aortic dissection is the most common aortic catastrophe, with an estimated annual incidence of 2.6 to 3.5 per 100,000 person-years.[2] The mean age of dissection as determined from 464 patients in the International Registry of Acute Aortic Dissection (IRAS) is 63 years and two-thirds of cases were in male individuals.[3] The most common predisposing factor is hypertension,[3] but patients younger than 40 years were less likely to have hypertension, and more likely to have a genetic or morphologic risk factor, such as bicuspid aortic valve, other genetic syndromes associated with aortopathy (eg, MFS), and/or previous aortic surgery.[4] The origin of ascending aortic dissections (type A) tends to be more proximal in younger patients at the sinuses of Valsalva and sinotubular junction.[4]

Aortic dissection classically occurs when a tear in the intima produces a separation of the intima from the media, creating a false lumen. The false lumen can propagate antegrade or retrograde, causing tamponade, aortic insufficiency, or compression or sheering of branch vessels with distal ischemia.[5]

Intramural Hematoma

Aortic IMH is a variant form of aortic dissection and can precede classic dissection.[2] IMH may occur as a primary event in hypertensive patients or may be caused by a penetrating ulcer or blunt chest trauma. Aortic IMH accounts for 5% to 20% of patients presenting with acute aortic syndromes.[6–10] IMH lacks an intimal tear and is thought to occur from a spontaneous rupture of the vasa vasorum, the blood vessels originating in the adventia that penetrate the outer half of the aortic media and supply blood to the outer aortic wall.[11] The hematoma can extend along the media of the aorta, and produce aortic wall rupture or aortic dissection.[11]

Penetrating Atherosclerotic Ulcer

Aortic ulcers initially just ulcerate the intima and are often asymptomatic. They can progress to penetrate into the media and lead to IMH, aortic dissection, or perforation.[12] Ulcers predominately affect the descending thoracic aorta, where atherosclerosis is most often encountered, and are principally a disease of elderly, hypertensive men.[13]

CONDITIONS ASSOCIATED WITH AORTIC DISEASE
Bicuspid Aortic Valve

Bicuspid aortic valve (BAV) is the most common congenital cardiac defect, affecting 0.5% to 2.0% of the general population, with a 3-to-1 prevalence in male versus female individuals.[14,15] BAV is heritable, with a prevalence of approximately 10% in first-degree relatives of an individual with a BAV.[16,17] BAV may develop progressive valve dysfunction (stenosis or regurgitation) or, less commonly, infective endocarditis. BAV disease is not confined to the valve leaflets, however, and is associated with an aortopathy. Compared with adults with a trileaflet aortic valve, patients with BAV have larger dimensions of the aortic sinuses and ascending aorta, abnormal aortic elasticity, and are at risk for aortic dilation and dissection.[18] Aortic dilation begins in childhood and is progressive.[19,20] Baseline aortic diameter is an important predictor of the rate of aortic expansion, which ranges between 0.2 and 1.9 mm per year in patients with BAV.[18,21,22]

BAV is common and consequently accounts for many of the cases of aortic emergencies, but the risk of such complications for any patient with BAV is actually low. Most cardiac complications in BAV cohorts involve valvular disease. Among 642 predominately male (86%) Canadian adults with BAV and a mean age of 35 years, 63% had normal or mildly abnormal valve function at baseline.[23] Over an average 9 years of follow-up, 25% experienced a primary cardiac event. These events were predominantly interventions on the aortic valve or ascending aorta, composed of 99 patients (15%) who had aortic valve surgery, 38 patients (6%) had an ascending aortic graft plus and an aortic valve replacement, and 5 patients (0.7%) required an aortic-root replacement. Eleven patients (2%) had an aortic complication: 5 dissections and 3 of these were in the ascending aorta. Independent predictors of an adverse cardiac event were age older than 30 and moderate or severe aortic valve dysfunction at baseline. Almost half (45%) of the whole cohort had dilation of either the aortic-root or ascending aorta at baseline probably contributing to the high overall event rate in this study, but the 10-year survival in the BAV group was not different from population estimates, however.

Similarly, a series of 212 asymptomatic adults with a BAV from Olmsted County, Minnesota, who had at most mild valve dysfunction and were followed for up to 20 years (mean follow-up of 15 years)[24] found significant cardiac morbidity with BAV, but mortality similar to the general population. Survival from time of diagnosis was 97% and 90% at 10 and 20 years, respectively.[24] Similarly, in the Canadian cohort, 10-year survival was 96%.[23]

A more recent publication from the Olmsted County cohort looked specifically at aortic complications in 416 adults with known BAV (mean age at diagnosis 35 years) followed for a mean of 16 years. Aortic dissection occurred in 2 patients, with an incidence of 3.1 cases per 10,000 person-years and an age-adjusted relative risk of 8.4. There were no dissections in patients with an aortic diameter smaller than 45 mm or in those with a normally functioning aortic valve.

Despite the high relative risk, the absolute incidence of aortic dissection on the basis of these 2 cohort studies remains very low.

Athletic training does not appear to accelerate the increase in aortic size in subjects with BAV. Yearly echocardiograms were performed in 88 athletes with BAV for 5 years. The yearly increase in the proximal ascending aorta was 0.98 mm.[25] This rate is comparable to that observed in nonathletes with BAV, which ranges among studies from 0.2 to 1.9 mm per year.[22]

Marfan Syndrome

Marfan syndrome (MFS) is an autosomal-dominant disorder of connective tissue with an estimated prevalence of 1 in 3000 to 5000 individuals and no predilection for either sex.[26] Approximately 25% of cases have no family history and represent de novo mutations. Cardinal features of MFS are abnormalities in the cardiovascular, ocular, and skeletal systems. In the most current "Revised Ghent Nosology" of 2010, greater weight is given to aortic dilation/dissection and ectopia lentis, family history of MFS, and genetic testing for mutations in the protein fibrillin-1. All other cardiovascular and ocular manifestations as well as manifestations in other organ systems of MFS, including skeletal, dura, skin, and lungs, contribute to a "systemic score," that assists in the diagnosis when aortic disease is present, but ectopia lentis is not.[27] Aortic dilation in these diagnostic criteria is defined as z-score of 2 or more, which has been criticized, because it may underestimate aortic-root dilation, especially in patients with large body surface area (BSA).[28] The most widely used formula for calculation of the z-score, endorsed by the American Society of Echocardiography,[29] was derived from the measurements of 35 children and 135 adults.[30] The formula assumes a linear relationship between BSA and aortic diameter. Healthy adults whose height exceeds the 95th percentile were underrepresented in this group, and the BSA-to-aortic diameter was extrapolated for those with high BSA. More recent studies suggest that the relationship of aortic-root size to BSA in very tall subjects is weaker and nonlinear and tends to plateau.[31,32] This is important in evaluating aortic size in patients with MFS because they are frequently tall and at or above the 95th percentile, and enlarged aortic size in this group may be inappropriately defined as normal based on the extrapolated data.

Aortic complications are the most life-threatening manifestations of MFS and consist of thoracic aortic aneurysms leading to dissections and/or rupture. Patients with MFS predominate among younger patients with aortic dissection. In the IRAS registry, 57% of patients younger than 40 years had MFS.[4] The aorta in MFS is stiffer and less distensible at all ages than normal aortas. The abnormal elastic properties appear to be directly related to the degree of aortic dilation.[33] Aortic-root dilation also occurs early in MFS. Among 160 patients with MFS diagnosed by the older Ghent criteria, the aortic-root was dilated in 35% by age 5 and in 68% by age 19.[34] Aortic dilation will be even more prevalent with the revised Ghent criteria because they require either aortic involvement or a family history of aortic involvement for the diagnosis.[27]

Ehlers-Danlos Syndrome Type IV, the Vascular Type

Vascular Ehlers-Danlos syndrome (EDS) is an autosomal-dominant defect in type III collagen synthesis due to mutations in the gene for type III procollagen (COL3A1). Approximately 50% of cases are due to de novo mutations. Vascular EDS is diagnosed when at least 2 of 4 major criteria are present: thin, translucent skin; arterial, intestinal, or uterine rupture; easy bruising; and a characteristic facial appearance (acrogeria). The diagnosis can be confirmed by observing that cultured fibroblasts synthesize abnormal type III procollagen or by identification of a mutation in COL3A1.

Vascular EDS is the most serious form of EDS because rupture, aneurysmal formation, and or dissections of major or minor arteries can occur.[35] Arterial rupture may be preceded by aneurysm, arteriovenous fistulae, or dissection, but also may occur de novo. Approximately 50% of the arterial ruptures occur in the thorax and abdomen, 25% in the head, and 25% in the extremities. Arterial events are the cause of most deaths in vascular EDS and reduce survival in these patients to a median age of 48 years.[35] Survival remains reduced because these events are largely unpredictable and the fragility of the tissue and vessel makes surgical repair difficult. Twenty-five percent of subjects experience a major vascular event or rupture of an internal organ by age 20, and more than 80% by age 40.[35]

Loeys-Dietz Syndrome

Loeys-Dietz syndrome (LDS) is an aortic aneurysm syndrome due to autosomal-dominant mutations of the transforming growth factor beta receptor genes 1 or 2 (TGFβR1 or TGFβR2). It is characterized by premature and aggressive aneurysms and dissections, hypertelorism (widely spaced in eyes) and a bifid uvula or cleft palate. LDS shares overlapping features with MFS and vascular EDS, including aortic-root dilation and skin and skeletal abnormalities. The vascular pathology in LDS is more aggressive, however. Arterial dilation and tortuosity occur earlier and progress more rapidly. Aortic-root dissections occur at smaller aortic-root dimensions compared with patients with MFS. Furthermore, whereas the arteriopathy in MFS is generally confined to the ascending aorta, aneurysmal dilation in LDS is more frequent in the abdominal aorta, and pelvic and intracranial vessels than with MFS. Median survival is 37 years.[36] Among 90 patients with LDS, 27 patients died. All deaths were vascular related and the leading cause was dissection of the thoracic (67%) or abdominal aorta (22%) or the cerebral arteries (7%).[36] These results are similar to EDS, but in contrast to MFS, dissection in LDS can occur without marked arterial dilation.

Determinates of Aortic-Root Size and Evaluation for Aortic Dilation

Age and height, weight, and BSA are key determinants of aortic-root dimensions in healthy individuals.[29,30,37–41] Aortic diameters indexed for BSA appear to predict most accurately the risk of dissection or rupture.[42] Height appears to be the most important of the anatomic determinants of aortic diameter,[43] and must be considered when evaluating subjects with very small or tall statures. For example, women with Turner syndrome (n = 166) have absolute aortic diameters similar to age-matched female controls (n = 26), but aortic size was significantly greater in the patients with Turner syndrome when indexed for BSA (1.89 ± 0.34 cm/m^2 vs 1.70 ± 0.16 cm/m^2, $P = .008$). Approximately 10% of women with Turner syndrome had absolute aortic dimension greater than the 95th percentile for healthy subjects, but 24% of women with Turner syndrome had aortic dimensions greater than the 95th percentile when indexed for BSA.[41] The most widely used nomogram[30] uses BSA to predict normal aortic diameter in individuals younger than 20, 20 to 40, and older than 40 years, but as mentioned, these equations assume linearity between BSA and aortic diameter. This may not be true in subjects who are in the greater than the 95th percentile for height, in whom the BSA-to–aortic diameter relationship seems to plateau.[31,32] Clinicians should therefore be cautious when evaluating the aortic-root in such subjects to avoid underestimating the increase in aortic-root dimensions. Being overweight also increases BSA but has less effect on aortic diameter, leading again to an underestimate of aortic dilation. Some advocate indexing aortic size by height,[41] but there are no large series defining normal ranges for this index. An additional problem is that the graphs are specific for children and young adults and are not continuous during the transition. Consequently, the same dimensions can be viewed differently by whether the patient is considered a child or a young adult.[30] This complicates management during the transition period. Gender and blood pressure also affect aortic-root size. Aortic dimensions are smaller in women[30,44] and increase with the mean diastolic blood pressure.[43,45]

Determinates of Aortic-Root Dimensions in Athletes

Aortic-root dimensions in athletes are influenced by the same factors as in the general population,[32,46] but could be affected by exercise training, given the hemodynamic stress on the aorta during exercise. We performed a meta-analysis including 23 studies to examine the effect of sports participation on aortic-root size. Meta-regression analysis of 5580 elite athletes and 727 sedentary controls[47] demonstrated that athletes have larger aortic-root diameters, especially at the sinuses of Valsalva. This effect is statistically significant but small because aortic diameters in athletes averaged only 3.2 mm larger than comparison subjects at the sinuses and only 1.6 mm larger at the aortic valve annulus. These differences are clinically insignificant and suggest that marked increases in aortic-root measurements in athletes should not be attributed to exercise training.

Most studies examining aortic-root dimensions in athletes are cross-sectional studies, and few studies matched athletes and controls for anthropometric parameters such as BSA and height. We therefore cannot exclude the possibility that some of the increase in aortic-root size may be due to the larger body size of athletes, and that exercise training has no effect.

Risk of Acute Aortic Syndrome with Exercise

The Laplace Law specifies that tension in a balloon can be estimated by the following:

$$\text{Tension} = \text{Pressure} \times \text{diameter/wall thickness}$$

The acute rise in systolic blood pressure that occurs during exercise increases wall stress and places athletes with aortic defects at risk for an acute aortic event. This concern is greatest for weightlifters, whose systolic blood pressure can exceed 300 mm Hg during exercise.[48] Aortic enlargement also increases wall tension, but enlargement is also associated with mechanical deterioration and loss of elasticity limiting the accommodation for increases in blood pressure.[49] A retrospective review examined 31 cases of acute aortic dissection during or immediately after weightlifting (n = 20) or other forms of physical activity. Thirty (97%) of the 31 cases were men, probably due to the twofold higher incidence of aortic dissection in men and the higher frequency of weightlifting in men.[50] Aortic imaging before the event was available in 26 patients, 22 of whom had aortic enlargement generally in the range of 4 to 5 cm (normal <4.0 cm). Only 2 of these patients were aware of their preexisting aortic dilation.

Prevalence of Aortic Dilation and Incidence of Acute Aortic Syndrome in Athletes

Approximately 1.6% of sudden cardiac deaths in athletes are due to acute aortic events, but few studies have examined the incidence of acute aortic syndromes in athletes. Japanese investigators determined aortic size in 1562 male and 367 female athletes aged 15 to 34 years. More than 20% of the athletes participated in basketball (mean height 179.9 ± 11.2 cm and BSA 1.92 ± 0.21 m^2) or volleyball (mean height 182.5 ± 11.8 and BSA 1.94 ± 0.19 m^2) and were taller than other athletes (mean height 171.0 ± 7.3 and BSA 1.75 ± 0.16 m^2). Seven (0.36%) had an aortic diameter larger than 40 mm, and 2 of these were diagnosed with MFS.[32] The aortic dilation was 47 mm or more in 5 athletes, and they were advised to discontinue sport participation. Three did, but 2 did not. One without MFS developed acute dissection of the ascending aorta immediately after exertion and 3 years after the initial diagnosis. He underwent emergent surgery and survived. The 2 athletes with aortic diameters of 42 and 46 mm continued full athletic participation for 3 and 6 years, respectively. Annual echocardiography revealed no further dilation.

Only 17 (1.3%) of 1300 male and 10 of 1017 female Italian athletes had aortic-root diameters of 40 mm or more or 34 mm, respectively.[51] None met diagnostic criteria for MFS, but were tall, averaging 188 ± 10 cm for men and 177 ± 1 cm for women in height. The men had large BSAs (2.17 ± 0.25 m^2). One athlete had a BAV. They all continued their athletic activities. There was a small, but significant increase in aortic-root dimensions from 40.9 mm ± 1.3–42.9 mm ± 3.6 mm (P<.01) in the men with initially enlarged aortas at a mean follow-up of 8 years. Interestingly, the largest increase in these men occurred after cessation of their athletic activities (41.9 mm ± 2.2 mm to 45.1 ± 4.1 mm, $P = .02$), whereas the increase was minimal (41.4 ± 1.7 mm to 41.9 ± 2.2 mm, $P = .04$) during their athletic careers when the aorta was exposed to the highest hemodynamic load. This suggests that the aortic dilation in these athletes is a pathologic process, a consequence of aging, a delayed effect of physical activity, or a combination of these factors. In contrast, there was no significant change in aortic-root diameter in the women athletes with initially large aortic dimensions at a mean follow-up of 9 years. No athlete with aortic dilation had an adverse cardiac event.

Screening of Athletes for Aortic Diseases

Catastrophic aortic events in athletes could potentially be prevented by screening echocardiography because most aortic events appear to be associated with aortic dilation. Such events are rare, however, so routine echocardiography for aortic assessment is not recommended. Athletes with the physical stigmata or family history of the connective tissue diseases associated with aortic disease should be evaluated by echocardiography. Computed tomography (CT) and cardiac MRI are more sensitive and specific for detecting and quantifying aortic-root dilation,[52,53] but are recommended only for assessing aortic dimensions in patients with BAV when the ascending aorta cannot be assessed by echocardiography[54] and in EDS Type IV and LDS because disease of the distal aorta is frequent in these syndromes.[55,56]

MANAGEMENT OF ATHLETES WITH AORTIC DISEASE
Aortic-Root Dilation

Our impression is that most sports clinicians restrict athletes with newly diagnosed aortic-root dilation of more than 40 to 45 mm from high-intensity activity as well as contact sports. In contrast, we are more liberal with tall athletes and also have generally allowed athletes with moderate aortic dilation to continue participation as long as there are no stigmata or family history of inherited aortic disease. We inform these athletes of the potential risk of continued participation and follow these athletes closely with echocardiography every 6 months for the first 2 years and then yearly thereafter. Our clinical experience is that most of these athletes do not dilate further, especially if they present with aortic dilation as adults. We are more cautious and restrictive with athletes younger than 21 because of concern that their aortic enlargement represents occult inherited disease. We also often perform exercise tests on these athletes to determine their exercise blood pressure response, and we treat athletes with aortic dilation with angiotensin converting enzyme (ACE) inhibitors or receptor blockers (ARB), especially if they demonstrate a hypertensive response to exertion. Athletes with aortic-root size greater than 45 mm should avoid high-intensity sport activities.

Bicuspid Aortic Valve

Guidelines on sports participation for athletes with BAV are based on the presence of valvular disease and/or aortic-root dilation. The presence of BAV in athletes without significant aortic regurgitation or stenosis and normal aortic-root dimensions (less than 40 mm or the equivalent when indexed for BSA in children and adolescents) does not limit the eligibility to practice sports, and these subjects may participate in all competitive sports without restrictions.[57] Management of these athletes consists mainly of surveillance by at least yearly transthoracic echocardiography (TTE) for progressive aortic valve dysfunction as well as aortic dilation. All patients with BAV should have both the aortic-root and ascending thoracic aorta evaluated.[58] If the aortic-root and ascending aorta above the sinotubular junction cannot be adequately visualized by echocardiography, noncontrast MRI or contrast CT is recommended.[54]

Current guidelines recommend that athletes with BAV and aortic-root dilation between 40 and 45 mm should be advised to participate only in low-intensity and moderate-intensity sports and avoid any contact sports; however, as discussed previously, we have generally been more liberal with such athletes, especially as adults. Only low-intensity sports are recommended when the aortic-root is larger than 45 mm,[57] and we have generally, but not always, followed these guidelines. Aortic-root repair is recommend for patients with BAV and an aortic diameter larger than 5.5 cm. Operative intervention also is reasonable when the aortic sinuses or ascending aorta is larger than 5.0 cm,[54] in those with a family history of aortic dissection and when there is dilation of 0.5 cm or more per year.[54] Short stature and small BSA also may trigger a recommendation for surgery at a smaller dimension.

Subjects with BAV and valvular dysfunction should follow the recommendations provided for athletes with aortic valvular disease. First-degree relatives of patients with BAV should be screened for the presence of BAV and thoracic aortic disease.[58]

Marfan Syndrome

Athletes with MFS are advised to avoid high-intensity exercise activities, including heavy weightlifting and contact sports.[59] They may participate in low-static and moderate-static and low-dynamic competitive sports if they do not have aortic-root dilation, moderate to severe mitral regurgitation, or a family history of dissection or sudden death. These athletes should undergo close surveillance with TTE repeated every 6 months.[59] All other athletes with MFS are advised to participate only in low-intensity activities.[59] Prophylactic aortic-root replacement is traditionally performed when the aorta is greater than or equal to 5 cm or earlier if growth exceeds 0.5 cm per year, or there is a family history of aortic dissection or progressive aortic regurgitation.[54]

Ehlers-Danlos Syndrome

Patients with vascular-type EDS should not engage in any competitive athletic activity because of the high incidence of major vascular events,[59] and the observation that vascular catastrophe can occur without previous vascular dilation.[35]

Loeys-Dietz Syndrome

The vascular disease in LDS is more aggressive than that in MFS, and aortic dissection can occur without marked arterial dilation, similar to EDS. LDS has not been addressed in available guidelines on sports participation, but in our opinion these patients should not participate in competitive sports activities.

Medical Therapy of Aortic-Root Dilation

Medical therapy seeks to reduce aortic dilation and events. Beta adrenergic blocking agents reduce the rate of aortic dilation, particularly in adults with MFS.[58,60] Beta blockers are therefore recommended in subjects with aortic-root dilation as well as BAV, MFS, EDS, and LDS. Alternatively, ACE inhibitors or ARBs can be used.[58] The beta blocker atenolol and the ARB losartan produce similar effects on the rate of aortic-root dilation over a 3-year period in children and young adults with MFS.[61] ACE inhibitors and ARBs are often better tolerated in athletes with aortic disease and are usually our initial choice in this population.

REFERENCES

1. Maron BJ, Haas TS, Murphy CJ, et al. Incidence and causes of sudden death in U.S. college athletes. J Am Coll Cardiol 2014;63:1636–43.
2. Tsai TT, Nienaber CA, Eagle KA. Acute aortic syndromes. Circulation 2005;112:3802–13.
3. Hagan PG, Nienaber CA, Isselbacher EM, et al. The International Registry of Acute Aortic Dissection (IRAD): new insights into an old disease. JAMA 2000;283:897–903.
4. Januzzi JL, Isselbacher EM, Fattori R, et al. Characterizing the young patient with aortic dissection: results from the International Registry of Aortic Dissection (IRAD). J Am Coll Cardiol 2004;43:665–9.
5. Meszaros I, Morocz J, Szlavi J, et al. Epidemiology and clinicopathology of aortic dissection. Chest 2000;117:1271–8.
6. Mohr-Kahaly S, Erbel R, Kearney P, et al. Aortic intramural hemorrhage visualized by transesophageal echocardiography: findings and prognostic implications. J Am Coll Cardiol 1994;23:658–64.
7. Nienaber CA, von Kodolitsch Y, Petersen B, et al. Intramural hemorrhage of the thoracic aorta. Diagnostic and therapeutic implications. Circulation 1995;92:1465–72.
8. Vilacosta I, San Roman JA, Ferreiros J, et al. Natural history and serial morphology of aortic intramural hematoma: a novel variant of aortic dissection. Am Heart J 1997;134:495–507.
9. Maraj R, Rerkpattanapipat P, Jacobs LE, et al. Meta-analysis of 143 reported cases of aortic intramural hematoma. Am J Cardiol 2000;86:664–8.
10. Song JK, Kim HS, Kang DH, et al. Different clinical features of aortic intramural hematoma versus dissection involving the ascending aorta. J Am Coll Cardiol 2001;37:1604–10.
11. Macura KJ, Corl FM, Fishman EK, et al. Pathogenesis in acute aortic syndromes: aortic dissection, intramural hematoma, and penetrating atherosclerotic aortic ulcer. AJR Am J Roentgenol 2003;181:309–16.
12. Braverman AC. Penetrating atherosclerotic ulcers of the aorta. Curr Opin Cardiol 1994;9:591–7.
13. Troxler M, Mavor AI, Homer-Vanniasinkam S. Penetrating atherosclerotic ulcers of the aorta. Br J Surg 2001;88:1169–77.
14. Hoffman JI, Kaplan S. The incidence of congenital heart disease. J Am Coll Cardiol 2002;39:1890–900.
15. Ward C. Clinical significance of the bicuspid aortic valve. Heart 2000;83:81–5.
16. Cripe L, Andelfinger G, Martin LJ, et al. Bicuspid aortic valve is heritable. J Am Coll Cardiol 2004;44:138–43.
17. Huntington K, Hunter AG, Chan KL. A prospective study to assess the frequency of familial clustering of congenital bicuspid aortic valve. J Am Coll Cardiol 1997;30:1809–12.
18. Michelena HI, Khanna AD, Mahoney D, et al. Incidence of aortic complications in patients with bicuspid aortic valves. JAMA 2011;306:1104–12.
19. Beroukhim RS, Kruzick TL, Taylor AL, et al. Progression of aortic dilation in children with a functionally normal bicuspid aortic valve. Am J Cardiol 2006;98:828–30.
20. Gurvitz M, Chang RK, Drant S, et al. Frequency of aortic root dilation in children with a bicuspid aortic valve. Am J Cardiol 2004;94:1337–40.
21. Shimada I, Rooney SJ, Pagano D, et al. Prediction of thoracic aortic aneurysm expansion: validation of formulae describing growth. Ann Thorac Surg 1999;67:1968–70 [discussion: 1979–80].

22. Tadros TM, Klein MD, Shapira OM. Ascending aortic dilatation associated with bicuspid aortic valve: pathophysiology, molecular biology, and clinical implications. Circulation 2009;119:880–90.
23. Tzemos N, Therrien J, Yip J, et al. Outcomes in adults with bicuspid aortic valves. JAMA 2008;300:1317–25.
24. Michelena HI, Desjardins VA, Avierinos JF, et al. Natural history of asymptomatic patients with normally functioning or minimally dysfunctional bicuspid aortic valve in the community. Circulation 2008;117:2776–84.
25. Galanti G, Stefani L, Toncelli L, et al. Effects of sports activity in athletes with bicuspid aortic valve and mild aortic regurgitation. Br J Sports Med 2010;44: 275–9.
26. Judge DP, Dietz HC. Marfan's syndrome. Lancet 2005;366:1965–76.
27. Loeys BL, Dietz HC, Braverman AC, et al. The revised Ghent nosology for the Marfan syndrome. J Med Genet 2010;47:476–85.
28. Radonic T, de Witte P, Groenink M, et al. Critical appraisal of the revised Ghent criteria for diagnosis of Marfan syndrome. Clin Genet 2011;80:346–53.
29. Lang RM, Bierig M, Devereux RB, et al. Recommendations for chamber quantification: a report from the American Society of Echocardiography's Guidelines and Standards Committee and the Chamber Quantification Writing Group, developed in conjunction with the European Association of Echocardiography, a branch of the European Society of Cardiology. J Am Soc Echocardiogr 2005;18:1440–63.
30. Roman MJ, Devereux RB, Kramer-Fox R, et al. Two-dimensional echocardiographic aortic root dimensions in normal children and adults. Am J Cardiol 1989;64:507–12.
31. Reed CM, Richey PA, Pulliam DA, et al. Aortic dimensions in tall men and women. Am J Cardiol 1993;71:608–10.
32. Kinoshita N, Mimura J, Obayashi C, et al. Aortic root dilatation among young competitive athletes: echocardiographic screening of 1929 athletes between 15 and 34 years of age. Am Heart J 2000;139:723–8.
33. Jeremy RW, Huang H, Hwa J, et al. Relation between age, arterial distensibility, and aortic dilatation in the Marfan syndrome. Am J Cardiol 1994;74:369–73.
34. Aburawi EH, O'Sullivan J. Relation of aortic root dilatation and age in Marfan's syndrome. Eur Heart J 2007;28:376–9.
35. Pepin M, Schwarze U, Superti-Furga A, et al. Clinical and genetic features of Ehlers-Danlos syndrome type IV, the vascular type. N Engl J Med 2000;342: 673–80.
36. Loeys BL, Schwarze U, Holm T, et al. Aneurysm syndromes caused by mutations in the TGF-beta receptor. N Engl J Med 2006;355:788–98.
37. Huwez FU, Houston AB, Watson J, et al. Age and body surface area related normal upper and lower limits of M mode echocardiographic measurements and left ventricular volume and mass from infancy to early adulthood. Br Heart J 1994;72:276–80.
38. Kaldararova M, Balazova E, Tittel P, et al. Echocardiographic measurements of the aorta in normal children and young adults. Bratisl Lek Listy 2007;108:437–41.
39. Nidorf SM, Picard MH, Triulzi MO, et al. New perspectives in the assessment of cardiac chamber dimensions during development and adulthood. J Am Coll Cardiol 1992;19:983–8.
40. Henry WL, Gardin JM, Ware JH. Echocardiographic measurements in normal subjects from infancy to old age. Circulation 1980;62:1054–61.
41. Matura LA, Ho VB, Rosing DR, et al. Aortic dilatation and dissection in Turner syndrome. Circulation 2007;116:1663–70.

42. Davies RR, Gallo A, Coady MA, et al. Novel measurement of relative aortic size predicts rupture of thoracic aortic aneurysms. Ann Thorac Surg 2006;81: 169–77.
43. Vasan RS, Larson MG, Levy D. Determinants of echocardiographic aortic root size. The Framingham heart study. Circulation 1995;91:734–40.
44. Francis GS, Hagan AD, Oury J, et al. Accuracy of echocardiography for assessing aortic root diameter. Br Heart J 1975;37:376–8.
45. Cuspidi C, Meani S, Valerio C, et al. Ambulatory blood pressure, target organ damage and aortic root size in never-treated essential hypertensive patients. J Hum Hypertens 2007;21:531–8.
46. D'Andrea A, Cocchia R, Riegler L, et al. Aortic root dimensions in elite athletes. Am J Cardiol 2010;105:1629–34.
47. Iskandar A, Thompson PD. A meta-analysis of aortic root size in elite athletes. Circulation 2013;127:791–8.
48. Mayerick C, Carre F, Elefteriades J. Aortic dissection and sport: physiologic and clinical understanding provide an opportunity to save young lives. J Cardiovasc Surg (Torino) 2010;51:669–81.
49. Koullias G, Modak R, Tranquilli M, et al. Mechanical deterioration underlies malignant behavior of aneurysmal human ascending aorta. J Thorac Cardiovasc Surg 2005;130:677–83.
50. Hatzaras I, Tranquilli M, Coady M, et al. Weight lifting and aortic dissection: more evidence for a connection. Cardiology 2007;107:103–6.
51. Pelliccia A, Di Paolo FM, De Blasiis E, et al. Prevalence and clinical significance of aortic root dilation in highly trained competitive athletes. Circulation 2010;122: 698–706, 3 p following 706.
52. Ocak I, Lacomis JM, Deible CR, et al. The aortic root: comparison of measurements from ECG-gated CT angiography with transthoracic echocardiography. J Thorac Imaging 2009;24:223–6.
53. Tsai SF, Trivedi M, Daniels CJ. Comparing imaging modalities for screening aortic complications in patients with bicuspid aortic valve. Congenit Heart Dis 2012;7: 372–7.
54. Nishimura RA, Otto CM, Bonow RO, et al. 2014 AHA/ACC guideline for the management of patients with valvular heart disease: a report of the American College of Cardiology/American Heart Association Task Force on Practice Guidelines. J Thorac Cardiovasc Surg 2014;148:e1–132.
55. Van Hemelrijk C, Renard M, Loeys B. The Loeys-Dietz syndrome: an update for the clinician. Curr Opin Cardiol 2010;25:546–51.
56. Pepin MG, Peter HB. Ehlers-Danlos syndrome type IV. In: Pagon RA, Adam MP, Ardinger HH, et al, editors. Gene reviews. Seattle (WA): University of Washington; 2011. Accessed January 6, 2015.
57. Bonow RO, Cheitlin MD, Crawford MH, et al. Task force 3: valvular heart disease. J Am Coll Cardiol 2005;45:1334–40.
58. Hiratzka LF, Bakris GL, Beckman JA, et al. 2010 ACCF/AHA/AATS/ACR/ASA/ SCA/SCAI/SIR/STS/SVM Guidelines for the diagnosis and management of patients with thoracic aortic disease. A Report of the American College of Cardiology Foundation/American Heart Association Task Force on Practice Guidelines, American Association for Thoracic Surgery, American College of Radiology, American Stroke Association, Society of Cardiovascular Anesthesiologists, Society for Cardiovascular Angiography and Interventions, Society of Interventional Radiology, Society of Thoracic Surgeons, and Society for Vascular Medicine. J Am Coll Cardiol 2010;55:e27–129.

59. Maron BJ, Ackerman MJ, Nishimura RA, et al. Task force 4: HCM and other cardiomyopathies, mitral valve prolapse, myocarditis, and Marfan syndrome. J Am Coll Cardiol 2005;45:1340-5.
60. Shores J, Berger KR, Murphy EA, et al. Progression of aortic dilatation and the benefit of long-term beta-adrenergic blockade in Marfan's syndrome. N Engl J Med 1994;330:1335-41.
61. Lacro RV, Dietz HC, Sleeper LA, et al. Atenolol versus Losartan in children and young adults with Marfan's syndrome. N Engl J Med 2014;371(22):2061-71.

Athletes with Implantable Cardioverter Defibrillators

Shiva P. Ponamgi, MD[a], Christopher V. DeSimone, MD, PhD[b], Michael J. Ackerman, MD, PhD[b,c],*

KEYWORDS

- Arrhythmia • Athlete • Bethesda Conference • Exercise
- Implanted cardioverter defibrillator (ICD) • Long QT syndrome
- Sudden cardiac death • European Society of Cardiology (ESC)

KEY POINTS

- Athletes with implantable cardioverter defibrillators (ICDs) are faced with many physical and psychological challenges posed by their passion to pursue exercise and training despite the restrictive recommendations based on expert opinion, rather than objective evidence.
- Current international guidelines (European Society of Cardiology and Bethesda Conference #36) for athletes with underlying heart disease recommend only moderate, leisure-time physical activity in patients with an ICD, thus making athletes with ICDs ineligible for most competitive sports. However, new North American guidelines are reassessing these 2005-based recommendations and a new set of 2013 disease-specific guidelines, such as those for patients with long QT syndrome, is embracing a shared decision-making approach to this issue rather than a default disqualification.
- The efficacy of ICDs in terminating a potentially lethal arrhythmia under the extreme conditions of competitive sports associated with metabolic and autonomic changes like catecholamine surges, dehydration, electrolyte derangements, and myocardial ischemia is unknown.
- There is preliminary data from registry-based studies and surveys demonstrating the relative safety of athletes engaging in vigorous physical activity or organized sporting activities.
- Inappropriate shocks from ICDs and potential damage to the integrity of the ICD system during engagement in intense physical activity or contact sports remain an area of concern for athletes and clinicians.

Dr DeSimone is supported by an NIH training grant #T32 HL007111.

Conflict of Interest: None (Dr S.P. Ponamgi, Dr C.V. DeSimone).

Dr M.J. Ackerman receives royalties from Transgenomic (Familion) and is a consultant for Boston Scientific, Gilead Sciences, Medtronic, and St. Jude Medical.

[a] Division of Hospital Internal Medicine, Mayo Clinic Health System–Austin, 1000 First Street Northwest, Austin, MN 55912, USA; [b] Division of Cardiovascular Medicine, Mayo Clinic, 200 First Street Southwest, Mary Brigh Building 4-506, Rochester, MN 55905, USA; [c] Mayo Clinic Windland Smith Rice Sudden Death Genomics Laboratory, 200 First Street Southwest, Guggenheim 5-01, Rochester, MN 55905, USA

* Corresponding author. Mayo Clinic, 200 First Street Southwest, Rochester, MN 55905.

E-mail address: Ackerman.Michael@mayo.edu

INTRODUCTION

The use of implantable cardioverter defibrillators (ICDs) for primary and secondary prevention of sudden cardiac death (SCD) has increased in the last 2 decades because of their proven efficacy in treating life-threatening cardiac arrhythmias.[1–3] The indications for ICDs in athletes are the same for those in the general population.[2,4] The athletic heart is faced with a milieu of increased emotional stress, hemodynamic changes, altered autonomic tone, and the potential for myocardial ischemia that can occur during vigorous physical exertion. Especially in athletes with a substrate of underlying cardiovascular disease, these factors may acutely and transiently increase the risk for SCD through initiation and perpetuation of life-threatening dysrhythmias.[5–8] These factors along with mandatory preparticipation screening recommended by the American Heart Association (AHA)[9] and the European Society of Cardiology (ESC)[10] for participation in most competitive sports have led to an increased recognition of athletes at risk for SCD,[11] and thus the issue of ICD therapy in these patients has come to the forefront. ICDs could be considered in athletes who are at increased risk of developing malignant arrhythmias, such as those with underlying electrical or structural cardiac abnormalities associated with hypertrophic cardiomyopathy (HCM), long QT syndrome (LQTS), Brugada syndrome (BrS), or arrhythmogenic right ventricular cardiomyopathy (ARVC).[12]

Current international guidelines[4,9,10,13] recommend only moderate, leisure-time physical activity in patients with an ICD, thus making athletes with ICDs ineligible for most competitive sports except those classified in North America as so-called class IA sports (billiards, bowling, cricket, curling, golf, and riflery) (**Fig. 1**).[14] Despite these very restrictive guidelines, many athletes with ICDs and normal left ventricular function have a strong passion to continue their participation in organized, and often high-intensity, sports, thereby posing a medical and ethical dilemma for the treating physician.[12] In this review, the current recommendations for athletes with ICDs, the major controversies that exist, the risks associated with ICDs, and the importance of shared decision-making between clinician and athlete are summarized.

EXAMINATION OF GUIDELINE-BASED RECOMMENDATIONS FOR ATHLETES AND ARRHYTHMIAS

The 2 most widely accepted guidelines used for determining the eligibility to participate in competitive sports are from (1) the United States: the 36th Bethesda Conference (BC #36), and (2) Europe: the ESC expert consensus document.[4,15,16] These documents were published in 2005 and contain recommendations made based on the available scientific data as well as individual and collective judgment and experience of the panel participants. Although these documents largely agree on their recommendations about athletic participation in patients with underlying cardiac disease, the discrepancies in their approach to the disqualification of athletes may be reflective of the very different cultural, social, and legal backgrounds existing in the United States and Europe.[17] These conflicting recommendations can be confusing to clinicians caring for athletes. Therefore, the commonly agreed on points from each of the guidelines are presented as well as the major disease-specific discrepancies from both expert panels are highlighted (**Table 1**).[4,15,16]

Overall General Recommendations Endorsed by Both the 36th Bethesda Conference and the European Society of Cardiology

1. Athletes with syncope or near syncope should not participate in sports where the likelihood of even a momentary loss of consciousness may be hazardous until the cause has been determined and treated, if necessary.

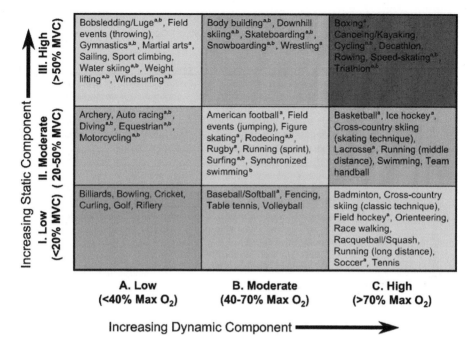

Fig. 1. Classification of sports. This classification is based on peak static and dynamic components achieved during competition. It should be noted, however, that higher values may be reached during training. The increasing dynamic component is defined in terms of the estimated percentage of maximal oxygen uptake (Max O$_2$) achieved and results in an increasing cardiac output. The increasing static component is related to the estimated percentage of maximal voluntary contraction (MVC) reached and results in an increasing blood pressure load. The lowest total cardiovascular demands (cardiac output and blood pressure) are shown in green and the highest in red. Blue, yellow, and orange depict low moderate, moderate, and high moderate total cardiovascular demands. [a] Danger of bodily collision. [b] Increased risk if syncope occurs. (*From* Mitchell JH, Haskell W, Snell P, et al. Task Force 8: classification of sports. J Am Coll Cardiol 2005;45(8):1366; with permission.)

2. Any athlete with a previously diagnosed arrhythmia should be re-evaluated every 6 to 12 months during training to determine if the conditioning process has affected the underlying arrhythmia.
3. Athletes on any anti-arrhythmic drug treatment to control their arrhythmia should be periodically checked for compliance with recommended therapy and for any recurrence of symptoms.
4. Abuse with drugs such as cocaine and ephedra may induce life-threatening arrhythmias and may need to be considered during evaluation of these athletes.
5. For some arrhythmias in athletes, an ablation approach may be preferred to drug therapy because catecholamines released during exercise may undermine the salutary effects of some antiarrhythmic agents. After such a successful ablation, return to athletics may be as quick as within a few days if repeated attempts at tachycardia induction during isoproterenol administration were unsuccessful. If no such testing was done, then a 2- to 4-week interval is recommended.
6. For athletes with ICDs, all moderate- and high-intensity sports are contraindicated and only class IA sports[14] are permitted because the efficacy with which these

Table 1
2005 Bethesda Conference #36 and 2005 European Society of Cardiology recommendations for participation in competitive sport

Condition	BC#36	ESC
HCM	Exclude athletes with probable or definitive clinical diagnosis from all competitive sports except perhaps class IA sports Genotype-positive/phenotype-negative athletes may still compete	Exclude all athletes irrespective of genotype or symptoms from all competitive sports A positive genetic test itself is self-sufficient for a comprehensive disqualification
ARVC	Exclude all athletes with probable or definitive diagnosis from all competitive sports except IA	Same as HCM
LQTS	Exclude any athlete with previous cardiac arrest or syncopal episode from competitive sports Asymptomatic LQTS athletes with overt QT prolongation restricted to IA sports Genotype-positive but phenotype-negative LQTS athletes given the OK to play	Same as HCM. All LQTS athletes from all sports period
SQTS	Exclude from all competitive sport except those of low intensity	—
BrS	Exclude from all competitive sport except those of low intensity (class IA)	Exclude from all competitive sport
Catecholaminergic polymorphic ventricular tachycardia	Exclude all patients with clinical diagnosis from competitive sport Genotype-positive/phenotype-negative patients may still compete in low-intensity sport (class IA)	Exclude all athletes irrespective of genotype or symptoms from all competitive sports

Adapted from Pugh A, Bourke JP, Kunadian V. Sudden cardiac death among competitive adult athletes: a review. Postgrad Med J 2012;88(1041):383; with permission.

devices will terminate a potentially lethal arrhythmia under the extreme conditions of competitive sports, with the associated metabolic and autonomic changes, and possible myocardial ischemia, is unknown.

7. Athletes who require anticoagulation should not participate in sports with a danger of bodily collision.
8. Athletes with ICDs/pacemakers should not engage in competitive sports with a danger of bodily collision/physical contact because such trauma may damage the ICD/pacemaker system.

It should be noted that the use of certain cardioactive drugs, such as β-adrenergic blocking agents, is banned in some competitive sports.

Arrhythmia-Specific Recommendations

The most important prognostic determinant of the arrhythmogenic potential in an athlete is the presence of underlying heart disease.[16,18–21] Specific recommendation points from the consensus documents (BC #36 and ESC) pertaining to major cardiac conditions are presented as follows:

Hypertrophic cardiomyopathy
Task Force 4 (36th Bethesda Conference)
1. Individuals with a positive genetic test but no clinical evidence of the disease (genotype-positive and phenotype-negative) are not precluded from participation in competitive sports.[22]
2. All other individuals irrespective of age, gender, phenotype, or symptoms, with probable or equivocal clinical diagnosis of HCM, can only participate in low-intensity (class IA) sports.

European Society of Cardiology
1. The ESC recommendations are more restrictive in patients with HCM and recommend only leisure-time or non-competitive sporting activities even in individuals with solely a positive genetic test.
2. Athletes with clinical or phenotypic evidence of HCM are restricted from ALL competitive sports, even the Bethesda Conference–sanctioned safe sports (class IA).

These recommendations by the ESC guidelines are based on the fact that there is a lack of sufficient data on the natural history of HCM in competitive athletes and the hypothesis that intense training and competitive sports can lead to activation of cellular pathways causing expression of the HCM phenotype (ie, left ventricular hypertrophy) and thereby lead to an increased risk of tachyarrhythmias and SCD in athletes with a predisposing gene abnormality.[23–25]

Arrhythmogenic right ventricular cardiomyopathy
Task Force 4 (36th Bethesda Conference)
Athletes with probable or definite diagnosis of ARVC should be excluded from most competitive sports, with the possible exception of those of low intensity (class IA).[22]

European Society of Cardiology
Athletes with ARVC should be excluded from all competitive sports including low intensity (class IA).

Ventricular flutter and ventricular fibrillation in athletes with ICDs
Common endorsements by both European Society of Cardiology and Task Force 7 (36th Bethesda Conference)
1. Athletes with conditions that result in cardiac arrest in the presence or absence of structural heart disease generally are treated with an ICD and cannot participate in any moderate- or high-intensity competitive sports or those that involve bodily contact.[4]
2. Athletes with ICDs and who have had no episodes of ventricular flutter or ventricular fibrillation (VF), but require device therapy may need to wait 6 months before engaging in class IA competitive sports.

Cardiac channelopathies
Long QT syndrome
  Task Force 7 (36th Bethesda Conference)
1. In athletes who are symptomatic (cardiac arrest or syncopal episodes), all competitive sports, except those in the class IA category, should be restricted irrespective of their QTc or underlying genotype.[4]

2. Asymptomatic patients with a baseline QT prolongation (QTc of 470 ms or more in male patients, 480 ms or more in female patients) should be restricted to class IA sports.
3. Asymptomatic patients with genetically proven type 3 LQTS (LQT3) that are currently restricted to class IA sports may be considered for more liberalization.
4. Asymptomatic athletes with genotype-positive/phenotype-negative LQTS may be allowed to participate in competitive sports.
5. Because of the strong association between swimming and LQT1, athletes with genotype-positive/phenotype-negative LQT1 should refrain from competitive swimming.

European Society of Cardiology
1. All patients with a confirmed diagnosis of congenital LQTS should be excluded from all competitive sports including those in class IA, irrespective of their genotype and symptoms.
2. Athletes with solely a positive genetic test should be excluded from all competitive sports.

Short QT syndrome
Task Force 7 (36th Bethesda Conference)
In all athletes with short QT syndrome (SQTS), participation in all competitive sports except those in class IA should be restricted.[4,26]

Catecholaminergic polymorphic ventricular tachycardia
Task Force 7 (36th Bethesda Conference)
1. Symptomatic patients without an ICD[27] are restricted to only class IA sports.[4]
2. Asymptomatic patients detected as part of familial screening with documented exercise- or isoproterenol-induced ventricular tachycardia (VT) should refrain from all competitive sports except possibly class IA activities.
3. In asymptomatic athletes with no inducible VT (genotype-positive and phenotype-negative), restrictions for competitive sports may be more relaxed.
4. As with LQT1, all patients with catecholaminergic polymorphic ventricular tachycardia should be restricted from competitive swimming.

Brugada syndrome
Task Force 7 (36th Bethesda Conference)
No clear association between exercise and SCD in patients with Brugada syndrome (BrS) has been thus far established, but due to the potential impact of hyperthermia in these patients, they are advised to refrain from all competitive sports except those in class IA.[4]

European Society of Cardiology
All patients with a confirmed diagnosis of BrS should be excluded from all competitive sports including class IA, irrespective of their genotype and symptoms.

Evidence and Reasons Behind the Recommendations for Athletic Restriction

The current recommendations by the ESC and BC #36 consensus documents restrict athletic participation in most competitive sports[4,28,29] for several reasons, these include (**Box 1**) the following:

1. Intense physical exertion increases the risk of SCD by almost 2.5 times in patients with underlying arrhythmogenic cardiac disease.[11]
2. ICD efficacy in terminating a potentially lethal arrhythmia under the extreme conditions of competitive sports, with the associated metabolic[30] and autonomic changes, as well as possible myocardial ischemia,[31] is unknown.[15,16]

> **Box 1**
> **Potential concerns faced by athletes with implantable cardioverter defibrillators during engagement in sporting activities**
>
> *Concerns in athletes with ICDs*
>
> Transient loss of consciousness causing serious injury/death during an ICD shock
>
> Damage to the integrity of the ICD/pacemaker system in athletes engaging in contact sports
>
> Lead fracture due to repeated arm movements and costoclavicular crush
>
> VT storm due to repeated shocks delivered during high catecholamine surge
>
> Unknown efficacy of ICD therapy in conditions associated with vigorous exercise
>
> Negative psychological impact due to fear of ICD shocks and sudden death
>
> High frequency of inappropriate shocks due to increased lead noise or T-wave oversensing
>
> Possibility of inducing ventricular arrhythmias if an inappropriate shock is delivered on the T wave

3. Sports with physical contact may result in damage to the ICD, thereby preventing its normal function.
4. In athletes with left-handed dominance, extreme arm movements can cause ICD lead fracture due to costoclavicular crush.[32]
5. A variety of conditions that occur during exercise, like sinus tachycardia, supraventricular tachycardia with rapid ventricular conduction, T wave oversensing during exercise, or noise due to lead failure, may lead to an increased frequency of inappropriate shocks in athletes with ICDs.[33]
6. The transient loss of consciousness from exercise-induced arrhythmias or inappropriate/appropriate ICD shocks may pose a serious risk of severe injury or death[34] to the athlete as well as to the spectators.[35]
7. Inappropriate shocks can have a negative psychological impact[36,37] on the athlete, which in turn can lead to SCD due to facilitation and destabilization of malignant ventricular arrhythmias by altering the tachycardia cycle length.[38]
8. Inappropriate shocks can also lead to ventricular arrhythmias if delivered on the T wave.
9. Catecholamines released during exercise may undermine the salutary effect of antiarrhythmic drugs and also exacerbate underlying conditions and may possibly lead to life-threatening VT storm and repeated shocks from the device.[35,39–41]

At the time of this article's submission (March 2015), the 2005 Bethesda Conference recommendations were being re-evaluated and updated with AHA/ACC–approved guidelines. The final approval from the respective societies has not yet been obtained and an estimated publication date has not yet been provided. As such, any departures from the 2005 recommendations are unknown at this time. There has been no announcement regarding the convening of and timing for a similar update to the 2005 ESC sports participation guidelines.

In addition, subsequent disease-specific guidelines, for example, the LQTS treatment guidelines from 2013, have indicated a shift away from a presumptive disqualification to a recommendation that embraces shared decision-making between an athlete and his or her physician.[42] In essence, for an athlete with LQTS who desires to remain a competitive athlete, the internationally sanctioned guidelines now stipulate that he or she should be evaluated by an LQTS expert in order to be well-diagnosed, risk-stratified, and treated, and in that setting, then be enabled to make a well-informed decision on how he or she would like to live their life.

CHALLENGING THE CURRENT RECOMMENDATIONS: IS IT REALLY EVIDENCE-BASED PRACTICE?
Lack of Data, Discrepancies in Guidance, and Acceptance in Clinical Practice

The expert committee formulating the 2005 guidelines acknowledged that these recommendations are largely based on individual and collective judgments and the experience of the panelists, and the evidence supporting them in the form of well-designed, scientifically acceptable studies was simply not present.[4,15] The European recommendations, being more restrictive compared with the American-based recommendations, allow athletes with ICDs to engage in only leisure-time activities with low to moderate intensity not involving body contact or collision.[28] These types of conflicting recommendations with respect to athletic participation in competitive sports from the above consensus statements, as well as the lack of data on the actual risk of sports in patients with ICDs, have resulted in these guidelines not being uniformly embraced by all practicing physicians.[43]

In fact, subsequent studies have documented the relative safety of athletes with ICDs participating in vigorous and competitive sports without physical injury or failure to terminate arrhythmias. These studies have also shown that ICD shock therapy during physical activity was no different during competition/exercise versus those occurring during other recreational activities.[37,43] Furthermore, these studies have also demonstrated the relative safety of exercise training in ICD patients during cardiac rehabilitation without any increase in shocks and also suggested an improved aerobic capacity in these patients.[44]

Clinician Perspectives: A Landmark Survey of the Landscape

Critical insight as to the thoughts of practicing clinicians on these guidelines was revealed by a survey involving all US physician members of the Heart Rhythm Society. Clinicians were asked about their recommendations to patients with respect to ICDs and sports participation, and these data revealed that a great variance from the guidelines existed. Only 10% of physicians recommended avoidance of all sports more vigorous than golf, 76% recommended avoidance of contact sports, and only 45% recommended avoidance of all competitive sports.[43] This survey also provided data about the adverse consequences of such athletic participation with 1% of physicians reporting injuries sustained by patients (all but 3 were minor); 5% were due to injury to the ICD system, and importantly, less than 1% had failure of ICD shocks to successfully terminate arrhythmias. The most common adverse event reported in this survey was lead damage attributed to repetitive-motion activities, most commonly weightlifting and golf, again contradicting the current recommendations.[15,16,43] In comparison, the relative risk of lead fracture reported by most other studies is about 0.4% to 4%.[45,46]

Survey data also reported that physicians noted a high rate of ICD shocks (both appropriate and inappropriate) in patients engaging in sports with up to 52% of them reporting ICD shocks in patients participating in vigorous exercises. These findings are not surprising because the risk of SCD may increase transiently by a factor of 14 to 45 in association with an episode of vigorous exertion,[7] thereby perpetuating malignant arrhythmias in these patients.[47] It must be noted that although these shocks are associated with a negative psychological impact[44] and quality of life,[48] restriction from sports participation also plays a major role in the mental well-being of these athletes. The survey also reported 2 cases of actual ICD shock failure during exercise; one of these was associated with known ethmozine-induced increase in defibrillation threshold, and the other shock failure was associated with exercise after very heavy alcohol consumption.

Implantable Cardioverter Defibrillator Sports Safety Registry

Contrary to the theoretic concerns and expectations by some for increased risk of danger to the host and damage to the device, the results from a multinational, prospective, observational registry of 372 athletes with ICDs participating in organized sports activities showed no deaths or shock-related injuries or generator malfunctions. In addition, the incidence of lead malfunction was not higher in athletes with ICDs compared with published rates in non-athletes.[37]

In line with the previously discussed survey-based study,[43] this prospective registry-based study reported an increased rate of appropriate and inappropriate shocks that occurred during physical activity. Also, 7 of the 8 ventricular storms recorded occurred during exercise.[37] Although these data provide some evidence to challenge the restrictive position of the previous guidelines with respect to the athlete with an ICD, a registry-based study is limited by many factors, such as (1) few patients had engaged in aggressive contact sports; (2) median time of enrollment was about 2 years (leading to survival or selection bias); and (3) the bias was associated with the study design of self-reporting and a self-selected group. Nevertheless, it has provided an observational signal to challenge previous opinion/experience-based renderings.

Another retrospective study, involving 130 athletes with LQTS who chose to continue their participation in competitive sports showed that 70 of the 130 athletes (54%) who were genotype-positive/phenotype-negative suffered no sport-related adverse events. Of the other 60 athletes with a genotype-positive/phenotype-positive profile, thereby participating contrary to both guidelines, only one athlete had a sporting-related adverse event with an appropriate shock.[49,50] The combination of these 2 aforementioned studies was cited by the newest LQTS-specific guidelines as the rationale for moving away from a one-size-fits-all disqualification from all competitive sports for all LQTS patients (the ESC 2005 position) to a position more consistent with the philosophy of individualized/personalized medicine and shared decision-making as admonished by Johnson and Ackerman in their Mayo Clinic study.[37,42,49,50]

Individual Factors: An Athlete's Perspective and Shared Clinical Decision-Making

When making recommendations, it is also important to take into account the individual athlete's perspective on what it would mean for them in terms of lifestyle change or quality of life when restricting them from a particular sporting activity. Physical activity and engaging in sports are known to promote psychological well-being in patients with heart disease apart from its well-recognized effect in reducing morbidity and mortality through various mechanisms.[51,52] On the contrary, the increased number of shocks associated with physical activity in these patients may also have profound psychological impact, subjecting them to fear of recurrent shocks and consequently reducing their sporting activities.[53] The previously discussed registry study of athletes with ICDs participating in organized sporting activity showed that about 30% of the patients who received a shock ended up stopping all sporting activities, underscoring the potential for adverse psychological sequelae of an ICD shock.[37]

Given the lack of substantial evidence supporting the Bethesda Conference and ESC recommendations for athletic participation in patients with ICDs, it is important to recognize patient/family autonomy and respect their rights to make a well-informed decision regarding continuation of athletics, thus paving the way for a shared decision-making engagement. Contrary to the myth that such shared decision-making is not possible, it is assumed that "all athletes will always choose to remain an athlete" has not been an observation at all over the past 15 years. Instead, it was shown that 1 in 5 athletes chose self-disqualification from competitive sports when given a choice after carefully explaining the individual risks and benefits of participation.[49]

PRACTICAL CONSIDERATIONS OF IMPLANTABLE CARDIOVERTER DEFIBRILLATORS IN ATHLETES
Single-Chamber Versus Dual-Chamber Implantable Cardioverter Defibrillators

Because inappropriate shocks are a major concern in athletes with ICDs who remain active, some electrophysiologists propose the use of a dual-chamber ICD over single-chamber device to improve the specificity of arrhythmia detection.[54] However, other studies have failed to show any significant difference in the incidence of inappropriate ICD shocks in patients with dual-chamber ICDs as compared with those with single-chamber devices.[55,56] Moreover, dual-chamber ICDs may lead to a higher incidence of early or late postoperative complications, along with increased complexity of implantation and follow-up.[57] In addition, athletes typically represent a generally younger population, and the fewer number of leads at initial implantation may help in reducing the number of leads that need extraction or replacement in the future, thus reducing the potential for long-term morbidity and mortality.[33] Accordingly, unless the underlying disease process may benefit from atrial pacing, the authors advise a single-lead ICD system for athletes.

Implantable Cardioverter Defibrillator Programming: Can We Reduce Inappropriate Shocks?

ICDs recognize malignant arrhythmias by closely monitoring the morphology and ventricular rate of the patient. This monitoring may in turn lead to a high frequency of inappropriate shocks in athletes because of the high incidence of faster heart rates (sinus tachycardia or supraventricular tachycardias), lead noise, or sensing issues during intense physical activity. Thus, one must be careful in activating lower thresholds in these patients because they may lead to an increase in inappropriate shocks. Programming additional differentiating parameters to improve the device's specificity in picking up ventricular arrhythmias (characterized by sudden onset, instability, and wide-complex morphology) has been suggested, but this may result in decreased sensitivity and so may be reserved as a second-line option in patients with a high frequency of inappropriate shocks.[33]

Certain ICD programming maneuvers have been attempted to decrease the rate of inappropriate shocks. These programming maneuvers include trying at least one attempt of antitachycardia pacing to stop arrhythmias in the VF zone while the device is charging,[58] increasing the VF zone threshold to greater than 210 to 220 beats per minute, and extending the detection time at these rates.[59] Apart from these measures, using long-term electrocardiogram recordings to calculate rate responsiveness during training and availing dual sensors (minute ventilation + activity) to help differentiate physical activities[60] may also have the potential to reduce the rate of inappropriate shocks in athletes with ICDs. If chronotropic incompetence or symptomatic bradycardia from the use of bradycardic drugs is suspected in these patients, atrioventricular sequential pacing through dual-chamber ICD is suggested to decrease symptoms from continued ventricular pacing.[33,60]

Subcutaneous Implantable Cardioverter Defibrillator

Due to various lead concerns in athletes with ICDs, there has been considerable interest in the newest generation subcutaneous ICD (S-ICD) systems.[61,62] Studies on S-ICDs indicate a high efficacy but relatively low specificity and this could translate to a significant increase in the number of inappropriate shocks in these individuals.[63] Another limitation to S-ICDs would be their inability to pace; therefore, these cannot be used in athletes with potentially pace-terminable arrhythmias. This area is clearly in need of further research and observation before further consideration in athletes as their primary source of shock therapy, which can literally be lifesaving.

Factors That May Help Reduce Risk in Athletes with Implantable Cardioverter Defibrillator Who Chose to Compete

It has been proposed that habitual exercise may decrease the risk of SCD during exercise by 7-fold, especially among people who exercise infrequently (ie, less than once a week).[7] The risk of SCD, however, appears to be independent of the level of athletic competition (ie, high school, college, or professional).[9] In these patients with ICDs, compliance with target heart rates may enable them to safely participate in physical exercise or training.[64] Monitoring and recognizing target heart rates may also decrease shocks that are due to sinus tachycardia.[54] Whether the use of mechanical barriers such as a Kevlar vest could decrease the risk associated with contact sports is unknown.[43] The use of β-blockers to counteract the catecholamine surge, ensuring adequate hydration, and electrolyte replacement during intense training and physical exertion may reduce the risk of SCD by decreasing the intrinsic arrhythmogenicity of the ventricular myocardium during a period of activity.[65] However, continued prospective/registry-based data are needed to further evaluate and validate these strategies.

SUMMARY

Athletes with predisposing cardiac disease for SCD represent a unique segment of the general population, who, despite their excellent physical condition, are at an increased risk of arrhythmias and SCD by the sheer virtue of the intensity and duration of the physical exercise they engage in. Current international recommendations preclude athletes with ICDs from participating in the vast majority of competitive sports. However, these guidelines are more than a decade old and are being reviewed, revised, and updated, and it is anticipated that the former "if in doubt, kick them out" position will be replaced increasingly with an individualized, shared decision-making approach. Although there are some preliminary data supporting the safety of athletes with ICDs when participating in organized sports, much progress is yet to be made to ensure safety in these patients, and larger trials and innovation are needed.

REFERENCES

1. Anvari A, Stix G, Grabenwoger M, et al. Comparison of three cardioverter defibrillator implantation techniques: initial results with transvenous pectoral implantation. Pacing Clin Electrophysiol 1996;19(7):1016–9.
2. Epstein AE, Dimarco JP, Ellenbogen KA, et al. ACC/AHA/HRS 2008 Guidelines for Device-Based Therapy of Cardiac Rhythm Abnormalities: Executive Summary: A Report of the American College of Cardiology/American Heart

Association Task Force on Practice Guidelines (Writing Committee to Revise the ACC/AHA/NASPE 2002 Guideline Update for Implantation of Cardiac Pacemakers and Antiarrhythmia Devices) Developed in Collaboration With the American Association for Thoracic Surgery and Society of Thoracic Surgeons. Heart Rhythm 2008;5(6):934–55.

3. van Rees JB, de Bie MK, Thijssen J, et al. Implantation-related complications of implantable cardioverter-defibrillators and cardiac resynchronization therapy devices: a systematic review of randomized clinical trials. J Am Coll Cardiol 2011; 58(10):995–1000.

4. Zipes DP, Ackerman MJ, Estes NA 3rd, et al. Task Force 7: arrhythmias. J Am Coll Cardiol 2005;45(8):1354–63.

5. Siscovick DS, Weiss NS, Fletcher RH, et al. The incidence of primary cardiac arrest during vigorous exercise. N Engl J Med 1984;311(14):874–7.

6. Giri S, Thompson PD, Kiernan FJ, et al. Clinical and angiographic characteristics of exertion-related acute myocardial infarction. JAMA 1999;282(18): 1731–6.

7. Albert CM, Mittleman MA, Chae CU, et al. Triggering of sudden death from cardiac causes by vigorous exertion. N Engl J Med 2000;343(19):1355–61.

8. Thompson PD, Franklin BA, Balady GJ, et al. Exercise and acute cardiovascular events placing the risks into perspective: a scientific statement from the American Heart Association Council on Nutrition, Physical Activity, and Metabolism and the Council on Clinical Cardiology. Circulation 2007;115(17):2358–68.

9. Maron BJ, Thompson PD, Ackerman MJ, et al. Recommendations and considerations related to preparticipation screening for cardiovascular abnormalities in competitive athletes: 2007 update: a scientific statement from the American Heart Association Council on Nutrition, Physical Activity, and Metabolism: endorsed by the American College of Cardiology Foundation. Circulation 2007;115(12): 1643–55.

10. Corrado D, Pelliccia A, Bjørnstad HH, et al. Cardiovascular pre-participation screening of young competitive athletes for prevention of sudden death: proposal for a common European protocol. Consensus Statement of the Study Group of Sport Cardiology of the Working Group of Cardiac Rehabilitation and Exercise Physiology and the Working Group of Myocardial and Pericardial Diseases of the European Society of Cardiology. Eur Heart J 2005;26:516–24.

11. Corrado D, Basso C, Rizzoli G, et al. Does sports activity enhance the risk of sudden death in adolescents and young adults? J Am Coll Cardiol 2003;42(11): 1959–63.

12. Lampert R, Cannom D. Sports participation for athletes with implantable cardioverter-defibrillators should be an individualized risk-benefit decision. Heart Rhythm 2008;5(6):861–3.

13. Corrado D, Basso C, Schiavon M, et al. Pre-participation screening of young competitive athletes for prevention of sudden cardiac death. J Am Coll Cardiol 2008;52(24):1981–9.

14. Mitchell JH, Haskell W, Snell P, et al. Task Force 8: classification of sports. J Am Coll Cardiol 2005;45(8):1364–7.

15. Maron BJ, Zipes DP. Introduction: eligibility recommendations for competitive athletes with cardiovascular abnormalities-general considerations. J Am Coll Cardiol 2005;45(8):1318–21.

16. Pelliccia A, Fagard R, Bjørnstad HH, et al. Recommendations for competitive sports participation in athletes with cardiovascular disease. A consensus document from the Study Group of Sports Cardiology of the Working Group of Cardiac

Rehabilitation and Exercise Physiology and the Working Group of Myocardial and Pericardial Diseases of the European Society of Cardiology. Eur Heart J 2005;26: 1422–45.

17. Pelliccia A, Zipes DP, Maron BJ. Bethesda Conference #36 and the European Society of Cardiology Consensus Recommendations revisited a comparison of U.S. and European criteria for eligibility and disqualification of competitive athletes with cardiovascular abnormalities. J Am Coll Cardiol 2008;52(24): 1990–6.
18. Maron BJ. Sudden death in young athletes. N Engl J Med 2003;349(11):1064–75.
19. Furlanello F, Bettini R, Cozzi F, et al. Ventricular arrhythmias and sudden death in athletes. Ann N Y Acad Sci 1984;427:253–79.
20. Corrado D, Basso C, Schiavon M, et al. Screening for hypertrophic cardiomyopathy in young athletes. N Engl J Med 1998;339(6):364–9.
21. Thiene G, Nava A, Corrado D, et al. Right ventricular cardiomyopathy and sudden death in young people. N Engl J Med 1988;318(3):129–33.
22. Maron BJ, Ackerman MJ, Nishimura RA, et al. Task Force 4: HCM and other cardiomyopathies, mitral valve prolapse, myocarditis, and Marfan syndrome. J Am Coll Cardiol 2005;45(8):1340–5.
23. Maron BJ, Shirani J, Poliac LC, et al. Sudden death in young competitive athletes. Clinical, demographic, and pathological profiles. JAMA 1996;276(3): 199–204.
24. Maron BJ. Hypertrophic cardiomyopathy: a systematic review. JAMA 2002; 287(10):1308–20.
25. Maron BJ, Shen WK, Link MS, et al. Efficacy of implantable cardioverter-defibrillators for the prevention of sudden death in patients with hypertrophic cardiomyopathy. N Engl J Med 2000;342(6):365–73.
26. Gaita F, Giustetto C, Bianchi F, et al. Short QT Syndrome: a familial cause of sudden death. Circulation 2003;108(8):965–70.
27. Sumitomo N, Harada K, Nagashima M, et al. Catecholaminergic polymorphic ventricular tachycardia: electrocardiographic characteristics and optimal therapeutic strategies to prevent sudden death. Heart 2003;89(1):66–70.
28. Heidbüchel H, Corrado D, Biffi A, et al. Recommendations for participation in leisure-time physical activity and competitive sports of patients with arrhythmias and potentially arrhythmogenic conditions. Part II: ventricular arrhythmias, channelopathies and implantable defibrillators. Eur J Cardiovasc Prev Rehabil 2006; 13(5):676–86.
29. Maron BJ, Chaitman BR, Ackerman MJ, et al. Recommendations for physical activity and recreational sports participation for young patients with genetic cardiovascular diseases. Circulation 2004;109(22):2807–16.
30. Medbo JI, Sejersted OM. Plasma potassium changes with high intensity exercise. J Physiol 1990;421:105–22.
31. Qin H, Walcott GP, Killingsworth CR, et al. Impact of myocardial ischemia and reperfusion on ventricular defibrillation patterns, energy requirements, and detection of recovery. Circulation 2002;105(21):2537–42.
32. Heidbuchel H. Implantable cardioverter defibrillator therapy in athletes. Cardiol Clin 2007;25(3):467–82, vii.
33. Heidbuchel H, Carre F. Exercise and competitive sports in patients with an implantable cardioverter-defibrillator. Eur Heart J 2014;35(44):3097–102.
34. Mohamed U, Gollob MH, Gow RM, et al. Sudden cardiac death despite an implantable cardioverter-defibrillator in a young female with catecholaminergic ventricular tachycardia. Heart Rhythm 2006;3(12):1486–9.

35. Suddath WO, Deychak Y, Varghese PJ. Electrophysiologic basis by which epinephrine facilitates defibrillation after prolonged episodes of ventricular fibrillation. Ann Emerg Med 2001;38(3):201–6.
36. Hegel MT, Griegel LE, Black C, et al. Anxiety and depression in patients receiving implanted cardioverter-defibrillators: a longitudinal investigation. Int J Psychiatry Med 1997;27(1):57–69.
37. Lampert R, Olshansky B, Heidbuchel H, et al. Safety of sports for athletes with implantable cardioverter-defibrillators: results of a prospective, multinational registry. Circulation 2013;127(20):2021–30.
38. Lampert R, Jain D, Burg MM, et al. Destabilizing effects of mental stress on ventricular arrhythmias in patients with implantable cardioverter-defibrillators. Circulation 2000;101(2):158–64.
39. Lombardi F, Malfatto G, Belloni A, et al. Effects of sympathetic activation on ventricular ectopic beats in subjects with and without evidence of organic heart disease. Eur Heart J 1987;8(10):1065–74.
40. Zouhal H, Jacob C, Delamarche P, et al. Catecholamines and the effects of exercise, training and gender. Sports Med 2008;38(5):401–23.
41. Sousa J, Kou W, Calkins H, et al. Effect of epinephrine on the efficacy of the internal cardioverter-defibrillator. Am J Cardiol 1992;69(5):509–12.
42. Priori SG, Wilde AA, Horie M, et al. HRS/EHRA/APHRS expert consensus statement on the diagnosis and management of patients with inherited primary arrhythmia syndromes: document endorsed by HRS, EHRA, and APHRS in May 2013 and by ACCF, AHA, PACES, and AEPC in June 2013. Heart Rhythm 2013;10(12):1932–63.
43. Lampert R, Cannom D, Olshansky B. Safety of sports participation in patients with implantable cardioverter defibrillators: a survey of heart rhythm society members. J Cardiovasc Electrophysiol 2006;17(1):11–5.
44. Isaksen K, Morken IM, Munk PS, et al. Exercise training and cardiac rehabilitation in patients with implantable cardioverter defibrillators: a review of current literature focusing on safety, effects of exercise training, and the psychological impact of programme participation. Eur J Prev Cardiol 2012;19(4):804–12.
45. Zipes DP, Roberts D. Results of the international study of the implantable pacemaker cardioverter-defibrillator. A comparison of epicardial and endocardial lead systems. The Pacemaker-Cardioverter-Defibrillator Investigators. Circulation 1995;92(1):59–65.
46. Kron J, Herre J, Renfroe EG, et al. Lead- and device-related complications in the antiarrhythmics versus implantable defibrillators trial. Am Heart J 2001;141(1):92–8.
47. Lampert R, Joska T, Burg MM, et al. Emotional and physical precipitants of ventricular arrhythmia. Circulation 2002;106(14):1800–5.
48. Schron EB, Exner DV, Yao Q, et al. Quality of life in the antiarrhythmics versus implantable defibrillators trial: impact of therapy and influence of adverse symptoms and defibrillator shocks. Circulation 2002;105(5):589–94.
49. Johnson JN, Ackerman MJ. Return to play? Athletes with congenital long QT syndrome. Br J Sports Med 2013;47(1):28–33.
50. Johnson JN, Ackerman MJ. Competitive sports participation in athletes with congenital long QT syndrome. JAMA 2012;308(8):764–5.
51. Graham I, Atar D, Borch-Johnsen K, et al. European guidelines on cardiovascular disease prevention in clinical practice: executive summary. Fourth Joint Task Force of the European Society of Cardiology and other societies on cardiovascular disease prevention in clinical practice (constituted by representatives of

nine societies and by invited experts). Eur J Cardiovasc Prev Rehabil 2007; 14(Suppl 2):E1–40.

52. Haskell WL, Lee IM, Pate RR, et al. Physical activity and public health: updated recommendation for adults from the American College of Sports Medicine and the American Heart Association. Med Sci Sports Exerc 2007;39(8):1423–34.

53. Berg SK, Moons P, Zwisler AD, et al. Phantom shocks in patients with implantable cardioverter defibrillator: results from a randomized rehabilitation trial (COPE-ICD). Europace 2013;15(10):1463–7.

54. Kolb C, Sturmer M, Sick P, et al. Reduced risk for inappropriate implantable cardioverter-defibrillator shocks with dual-chamber therapy compared with single-chamber therapy: results of the randomized OPTION study. JACC Heart Fail 2014;2(6):611–9.

55. Deisenhofer I, Kolb C, Ndrepepa G, et al. Do current dual chamber cardioverter defibrillators have advantages over conventional single chamber cardioverter defibrillators in reducing inappropriate therapies? A randomized, prospective study. J Cardiovasc Electrophysiol 2001;12(2):134–42.

56. Sinha AM, Stellbrink C, Schuchert A, et al. Clinical experience with a new detection algorithm for differentiation of supraventricular from ventricular tachycardia in a dual-chamber defibrillator. J Cardiovasc Electrophysiol 2004;15(6):646–52.

57. Connolly SJ, Kerr CR, Gent M, et al. Effects of physiologic pacing versus ventricular pacing on the risk of stroke and death due to cardiovascular causes. Canadian Trial of Physiologic Pacing Investigators. N Engl J Med 2000;342(19): 1385–91.

58. Wathen MS, DeGroot PJ, Sweeney MO, et al. Prospective randomized multicenter trial of empirical antitachycardia pacing versus shocks for spontaneous rapid ventricular tachycardia in patients with implantable cardioverter-defibrillators: Pacing Fast Ventricular Tachycardia Reduces Shock Therapies (PainFREE Rx II) trial results. Circulation 2004;110(17):2591–6.

59. Moss AJ, Schuger C, Beck CA, et al. Reduction in inappropriate therapy and mortality through ICD programming. N Engl J Med 2012;367(24):2275–83.

60. Israel CW, Hohnloser SH. Current status of dual-sensor pacemaker systems for correction of chronotropic incompetence. Am J Cardiol 2000;86(9A):86K–94K.

61. Olde Nordkamp LR, Knops RE, Bardy GH, et al. Rationale and design of the PRAETORIAN trial: a Prospective, RAndomizEd comparison of subcuTaneOus and tRansvenous ImplANtable cardioverter-defibrillator therapy. Am Heart J 2012;163(5):753–60.e2.

62. Bardy GH, Smith WM, Hood MA, et al. An entirely subcutaneous implantable cardioverter-defibrillator. N Engl J Med 2010;363(1):36–44.

63. Weiss R, Knight BP, Gold MR, et al. Safety and efficacy of a totally subcutaneous implantable-cardioverter defibrillator. Circulation 2013;128(9):944–53.

64. Vanhees L, Kornaat M, Defoor J, et al. Effect of exercise training in patients with an implantable cardioverter defibrillator. Eur Heart J 2004;25(13):1120–6.

65. Sejersted OM, Sjogaard G. Dynamics and consequences of potassium shifts in skeletal muscle and heart during exercise. Physiol Rev 2000;80(4):1411–81.

Sports and Exercise in Athletes with Hypertrophic Cardiomyopathy

Craig Alpert, MD[a], Sharlene M. Day, MD[b], Sara Saberi, MD, MS[c],*

KEYWORDS

- Hypertrophic cardiomyopathy • Exercise • Exercise paradox
- Sudden cardiac death • Bethesda conference • Automated external defibrillator

KEY POINTS

- Hypertrophic cardiomyopathy (HCM), characterized by ventricular hypertrophy and relaxation abnormalities, is the most common genetic cardiovascular disease and among the leading causes of sudden cardiac death in young athletes.
- Current guidelines of both American and European cardiology societies recommend that patients with HCM refrain from all but low-intensity sports independent of implantable cardioverter-defibrillator (ICD) use.
- Despite theoretic concerns that exercise can increase the risk of SCD, many patients with HCM have safely participated in physical activity.
- Improved quantification of risk of a given individual for a given activity, coupled with better emergency preparedness, may allow most patients with HCM to participate in physical activity in a safe manner.

Life changed all too quickly for Nick Knapp in the fall of 1994.[1] A standout forward on the high school basketball team, he had previously accepted a full scholarship to Northwestern University. During a preseason pickup game in his senior year, however, he collapsed on the basketball court because of a ventricular fibrillation (VF) arrest.[2] He received shock twice and was intubated in the field and went on to make a

Funding sources: Dr C. Alpert, nil; Dr S.M. Day, NIH R01 GRANT11572784; Dr S. Saberi, AHA Award 11CRP7510001, MICHR UL1TR000433.

Conflict of interest: Nil.

[a] Division of Cardiovascular Medicine, Department of Internal Medicine, 2381 Frankel Cardiovascular Center, University of Michigan School of Medicine, 1500 East Medical Center Drive, Suite 5853, Ann Arbor, MI 48109-0366, USA; [b] Division of Cardiovascular Medicine, Department of Internal Medicine, Frankel Cardiovascular Center, University of Michigan School of Medicine, 1150 West Medical Center Drive, 7301 MSRBIII, Ann Arbor, MI 48109-5644, USA; [c] Division of Cardiovascular Medicine, Department of Internal Medicine, Frankel Cardiovascular Center, University of Michigan School of Medicine, Suite 2364, 1500 East Medical Center Drive, Ann Arbor, MI 48109-5853, USA

* Corresponding author.

E-mail address: saberis@med.umich.edu

remarkable recovery. Subsequent workup yielded a new diagnosis of HCM, and he was outfitted with an ICD within 10 days. Although he matriculated the following fall, Northwestern University failed to share his optimism. Team physicians judged Knapp to be medically ineligible, effectively launching a protracted legal battle that would rage on for more than a year. If you were the judge, how would you rule? Careful review of the current guidelines, as well as the evidence behind them, should help you to reach a decision.

HYPERTROPHIC CARDIOMYOPATHY: EPIDEMIOLOGY, PATHOPHYSIOLOGY, DIAGNOSIS, CLINICAL COURSE, AND TREATMENT

HCM is the most common genetic cardiovascular disease, affecting 1 in 500 people and characterized by ventricular hypertrophy and relaxation abnormalities (**Fig. 1**).[3] The disease is not only common but also nondiscriminating; it afflicts patients around the world irrespective of geography, sex, ethnicity, and race.[4–7] It is also a leading cause of sudden cardiac death (SCD) in young athletes younger than 40 years.[8] Although shrouded in mystery for decades after its initial description more than 65 years ago, and known by several misnomers along the way, HCM is now recognized to be a treatable condition in terms of reducing symptom burden and preventing SCD.

HCM is inherited in an autosomal dominant manner. Hundreds of mutations have been cataloged across more than 12 genes that encode proteins of the cardiac

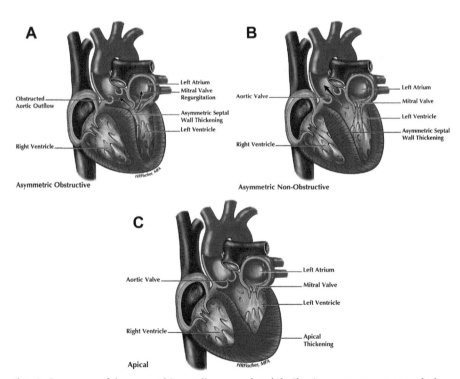

Fig. 1. Spectrum of hypertrophic cardiomyopathy. (*A*) Classic reverse-curve morphology causing outflow tract obstruction. (*B*) Example of asymmetric hypertrophy morphology (neutral septum) not associated with outflow obstruction. (*C*) Apical variant hypertrophic cardiomyopathy.

sarcomere, most commonly myosin-binding protein C (MYBPC3) and beta-myosin heavy chain (MYH7).[6] Although HCM is considered a monogenic disease, it is heterogeneous with respect to clinical disease severity marked by variable courses and prognoses, even within a single family sharing an identical mutation. Furthermore, the widespread availability of clinical genetic testing has revealed a new cohort of individuals who carry a gene mutation yet lack any evidence of clinical disease (referred to as genotype positive–phenotype negative).[9,10]

Diagnosis of HCM relies on history, physical examination, electrocardiography (ECG), imaging, and sometimes genetic testing. A personal or family history of either syncope or SCD can be informative. Physical examination may reveal a systolic murmur characteristic of outflow obstruction or may show normal results.[11] An ECG may show high voltages or repolarization abnormalities. Echocardiography typically demonstrates a nondilated, hypertrophied, hyperdynamic left ventricle (LV) in the absence of hypertension, aortic stenosis, or any other systemic disease that may otherwise explain the hypertrophy. There may also be systolic anterior motion of the mitral valve that can result in outflow tract obstruction.

HCM can be complicated by SCD, heart failure, or cardioembolic stroke resulting from atrial fibrillation (AF), which affects up to 28% of patients with HCM.[12] Treatment options for HCM include ICDs to prevent SCD, as well as medications, percutaneous alcohol septal ablation, or surgical myectomy to reduce symptomatic outflow tract obstruction. Rate- or rhythm-control strategies, including radiofrequency ablation along with anticoagulation, are used in the management of AF. However, many patients have a normal life expectancy, as the average mortality rate for individuals afflicted with HCM roughly equals that of the US population.[6]

THE BIRTH OF GUIDELINES: BETHESDA AND BEYOND

In 1985, the American College of Cardiology (ACC) sponsored the 16th Bethesda Conference, which outlined for the first time consensus recommendations to govern the participation of patients with HCM in competitive sports.[13] Underlying its mission was the assumption that intensive physical activity could provoke SCD and, conversely, that limiting such activity could mitigate that risk. Although the committee made use of published data and clinical experience, it also freely acknowledged its reliance on a "common sense approach to the art of the practice of medicine." These initial guidelines considered patients with HCM with markedly abnormal wall thickness, significant outflow tract obstruction, a history of syncope or arrhythmias, or a family history of SCD to be at higher risk and unilaterally advised against participation in "any competitive sports." Medical or surgical treatment to alter the patients' physiology did not downgrade the assigned risk in the eyes of the committee.

Just 9 years later, the committee reconvened at the 26th Bethesda Conference and generalized its recommendations to any patient with an "unequivocal" diagnosis of HCM.[14] It opened a new opportunity for such a patient to compete in "low-intensity" sports and exempted the newly emerging cohort of genotype positive–phenotype negative individuals from any restrictions.

Finally, in 2005, the 36th Bethesda Conference Task Force further revised its recommendations, specifying that patients with an ICD must be restricted in a manner identical to those without one.[15]

Although the Bethesda Conferences clearly outlined the expert consensus regarding participation of patients with HCM viewed as elite athletes in competitive sports, there was no comparable statement guiding everyday physical activity and recreational sports until 2004, when the American Heart Association (AHA) commissioned such a consensus document.[16] There, the committee categorized the most common sports by 1 of 3 levels of intensity, which then dictated the recommendation. It also provided general advice to patients with HCM that applied to all sports across all levels of intensity.

COMPARISONS TO EUROPEAN GUIDELINES

Although the initial recommendations were made in the United States, the European Society of Cardiology (ESC) followed soon thereafter with similar documents guiding participation of patients with various types of heart disease in both competitive and recreational sports.[17,18] The guidelines were nearly identical, save for recommendations for genotype positive–phenotype negative individuals. The ESC opted to include these individuals among the at-risk population and recommended activity restrictions, whereas the American committee argued that they should be exempt from restrictions given insufficient evidence of elevated risk.[19]

Although broader guidelines for HCM management have been published by the Heart Rhythm Society (HRS), ACC, and ESC, they all defer to the Bethesda Conference or its European analogs with regard to physical activity and sports participation.[20–22]

THE EVIDENCE BEHIND THE GUIDELINES

Estimates of the proportion of SCD in athletes attributable to HCM vary widely. The US National Registry of Sudden Death in Athletes, which builds its database from review of public records, reports that HCM underlies 36% of SCD.[7,8,23] Another study using a similar approach to analyze deaths of high school and college athletes identified half of SCDs as being due to HCM.[24] In stark contrast, a mandatory reporting system implemented in Northern Italy studying competitive athletes noted only 2% incidence of HCM among its SCD cases, with most being instead attributed to arrhythmogenic right ventricular cardiomyopathy.[25] Furthermore, HCM was responsible for only 6% of nontraumatic sudden death in young US military recruits and only 4% of young adults suffering SCD during exercise in King County, Washington.[26,27] Such variation is not unique to athletes and is mirrored in the general young adult population as well.[28]

Several factors contribute to the variation in the incidence and causes of SCD, among them geographic diversity and unique regional preparticipation screening methods, inconsistent definitions of the competitive athlete, disparate autopsy adjudications, and heterogeneous demographics such as age, sex, race, and ethnicity. Furthermore, the absolute number of events in any given study is fairly small. Nevertheless, sufficient data exist to calculate the relative incidence of SCD among patients with HCM, which is very low.[29] Based on published reports of the incidence of SCD among athletes and the known prevalence of HCM, it is estimated that the risk of SCD for athletes with HCM competing in sports is in the range of 0.03% to 0.1% per year.[23,30,31]

THE CAUSE OF SUDDEN CARDIAC DEATH IN HYPERTROPHIC CARDIOMYOPATHY IS ROOTED IN AN ELECTRICALLY UNSTABLE SUBSTRATE

The precise mechanism of SCD in patients with HCM is presumed to be ventricular tachyarrhythmias, which develop as a direct result of structural abnormalities.[32] At the cellular level, hypertrophied myocytes are associated with prolonged repolarization of transmembrane action potentials.[33] In addition, both the composition and distribution of ion channels seen in typical myocytes are deranged in hypertrophied cells.[34] When such hypertrophy occurs with regional variation, it conceivably generates islands of altered electrical currents that in turn may contribute to a proarrhythmic substrate.[34] At the histologic level, the myocardial disarray that defines the disease may similarly disrupt normal electrical circuitry and induce malignant arrhythmias.

Some have argued that the risk for electrical instability is due to more than just the intrinsically proarrhythmic cardiac tissue. Repetitive microvascular ischemia, which over time generates scarring, provides a nidus for reentrant ventricular arrhythmias that only compounds the risk.[35,36] This may help to explain why marked LV wall thickness independently predicts incidence of ventricular arrhythmia, as replacement fibrosis has been shown to correlate linearly with septal thickness.[36]

DOES EXERCISE INCREASE THE RISK OF SUDDEN CARDIAC DEATH IN HYPERTROPHIC CARDIOMYOPATHY?

Given the underlying structural predisposition to rogue electrical currents in these patients, any external stress to such a system could understandably have catastrophic outcomes. Physical activity can alter blood volume, electrolytes, metabolism, catecholamine levels, and autonomic tone, any of which may contribute to a heightened risk of ventricular arrhythmias.[37] Nevertheless, in a study of patients with HCM undergoing treadmill or bicycle ergometer exercise testing, only 3 of 1380 developed exercise-induced VF.[38] In addition, retrospective studies have shown that among patients with HCM, only a small fraction of SCD (16%–30%) occurs with significant exertion.[27,39] Furthermore, HCM seems to contribute equally to the risk of SCD whether death occurs during exercise or not.[27] These studies suggest that the risk of SCD associated with exercise is grossly overestimated in practice.

There is also a hypothetical consideration that vigorous exercise could promote the progression of the underlying HCM disease process through myocardial ischemia or the development of LV systolic or diastolic dysfunction.[40–42] High-intensity exercise training has also been shown to promote the development of AF, and athletes with HCM may be more predisposed than athletes with a structurally normal heart.[43,44] However, there are no data that support the concept that vigorous or even competitive physical activity has any detrimental effects on the myocardial structure or function in individuals with HCM.

Finally, it is worth mentioning that the risk of SCD in HCM as it relates to the intensity of an activity has not been well studied. It seems logical that mild or even moderate recreational exercise for the purpose of physical fitness would carry a lower risk of SCD than vigorous training for competition. The guidelines do acknowledge this assumption and use this rationale to stratify common activities by intensity level to modify recommendations. Further study in this area is especially necessary given that it is arguably recreational activity, not competitive sports, that is more relevant to the HCM population at large. Investigation into age as a risk factor is also necessary, as there are no data about the risk of SCD for master's level competitive or recreational athletes.

THE EXERCISE PARADOX IN HYPERTROPHIC CARDIOMYOPATHY

Many have written of the so-called exercise paradox among adults, struggling to reconcile the many known cardioprotective benefits of physical activity with the attributed increase in risk for SCD.[45] Exercise has long been embraced by the scientific community as a means of decreasing cardiovascular morbidity and mortality and has been championed by countless organizations as a public health initiative.[46–49] Furthermore, exercise capacity is strongly correlated with longevity.[50] Although exercise can transiently increase the risk of SCD, habitual exercise progressively decreases the risk of SCD over time.[51–56] Different doses of habitual exercise may even have variable effects on all-cause mortality.[57]

Does such a paradox extend to patients with HCM as well? Although vigorous exercise may trigger SCD, studies suggest that exercise may also benefit the underlying pathophysiology of HCM. In one compelling study in a mouse model of HCM, routine exercise before the development of the HCM phenotype prevented subsequent fibrosis, myocyte disarray, and induction of markers of hypertrophy.[58] Similarly, among mice already expressing the HCM phenotype, such exercise effectively reversed the architectural disarray and induction of markers of hypertrophy. These changes were postulated to be mediated through alterations in apoptosis as well as improved metabolic matching.[59] It is conceivable that such changes take place in humans as well. Finally, regular exercise increases vagal tone, which may actually neutralize the very electrical substrate that predisposes patients with HCM to elevated risk in the first place.[55] Through this mechanism, routine exercise may decrease the risk of SCD in patients with HCM much as it does among the general population.

Restriction from physical activity may cause other detrimental long-term consequences. Perhaps reflective of such restriction, patients with HCM relative to those without the diagnosis have a statistically significant higher body mass index, which in and of itself has been tied to increased cardiovascular morbidity and mortality.[60] In addition, physical activity has been shown to improve quality of life and self-reported health status and to decrease the frequency of hospitalizations and overall mortality in a similar cohort, those with chronic heart failure.[61–64] Presumably, patients restricted from activity must forfeit these associated benefits. Studies have already documented that the quality of life among athletes restricted from sports for health considerations is significantly lower than that of nonathletes.[65] Patients with HCM also readily admitted that restriction from sports negatively affected their emotional well-being.[60] Such patients frequently feel ostracized, especially during young adulthood when sport participation is intertwined with socialization. Abrupt removal following a new diagnosis may be particularly traumatic. Moreover, the restriction not only limits activities of leisure but also dictates occupational choices and in so doing potentially affects socioeconomic status as well.[60]

CHALLENGING THE GUIDELINES

A substantial proportion of patients with HCM continue to compete at a high-intensity level, often perhaps against medical advice. Of 897 patients with HCM surveyed in one particular study, 63% reported having participated in competitive athletics, often in multiple sports.[60] Case reports and case series abound that identify upper echelon athletes competing at extreme levels only to later be diagnosed with HCM.[66,67] It therefore stands to reason that unilateral restriction of all patients with HCM from vigorous or competitive activity may be excessive. One need look no further than the guidelines for ICD implantation to appreciate that all patients with HCM are clearly not at equivalent risk for SCD.

DEFINING THE HIGH-RISK COHORT
Stratification by Genetics

There has been considerable interest to risk stratify patients with HCM based on their particular genetic mutation. Lending further hope was the fact that such strategies had been successfully implemented in other inherited diseases that similarly predispose to SCD, such as long-QT syndrome.[68] Several studies successfully identified a limited number of genetic defects of a particularly malignant variety.[69–71] However, this once promising approach has ultimately been thwarted by an unanticipated volume of unique mutations as well as the inconsistent correlation between genotype and phenotype.[10,70,72] At least for the time being, genetics does not typically affect risk stratification for athletes with HCM.

Stratification by Patient and Sport Characteristics

Although patients diagnosed with HCM comprise a diverse patient population with respect to geography, sex, ethnicity, and race, there do seem to be certain patterns emerging among the subset of young athletes with HCM who suffer SCD. Relative to the general population of patients with HCM, those experiencing SCD are overwhelmingly male and African American.[7,8,23,24,30,73–75] It has been suggested that such factors may confer an elevated risk by means of disproportionately increased training-induced ventricular hypertrophy, which is common to both cohorts.[74]

Not only are certain demographics thought to be at higher risk for SCD, but certain sports are also thought to confer greater risk. Basketball consistently confers the highest additional risk, although football, swimming, lacrosse, cross-country, and water polo also are associated with elevated incidence of SCD.[30,73] When quantifying risk among National Collegiate Athletic Association athletes, those in Division I had higher rates of SCD than those in Division II and Division III, perhaps suggesting a relationship to the intensity or duration of training or the level of competition.[30]

Stratification by Clinical Phenotype: History and Diagnostic Testing

Roughly half of young adults who died of SCD have preceding symptoms such as chest discomfort or syncope, and 16% have a family history of SCD.[28,39] Clinical features that are associated with an independent increased risk of SCD besides syncope and positive family history of SCD include significant left ventricular hypertrophy, nonsustained ventricular tachycardia, and abnormal blood pressure response to exercise.[76,77] Therefore, these are the risk factors used at present to determine which patients are eligible for ICD implantation for primary prevention (**Box 1**).[78,79] The presence of even 1 risk factor is potentially worrisome. In a cohort of 506 patients with HCM treated with ICDs, more than one-third received appropriate defibrillation despite having just 1 of those 5 risk factors.[80] Beyond these major risk factors,

---

Box 1
Indications for ICD therapy

Indications for ICD implantation in patients with HCM (class IIa; level of evidence, C)

ICD implantation is reasonable for patients with HCM who have one or more of the following major risk factors for SCD:

- Prior cardiac arrest
- Spontaneous sustained ventricular tachycardia (VT)
- Spontaneous nonsustained VT
- Family history of SCD
- Syncope
- Maximal LV wall thickness 30 mm or more
- Abnormal blood pressure response to exercise

Adapted from Tracy CM, Epstein AE, Darbar D, et al. 2012 ACCF/AHA/HRS focused update of the 2008 guidelines for device-based therapy of cardiac rhythm abnormalities: a report of the American College of Cardiology Foundation/American Heart Association Task Force on Practice Guidelines. J Am Coll Cardiol 2012;60(14):1297–313.

consideration should also be given to the presence of left ventricular outflow tact obstruction, AF, age less than 60 years, left atrial enlargement, late gadolinium enhancement on cardiac MRI, and history of alcohol septal ablation, although the increment in absolute risk for each remains less robustly defined.[11,44,80–83] Among patients undergoing successful surgical septal myectomy, although long-term survival approached that of the general population, the risk of SCD persisted after the treatment (**Table 1**).[84,85] However, a significant challenge is the lack of data correlating baseline risk of SCD and risk of SCD with exercise, which could theoretically supersede traditional risk factors. These questions can be answered only with large prospective registries.

Notably absent among the aforementioned risk factors is any finding on ECG, which, although possibly useful as a screening test for HCM, does not further subdivide patients with HCM into groups of lower or higher risk.[86] In addition, arrhythmia induction during an electrophysiologic study, once thought meaningful, similarly does not help with risk stratification.[15,80]

Thus, it would seem that a model could be developed to incorporate features of a patient's demographic, type of athletic activity, and clinical phenotype to render a more individualized risk assessment. Such information could be obtained from careful history, physical examination, echocardiography, and exercise stress testing. Not only can exercise stress testing be done safely in patients with HCM, but in addition to revealing hemodynamic response to exercise, it can provide further diagnostic and prognostic information, such as functional capacity, resting and dynamic outflow obstruction, and inducibility of arrhythmias during exercise, which itself was shown to be a strong predictor of SCD.[29,38,87–94]

Stratification by Presence of Implantable Cardioverter-Defibrillator

Although ICDs are uncontested in their ability to minimize the risk of SCD, what remains more controversial is whether or not the presence of an ICD should allow a patient with

Table 1
Risk factors for SCD in HCM

Major Risk Factors	Hazard Ratio	95% Confidence Interval
Nonsustained ventricular tachycardia	2.89	2.21–3.58
Family history of SCD	1.27	1.16–1.38
Abnormal blood pressure response to exercise	1.30	0.64–1.96
Unexplained syncope	2.68	0.97–4.38
Maximal LV wall thickness ≥30 mm	3.1	1.81–4.40
Other Possible Risk Factors		
Young age		
LV outflow tract obstruction		
Atrial fibrillation		
Left atrial enlargement		
Fractionation of paced ventricular electrograms		
Myocardial ischemia		
Genetic mutations		
LV apical aneurysm		

Adapted from O'Mahony C, Elliott PM. Prevention of sudden cardiac death in hypertrophic cardiomyopathy. Heart 2014;100(3):254–60.

HCM to resume competitive athletics. Concern for this patient group is founded on 3 main premises, namely, the device fails to recognize and treat fatal arrhythmias, it incorrectly recognizes and treats nonlethal rhythms, and defibrillation, be it appropriate or inappropriate, may subject the athlete and others in the vicinity to significant trauma.[15,95] Physicians have also voiced concern that the device and its leads are at significant risk for damage, particularly in contact sports, and that malfunction could ensue with unacceptable frequency. There is additional hypothetical concern that exercise-induced physiologic changes (ie, alterations in electrolytes, autonomic tone, myocardial oxygenation, and neurohormonal milieu) could increase the defibrillation threshold and also interfere with device function. As a result, the North American Society of Pacing and Electrophysiology (NASPE), the immediate predecessor to HRS, agreed with guidelines put forth at the Bethesda Conference that patients with an ICD limit athletic participation to low-intensity sports, such as golf or bowling, which pose little risk to the device, so long as 6 months has elapsed since device implantation.[20]

Despite such reasonable concerns, however, patients have continued to participate in athletics even with an ICD in place. When surveyed, more than 40% of electrophysiologists reported having at least one of their patients with an ICD participate in competitive athletics with minimal adverse events.[96] Subsequently, a prospective, multinational registry was developed to examine the safety of athletic participation in patients with an ICD. Among 372 patients with an ICD, including 65 with HCM, followed up for a median of 31 months, there were no deaths, resuscitated arrests, or defibrillation-related injuries despite participation in high-intensity competitive sports.[95] About 21% of this patient population received a shock from their device, and 73% of these shocks occurred during physical activity. About 13% experienced a shock appropriately and 11%, inappropriately. Yet, among those with HCM and an ICD, only 1 of the 65 patients received a shock during competition or practice. Perhaps most telling of all, most athletes who received a shock during competition chose to continue playing after the shock.[95] A total of 13 definite and 14 possible lead malfunctions were reported, which translates into event rates comparable with those of nonathlete populations. Thus, theoretic concerns about competing with an ICD are now being questioned.

It is conceivable, much as the NASPE committee anticipated, that allowing patients with an ICD to participate in sports might increase demand for an ICD in patients for whom the device is not otherwise indicated. It may also lead to displays of moral hazard, whereby an athlete feels so protected by the device that he or she intentionally takes on greater risk as a result.

Such findings also raise a separate question as to whether athletes, including those with HCM, could preferentially undergo leadless, subcutaneous ICD implantation to minimize risks attributable to activity-induced lead malfunction. At present, there are insufficient data to answer that question.[97,98]

OTHER AVENUES OF PREVENTION

Although risk stratification, be it by genetic mutation, patient demographic, or clinical presentation, allows a clinician to identify many patients at increased risk of SCD and respond by restricting activities and/or implanting an ICD, such a strategy will inevitably fail to prevent SCD entirely. A substantial proportion of patients with SCD due to HCM are actually asymptomatic until an episode of SCD, posing a major challenge for prevention efforts.[8,39,99] In some cases, these patients escape diagnosis until the sentinel event. In others, the patients are diagnosed but then deemed to be at low risk for SCD and permitted to compete without necessary safeguards. To address the first cohort, preparticipation screening may facilitate the diagnosis of new cases of HCM before initiation of athletic activity. This topic is discussed in detail in other articles in this issue.

Emergency Preparedness

It is unrealistic to assume that all SCD can effectively be eliminated by risk stratification and screening. For now, the goal is simply to minimize the frequency with which it occurs and maximize the resuscitative efforts in place to assure survival when it does. Studies have shown that survival rates following SCD decline rapidly over time, on the order of 7% to 10% for each minute defibrillation is delayed.[100] Therefore, the AHA recommends that an automated external defibrillator (AED) be present at any school in which an emergency medical services (EMS) call-to-shock time of 5 minutes or less cannot be achieved more than 90% of the time.[101] In addition to having the requisite equipment, every school or institution sponsoring athletic activities should have an emergency action plan (EAP) that is developed in concert with local EMS personnel and reviewed annually. Appropriate education and training should be made available to all involved personnel, including coaches, families, fellow athletes, and staff. Similar recommendations from the AHA exist for health and fitness facilities, whereby drills should be practiced every 3 months.[102] The benefits of preparedness are clear. When immediate bystander cardiopulmonary resuscitation is initiated, and defibrillation occurs within 3 to 5 minutes of witnessed out-of-hospital collapse, survival rates range from 41% to 74%, which are well more than rates in the absence of such interventions.[103] Thus, schools with an AED on-site, as well as schools with an EAP, demonstrate an improved SCD survival rate compared with those lacking such resources.[104]

MEDICAL-LEGAL IMPLICATIONS

SCD is invariably devastating to a treating physician, yet it often carries legal implications. Athletes and their families have brought litigation against physicians for what was perceived to be inappropriate clearance.[105] On the other hand, athletes have also sued physicians for inappropriately restricting them from competition.[106] Unfortunately, limited by the lack of established legal precedent, most cases has been settled over the years.

Guidelines certainly provide a helpful framework to providers charged with making such decisions, but in the end, they are only a framework. Given that disease severity and risk in HCM are so highly variable, an individualized treatment plan is critical and depends on a strong doctor-patient relationship. Using the art of medicine, physicians can and should tailor recommendations to an individual patient. As in everyday practice, a physician is charged only with providing customary, accepted, or reasonable medical practice and is not liable for the morbidity or mortality caused by a previously undiagnosed condition that evaded customary medical practice.[75]

Patient autonomy, including the right of an individual to accept or refuse treatment, is maintained in the doctor-athlete relationship, so long as the individual is competent and sufficiently informed of the associated risks. However, the legal system often defers to the expertise of the treating physician in recognition of the fact that athletes are not always able to distinguish worrisome signs or symptoms from the normal physiologic stress of competing. On occasion, athletes have invoked their autonomy and signed waivers of liability. Ultimately, however, the decision of whether the waiver is honored is made by the overarching organization.[1,23,35] Thus, it is not uncommon for an athlete barred from competing in one particular circumstance to find another outlet willing to accommodate him or her.[1,107]

SHOULD HE BE ALLOWED TO PLAY? THE CASE OF NICHOLAS KNAPP

Nick Knapp dreamed of playing college basketball. When team physicians at Northwestern University declared him ineligible because of a history of HCM and recent aborted SCD for which an ICD was placed, he took them to court. Although the initial ruling was in favor of Knapp, Northwestern University subsequently won the appeal.[106] Knapp then enrolled at another Division I university that allowed him to compete despite his medical history. After a successful career spanning more than 3 years, his device appropriately fired again during a practice, and his basketball career came to an end.

FUTURE DIRECTIONS

The current understanding of HCM and its associated risk of SCD has evolved tremendously since the disease was first characterized more than 60 years ago. Furthermore, with the advent of the ICD and AED, SCD in an athlete can now often be aborted successfully. Yet the goal of eliminating SCD entirely remains, and the significant gaps in knowledge provide ample opportunities for continued exploration. Clinical trials in the HCM population are underway, including some that hope to establish the safety and benefit of moderate-intensity exercise in the form of a structured exercise training program.[108,109] So-called molecular autopsies are being performed to help identify phenotypically elusive SCD to further the understanding of SCD and improve risk stratification.[110] Moving forward, comprehensive national and international registries must also be formed to generate, organize, and curate data for analysis.

SUMMARY

Contemporary guidelines freely admit to taking a necessarily conservative stance because high-quality evidence on which to base its recommendations is lacking. Yet many patients with HCM choose to continue to compete and enjoy all of the physical and mental benefits of athletics.[66,67] Ongoing research will further refine the guidelines so that the benefits to be enjoyed by many are no longer forfeited to avoid the potential harm of a select few.

REFERENCES

1. Maron BJ, Mitten MJ, Quandt EF, et al. Competitive athletes with cardiovascular disease—the case of Nicholas Knapp. N Engl J Med 1998;339(22):1632–5.
2. Haugh D. Knapp still puts his heart into it. Chicago: Tribune; 2010.
3. Maron BJ. Hypertrophic cardiomyopathy: a systematic review. JAMA 2002; 287(10):1308–20.
4. Maron BJ. Hypertrophic cardiomyopathy: an important global disease. Am J Med 2004;116(1):63–5.
5. Olivotto I, Maron MS, Adabag AS, et al. Gender-related differences in the clinical presentation and outcome of hypertrophic cardiomyopathy. J Am Coll Cardiol 2005;46(3):480–7.
6. Maron BJ, Maron MS. Hypertrophic cardiomyopathy. Lancet 2013;381(9862): 242–55.
7. Maron BJ, Carney KP, Lever HM, et al. Relationship of race to sudden cardiac death in competitive athletes with hypertrophic cardiomyopathy. J Am Coll Cardiol 2003;41(6):974–80.
8. Maron B, Shirani J, Poliac LC, et al. Sudden death in young competitive athletes. Clinical, demographic, and pathological profiles. JAMA 1996;276(3):199–204.

9. Towbin JA. Molecular genetic basis of sudden cardiac death. Pediatr Clin North Am 2004;51(5):1229–55.
10. Sylvester J, Seidenberg P, Silvis M. The dilemma of genotype positive-phenotype negative hypertrophic cardiomyopathy. Curr Sports Med Rep 2014;13(2):94–9.
11. Maron MS, Olivotto I, Betocchi S, et al. Effect of left ventricular outflow tract obstruction on clinical outcome in hypertrophic cardiomyopathy. N Engl J Med 2003;348(4):295–303.
12. Olivotto I, Maron B, Cecchi F. Clinical significance of atrial fibrillation in hypertrophic cardiomyopathy. Curr Cardiol Rep 2001;3(2):141–6.
13. Mitchell JH, Maron BJ, Epstein SE. 16th Bethesda Conference: cardiovascular abnormalities in the athlete: recommendations regarding eligibility for competition. October 3-5, 1984. J Am Coll Cardiol 1985;6(6):1186–232.
14. Maron BJ, Mitchell JH. 26th Bethesda Conference: recommendations for determining eligibility for competition in athletes with cardiovascular abnormalities. J Am Coll Cardiol 1994;24(4):845–7.
15. Maron B, Ackerman MJ, Nishimura RA, et al. Task Force 4: HCM and other cardiomyopathies, mitral valve prolapse, myocarditis, and Marfan syndrome. J Am Coll Cardiol 2005;45(8):1340–5.
16. Maron BJ, Chaitman BR, Ackerman MJ, et al. Recommendations for physical activity and recreational sports participation for young patients with genetic cardiovascular diseases. Circulation 2004;109(22):2807–16.
17. Pelliccia A, Fagard R, Bjørnstad HH, et al. Recommendations for competitive sports participation in athletes with cardiovascular disease. A consensus document from the Study Group of Sports Cardiology of the Working Group of Cardiac Rehabilitation and Exercise Physiology and the Working Group of Myocardial and Pericardial Diseases of the European Society of Cardiology. Eur Heart J 2005;26:1422–45.
18. Pelliccia A, Corrado D, Bjørnstad HH, et al. Recommendations for participation in competitive sport and leisure-time physical activity in individuals with cardiomyopathies, myocarditis and pericarditis. Eur J Cardiovasc Prev Rehabil 2006; 13(6):876–85.
19. Pelliccia A, Zipes DP, Maron BJ. Bethesda Conference #36 and the European Society of Cardiology consensus recommendations revisited: a comparison of U.S. and European criteria for eligibility and disqualification of competitive athletes with cardiovascular abnormalities. J Am Coll Cardiol 2008;52(24):1990–6.
20. Estes NA, Link MS, Cannom D, et al. Report of the NASPE policy conference on arrhythmias and the athlete. J Cardiovasc Electrophysiol 2001;12(10):1208–19.
21. Members WC, Maron BJ, Bonow RO, et al. 2011 ACCF/AHA guideline for the diagnosis and treatment of hypertrophic cardiomyopathy: a report of the American College of Cardiology Foundation/American Heart Association Task Force on practice guidelines. Circulation 2011;124:e783–831.
22. Authors/Task Force Members, Elliott PM, Anastasakis A, et al. 2014 ESC guidelines on diagnosis and management of hypertrophic cardiomyopathy: the Task Force for the Diagnosis and Management of Hypertrophic Cardiomyopathy of the European Society of Cardiology (ESC). Eur Heart J 2014;35(39):2733–79.
23. Maron BJ, Doerer JJ, Haas TS, et al. Sudden deaths in young competitive athletes: analysis of 1866 deaths in the United States, 1980–2006. Circulation 2009; 119(8):1085–92.
24. Van Camp S, Bloor CM, Mueller FO, et al. Nontraumatic sports death in high school and college athletes. Med Sci Sports Exerc 1995;27(5):641–7.

25. Corrado D, Basso C, Rizzoli G, et al. Does sports activity enhance the risk of sudden death in adolescents and young adults? J Am Coll Cardiol 2003; 42(11):1959–63.
26. Eckart RE, Scoville SL, Campbell CL, et al. Sudden death in young adults: a 25-year review of autopsies in military recruits. Ann Intern Med 2004;141(11):829–34.
27. Meyer L, Stubbs B, Fahrenbruch C, et al. Incidence, causes, and survival trends from cardiovascular-related sudden cardiac arrest in children and young adults 0 to 35 years of age: a 30-year review. Circulation 2012;126(11):1363–72.
28. Liberthson RR. Sudden death from cardiac causes in children and young adults. N Engl J Med 1996;334(16):1039–44.
29. Day SM. Exercise in hypertrophic cardiomyopathy. J Cardiovasc Transl Res 2009;2(4):407–14.
30. Harmon KG, Asif IM, Klossner D, et al. Incidence of sudden cardiac death in National Collegiate Athletic Association athletes. Circulation 2011;123(15):1594–600.
31. Harmon KG, Drezner JA, Maleszewski JJ, et al. Pathogeneses of sudden cardiac death in National Collegiate Athletic Association athletes. Circ Arrhythm Electrophysiol 2014;7(2):198–204.
32. Maron BJ, Shen WK, Link MS, et al. Efficacy of implantable cardioverter–defibrillators for the prevention of sudden death in patients with hypertrophic cardiomyopathy. N Engl J Med 2000;342(6):365–73.
33. Cameron JS, Myerburg RJ, Wong SS, et al. Electrophysiologic consequences of chronic experimentally induced left ventricular pressure overload. J Am Coll Cardiol 1983;2(3):481–7.
34. Myerburg RJ. Scientific gaps in the prediction and prevention of sudden cardiac death. J Cardiovasc Electrophysiol 2002;13(7):709–23.
35. Maron BJ. Sudden death in young athletes. N Engl J Med 2003;349(11):1064–75.
36. Basso C, Thiene G, Corrado D, et al. Hypertrophic cardiomyopathy and sudden death in the young: pathologic evidence of myocardial ischemia. Hum Pathol 2000;31(8):988–98.
37. Maron BJ. Cardiovascular risks to young persons on the athletic field. Ann Intern Med 1998;129(5):379–86.
38. Gimeno JR, Tomé-Esteban M, Lofiego C, et al. Exercise-induced ventricular arrhythmias and risk of sudden cardiac death in patients with hypertrophic cardiomyopathy. Eur Heart J 2009;30:2599–605.
39. Maron BJ, Olivotto I, Spirito P, et al. Epidemiology of hypertrophic cardiomyopathy–related death: revisited in a large non–referral-based patient population. Circulation 2000;102(8):858–64.
40. Pelliccia F, Cianfrocca C, Pristipino C, et al. Cumulative exercise-induced left ventricular systolic and diastolic dysfunction in hypertrophic cardiomyopathy. Int J Cardiol 2007;122(1):76–8.
41. Sakata K, Ino H, Fujino N, et al. Exercise-induced systolic dysfunction in patients with non-obstructive hypertrophic cardiomyopathy and mutations in the cardiac troponin genes. Heart 2008;94(10):1282–7.
42. Ashrafian H, Watkins H. Exercise-induced ventricular dysfunction in hypertrophic cardiomyopathy: stunning by any other name? Heart 2008;94(10):1251–3.
43. Abdulla J, Nielsen JR. Is the risk of atrial fibrillation higher in athletes than in the general population? A systematic review and meta-analysis. Europace 2009; 11(9):1156–9.
44. Siontis KC, Geske JB, Ong K, et al. Atrial fibrillation in hypertrophic cardiomyopathy: prevalence, clinical correlations, and mortality in a large high-risk population. J Am Heart Assoc 2014;3:e001002.

45. Maron BJ. The paradox of exercise. N Engl J Med 2000;343(19):1409–11.
46. Thompson PD, Franklin BA, Balady GJ, et al. Exercise and acute cardiovascular events: placing the risks into perspective: a scientific statement from the American Heart Association Council on Nutrition, Physical Activity, and Metabolism and the Council on Clinical Cardiology. Circulation 2007;115(17):2358–68.
47. Office of Disease Prevention and Health Promotion 2008 physical activity guidelines for Americans. Available at: http://www.health.gov/paguidelines/guidelines/summary.aspx. Accessed December 24, 2014.
48. Physical activity and cardiovascular health. NIH consensus development panel on physical activity and cardiovascular health. JAMA 1996;276(3):241–6.
49. Fletcher GF, Balady G, Blair SN, et al. Statement on exercise: benefits and recommendations for physical activity programs for all Americans: a statement for health professionals by the Committee on Exercise and Cardiac Rehabilitation of the Council on Clinical Cardiology, American Heart Association. Circulation 1996;94(4):857–62.
50. Kokkinos P, Myers J, Kokkinos JP, et al. Exercise capacity and mortality in black and white men. Circulation 2008;117(5):614–22.
51. Morris JN, Chave SP, Adam C, et al. Vigorous exercise in leisure-time and the incidence of coronary heart-disease. Lancet 1973;301(7799):333–9.
52. Morris JN, Everitt MG, Pollard R, et al. Vigorous exercise in leisure-time: protection against coronary heart disease. Lancet 1980;316(8206):1207–10.
53. Paffenbarger RS, Hale WE. Work activity and coronary heart mortality. N Engl J Med 1975;292(11):545–50.
54. Garcia-Palmieri MR, Costas R Jr, Cruz-Vidal M, et al. Increased physical activity: a protective factor against heart attacks in Puerto Rico. Am J Cardiol 1982;50(4):749–55.
55. Albert CM, Mittleman MA, Chae CU, et al. Triggering of sudden death from cardiac causes by vigorous exertion. N Engl J Med 2000;343(19):1355–61.
56. Siscovick DS, Weiss NS, Fletcher RH, et al. The incidence of primary cardiac arrest during vigorous exercise. N Engl J Med 1984;311(14):874–7.
57. Schnohr P, O'Keefe JH, Marott JL, et al. Dose of jogging and long-term mortality: the Copenhagen City Heart Study. J Am Coll Cardiol 2015;65(5):411–9.
58. Konhilas JP, Watson PA, Maass A, et al. Exercise can prevent and reverse the severity of hypertrophic cardiomyopathy. Circ Res 2006;98(4):540–8.
59. Watson PA, Reusch JE, McCune SA, et al. Restoration of CREB function is linked to completion and stabilization of adaptive cardiac hypertrophy in response to exercise. Am J Physiol Heart Circ Physiol 2007;293:H246–59.
60. Reineck E, Rolston B, Bragg-Gresham JL, et al. Physical activity and other health behaviors in adults with hypertrophic cardiomyopathy. Am J Cardiol 2013;111(7):1034–9.
61. Flynn KE, Piña IL, Whellan DJ, et al. Effects of exercise training on health status in patients with chronic heart failure: HF-ACTION randomized controlled trial. JAMA 2009;301(14):1451–9.
62. O'Connor CM, Whellan DJ, Lee KL, et al. Efficacy and safety of exercise training in patients with chronic heart failure: HF-ACTION randomized controlled trial. JAMA 2009;301(14):1439–50.
63. van Tol BA, Huijsmans RJ, Kroon DW, et al. Effects of exercise training on cardiac performance, exercise capacity and quality of life in patients with heart failure: a meta-analysis. Eur J Heart Fail 2006;8(8):841–50.
64. Piepoli MF, Davos C, Francis DP, et al. Exercise training meta-analysis of trials in patients with chronic heart failure (ExTraMATCH). BMJ 2004;328:189.

65. McAllister DR, Motamedi AR, Hame SL, et al. Quality of life assessment in elite collegiate athletes. Am J Sports Med 2001;29(6):806–10.
66. Wilson M, Chandra N, Papadakis M, et al. Hypertrophic cardiomyopathy and ultra-endurance running - two incompatible entities? J Cardiovasc Magn Reson 2011;13(1):77.
67. Maron BJ, Klues HG. Surviving competitive athletics with hypertrophic cardio-myopathy. Am J Cardiol 1994;73(15):1098–104.
68. Priori SG, Schwartz PJ, Napolitano C, et al. Risk stratification in the long-QT syndrome. N Engl J Med 2003;348(19):1866–74.
69. Watkins H, Rosenzweig A, Hwang DS, et al. Characteristics and prognostic implications of myosin missense mutations in familial hypertrophic cardiomyopathy. N Engl J Med 1992;326(17):1108–14.
70. Ackerman MJ, VanDriest SL, Ommen SR, et al. Prevalence and age-dependence of malignant mutations in the beta-myosin heavy chain and troponin T genes in hypertrophic cardiomyopathy: a comprehensive outpatient perspective. J Am Coll Cardiol 2002;39(12):2042–8.
71. Richard P, Charron P, Carrier L, et al. Hypertrophic cardiomyopathy: distribution of disease genes, spectrum of mutations, and implications for a molecular diagnosis strategy. Circulation 2003;107(17):2227–32.
72. Van Driest SL, Ackerman MJ, Ommen SR, et al. Prevalence and severity of "benign" mutations in the β-myosin heavy chain, cardiac troponin T, and α-tropomyosin genes in hypertrophic cardiomyopathy. Circulation 2002; 106(24):3085–90.
73. Maron BJ, Pelliccia A. The heart of trained athletes: cardiac remodeling and the risks of sports, including sudden death. Circulation 2006;114(15):1633–44.
74. Rowland T. Sudden unexpected death in young athletes: reconsidering "hypertrophic cardiomyopathy". Pediatrics 2009;123(4):1217–22.
75. Maron BJ, Friedman RA, Kligfield P, et al. Assessment of the 12-lead electrocardiogram as a screening test for detection of cardiovascular disease in healthy general populations of young people (12-25 years of age): a scientific statement from the American Heart Association and the American College of Cardiology. J Am Coll Cardiol 2014;64(14):1479–514.
76. O'Mahony C, Elliott PM. Prevention of sudden cardiac death in hypertrophic cardiomyopathy. Heart 2014;100(3):254–60.
77. Elliott PM, Poloniecki J, Dickie S, et al. Sudden death in hypertrophic cardiomyopathy: identification of high risk patients. J Am Coll Cardiol 2000; 36(7):2212–8.
78. Tracy CM, Epstein AE, Darbar D, et al. 2012 ACCF/AHA/HRS focused update of the 2008 guidelines for device-based therapy of cardiac rhythm abnormalities: a report of the American College of Cardiology Foundation/American Heart Association Task Force on Practice Guidelines. J Am Coll Cardiol 2012;60(14): 1297–313.
79. Christiaans I, van Engelen K, van Langen IM, et al. Risk stratification for sudden cardiac death in hypertrophic cardiomyopathy: systematic review of clinical risk markers. Europace 2010;12:313–21.
80. Maron BJ, Spirito P. Implantable defibrillators and prevention of sudden death in hypertrophic cardiomyopathy. J Cardiovasc Electrophysiol 2008;19(10): 1118–26.
81. Maron BJ, Rowin EJ, Casey SA, et al. Risk stratification and outcome of patients with hypertrophic cardiomyopathy ≥60 years of age. Circulation 2013;127(5): 585–93.

82. Spirito P, Autore C, Formisano F, et al. Risk of sudden death and outcome in patients with hypertrophic cardiomyopathy with benign presentation and without risk factors. Am J Cardiol 2014;113(9):1550–5.
83. O'Hanlon R, Grasso A, Roughton M, et al. Prognostic significance of myocardial fibrosis in hypertrophic cardiomyopathy. J Am Coll Cardiol 2010;56(11):867–74.
84. Ommen SR, Maron BJ, Olivotto I, et al. Long-term effects of surgical septal myectomy on survival in patients with obstructive hypertrophic cardiomyopathy. J Am Coll Cardiol 2005;46(3):470–6.
85. Rothman RD, Richard D, Safiia MA, et al. Risk stratification for sudden cardiac death after septal myectomy. J Cardiol Cases 2011;3:e65–7.
86. Chaitman BR. An electrocardiogram should not be included in routine preparticipation screening of young athletes. Circulation 2007;116(22):2610–4 [discussion: 2615].
87. Bunch TJ, Chandrasekaran K, Ehrsam JE, et al. Prognostic significance of exercise induced arrhythmias and echocardiographic variables in hypertrophic cardiomyopathy. Am J Cardiol 2007;99(6):835–8.
88. Maron MS, Olivotto I, Zenovich AG, et al. Hypertrophic cardiomyopathy is predominantly a disease of left ventricular outflow tract obstruction. Circulation 2006;114(21):2232–9.
89. Shah JS, Esteban MT, Thaman R, et al. Prevalence of exercise-induced left ventricular outflow tract obstruction in symptomatic patients with non-obstructive hypertrophic cardiomyopathy. Heart 2008;94(10):1288–94.
90. Vaglio JC Jr, Ommen SR, Nishimura RA, et al. Clinical characteristics and outcomes of patients with hypertrophic cardiomyopathy with latent obstruction. Am Heart J 2008;156(2):342–7.
91. Prasad K, Williams L, Campbell R, et al. Episodic syncope in hypertrophic cardiomyopathy: evidence for inappropriate vasodilation. Heart 2008;94(10):1312–7.
92. Sadoul N, Prasad K, Elliott PM, et al. Prospective prognostic assessment of blood pressure response during exercise in patients with hypertrophic cardiomyopathy. Circulation 1997;96(9):2987–91.
93. Frenneaux MP, Counihan PJ, Caforio AL, et al. Abnormal blood pressure response during exercise in hypertrophic cardiomyopathy. Circulation 1990; 82(6):1995–2002.
94. Drinko JK, Nash PJ, Lever HM, et al. Safety of stress testing in patients with hypertrophic cardiomyopathy. Am J Cardiol 2004;93(11):1443–4.
95. Lampert R, Olshansky B, Heidbuchel H, et al. Safety of sports for athletes with implantable cardioverter-defibrillators: results of a prospective, multinational registry. Circulation 2013;127(20):2021–30.
96. Lampert R, Cannom D, Olshansky B. Safety of sports participation in patients with implantable cardioverter defibrillators: a survey of Heart Rhythm Society members. J Cardiovasc Electrophysiol 2006;17(1):11–5.
97. Baez-Escudero JL, Beshai JF, Burke MC. Use of a primary prevention totally subcutaneous defibrillator in hypertrophic cardiomyopathy. Circ Arrhythm Electrophysiol 2010;3(5):560–1.
98. Olde Nordkamp LR, Warnaars JL, Kooiman KM, et al. Which patients are not suitable for a subcutaneous ICD: incidence and predictors of failed QRS-T-wave morphology screening. J Cardiovasc Electrophysiol 2014;25(5):494–9.
99. Maron BJ, Estes NA 3rd, Maron MS, et al. Primary prevention of sudden death as a novel treatment strategy in hypertrophic cardiomyopathy. Circulation 2003; 107(23):2872–5.

100. Drezner JA, Courson RW, Roberts WO, et al. Inter-association Task Force recommendations on emergency preparedness and management of sudden cardiac arrest in high school and college athletic programs: a consensus statement. Heart Rhythm 2007;4(4):549–65.
101. Guidelines 2000 for Cardiopulmonary Resuscitation and Emergency Cardiovascular Care. Part 4: the automated external defibrillator: key link in the chain of survival. The American Heart Association in Collaboration with the International Liaison Committee on Resuscitation. Circulation 2000;102(Suppl 1):I60–76.
102. Balady GJ, Chaitman B, Driscoll D, et al. Recommendations for cardiovascular screening, staffing, and emergency policies at health/fitness facilities. Circulation 1998;97(22):2283–93.
103. Link MS, Atkins DL, Passman RS, et al. Part 6: electrical therapies: automated external defibrillators, defibrillation, cardioversion, and pacing: 2010 American Heart Association guidelines for cardiopulmonary resuscitation and emergency cardiovascular care. Circulation 2010;122(18 Suppl 3):S706–19.
104. Drezner JA, Toresdahl BG, Rao AL, et al. Outcomes from sudden cardiac arrest in US high schools: a 2-year prospective study from the National Registry for AED use in sports. Br J Sports Med 2013;47(18):1179–83.
105. Mitten MJ. Team physicians and competitive athletes: allocating legal responsibility for athletic injuries. University of Pittsburgh Law Review, 1993-1994. 55. p. 129–69.
106. Nicholas Knapp v Northwestern University. Available at: http://cehdclass.gmu.edu/jkozlows/knapp.htm. Accessed December 26, 2014.
107. CardioSource, ACCEL: Athletes with an ICD should be able to participate in sports: contemporary debates in ICD therapy.
108. University of Michigan. A randomized trial of moderate intensity exercise training in hypertrophic cardiomyopathy (RESET-HCM). ClinicalTrials.gov [Internet]. Bethesda (MD): National Library of Medicine (US); 2000. Available at: http://clinicaltrials.gov/show/NCT01127061. Accessed February 27, 2015.
109. Sheba Medical Center. Exercise training in patients with hypertrophic cardiomyopathy. ClinicalTrials.gov [Internet]. Bethesda (MD): National Library of Medicine (US); 2000. Available at: http://clinicaltrials.gov/show/NCT01518114. Accessed February 27, 2015.
110. Brown E. Clinical trial seeks answers to sudden deaths of healthy young people. Los Angeles Times 2014. Available at: http://www.latimes.com/local/california/la-me-genome-sudden-death-20141210-story.html#page=1. Accessed December 19, 2014.

Legal and Ethical Issues in the Cardiovascular Care of Elite Athletes

Michael S. Emery, MD[a,b,]*, Eric F. Quandt, JD[c]

KEYWORDS

• Cardiovascular • Athletes • Legal • Ethics

KEY POINTS

• The courts generally recognize national guidelines as good medical practice; however, they are not conclusive evidence of the medical or legal standard of care.

• Temporary restriction and referral to a specialist is prudent when the suspicion of a cardiovascular condition arises.

• The ultimate decision on return to play is at the discretion of the team physician.

• The evaluation and management of a professional athlete has several distinct differences from a collegiate or high school athlete that may alter the athlete–physician relationship.

INTRODUCTION

There continues to be growing support for more specialized cardiovascular care of competitive and elite athletes. Most of this concerns the identification of an underlying, potentially asymptomatic cardiovascular condition that could place the unsuspecting athlete at risk for sudden cardiac arrest (SCA) or sudden cardiac death (SCD). Although these are rare events in athletes ranging from approximately 0.24 to 0.7 per 100,000 athlete-years[1–3] to 1 in 44,000 per athlete-year in National Collegiate Athletic Association (NCAA) athletes,[4] they are devastating to the athlete, their family, and the local community.

There are a variety of cardiac conditions responsible for SCA/SCD in athletes. These conditions differ depending on the age of the athlete with primarily unsuspected congenital cardiac conditions predominating in young athletes[2] and ischemic heart disease in older athletes.[5] The American Heart Association (AHA) 14-point preparticipation history and physical[6] and the fourth edition of the preparticipation physical evaluation (PPE) monograph[7] are the standard in the United States for screening

[a] Sports Cardiology Program, Greenville Health System, Greenville, SC, USA; [b] Department of Medicine, University of South Carolina School of Medicine Greenville, PO Box 8795, Greenville, SC 29604, USA; [c] Scharf Banks Marmor LLC, 333 West Wacker Drive, Suite 450, Chicago, IL 60606, USA
* Corresponding author. Sports Cardiology Program, Greenville Health System, Greenville, SC.
E-mail address: docemery02@gmail.com

Clin Sports Med 34 (2015) 507–516
http://dx.doi.org/10.1016/j.csm.2015.02.004
0278-5919/15/$ – see front matter © 2015 Elsevier Inc. All rights reserved.

athletes for underlying cardiac conditions before participating in competitive athletics. Although adding an electrocardiogram (ECG) and/or an echocardiogram is controversial, it is being performed by multiple nonprofit organizations, universities, and professional leagues in the United States. Return to play for the athlete with either symptoms of potential cardiac disease, an abnormal screen (PPE and/or ECG) or with established cardiac disease have been outlined by the 36th Bethesda Guidelines,[8] which have established legal precedence.

With the increasing presence of medical professionals in the cardiovascular care of athletes, there is a rising concern about the ethical and legal implications of screening, restricting, and disqualifying athletes. Whether this is at the youth/high school, collegiate, or professional levels, a number of considerations can be made.

UNDERSTANDING LEGAL STANDARDS

Providing health care to athletes raises the potential for liabilities and may represent a different patient population than the "average" cardiology patient. There is no national standard of care in providing professional medical services to athletes; therefore, health care providers should be aware of the standard of care applicable to them in their particular state as defined by the courts in that state and under applicable regulations and statutes. Although there exist common principles among the laws of each state, differences can arise. As a general proposition, licensed physicians are held to the standard of care of possessing and applying the knowledge ordinarily used by reasonably well-qualified physicians in providing professional services under same or similar circumstances. Additionally, individuals within a profession who specialize may be held to an even higher standard of care. Thus, professional negligence by a cardiologist may be determined by the failure to do something that a reasonably careful cardiologist would do under the same or similar circumstances. However, there is latitude in the scope of what may be reasonable under any specific set of circumstances because individualized clinical judgment plays a key role. Generally, a physician's responsibility is to conform to accepted, customary, or reasonable medical practice. Courts have recognized that guidelines established by national medical associations are evidence of good medical practice; however, they are not conclusive evidence of the medical or legal standard of care. Additionally, it is important to provide sports participation recommendations both from a short- and long-term perspective, congruent with an athlete's medical best interests.

"Good Samaritan" laws are statutes designed to protect individuals from civil liability for acting negligently while providing voluntary emergency care. From state to state, Good Samaritan laws vary greatly as to the categories of people protected and circumstances in which they apply. Most states only provide immunity for persons who render care in an emergency, at the scene of an emergency, and without compensation. Voluntarily providing medical services, such as performing ECG screening programs, probably would not meet the requisite criteria. In such cases, the physician should request coverage under an insurance policy for the voluntary services rendered.

EVIDENCE OF THE STANDARD

The determination of whether there exists a deviation from the standard of care, that is, professional negligence, will be made by the trier of fact, which could be a judge, but often is determined by a jury. The jury hears the evidence and then is given specific instructions from the judge. Generally, lay juries are instructed that they must consider the expert testimony from the professional health care witnesses on the stand in making the determination of any deviation from the standard of care. In other words, such determinations are not made from their own knowledge and experiences. Hence, trials often revolve around the so-called battle of the experts. The opinions of the experts are based on their own education, knowledge, and experience in the relative field, but may also be based on published medical literature, bylaws, rules, regulations, policies, and procedures. The extent to which this evidence is adduced during trial can vary from state to state.

As an example, on the collegiate level, it is important to note the NCAA Sports Medicine Handbook.[9] As stated in the preface, "appropriate care and treatment of student-athletes must be based on the clinical judgment of the institution's team physician or athletic health care team that is consistent with sound principles of sports medicine care. These recommendations provide guidance for an institution's athletics administrators and sports medicine staff in protecting student-athletes health and safety, but do not establish any rigid requirements that must be followed in all cases." This handbook consists of "guidelines…and guidelines may constitute some evidence of the legal standard of care."

Differences may apply at alternate levels of competition with some potential variability between high school, youth athletic leagues, and even professional sports. At the high school level, the National Federation of State High School Associations publishes its own Sports Medicine Handbook.[10] The professional level is considerably more variable, not only between sports, but between individual teams within the same sport, and attention needs to be paid to those specific rules, regulations, policies, and procedures. This type of information not only might be used by the various independent expert witnesses at trial, but may also be used during the direct and cross-examination of the individual defendant physician on the witness stand.

ELITE ATHLETES VERSUS THE NORMAL PATIENT POPULATION

Consideration needs to be given to differences that may exist in providing professional medical services to an elite athlete as opposed to the "normal" patient population. In the latter population, the patient may be very willing and specific in offering details about their subjective complaints, symptoms, and so on. However, it is the desire of the elite athlete to compete—to participate in their respective sport—and they may not be as forthcoming. For example, situations may arise when attempting to take a history or elicit subjective complaints from an athlete when they may not be as willing to detail their history or complaint as a nonathletic patient. Hence, particular attention needs to be paid to the physical examination, screenings, prior medical records, or any other medical information that may raise a "red flag" in the mind of the health care professional. This care may in turn lead to making additional inquiries to understand the complete set of medical facts relied on in arriving at medical conclusions and using reasonable clinical judgment. Obviously, concerns of physician–patient confidentiality are of paramount importance; however, when necessary, careful consideration may need to be undertaken to obtain additional important factual information in consultation with appropriate professionals knowledgeable about confidentiality issues within their respective states.

Finally, providers should be aware of competing interests in situations surrounding eligibility/disqualification decisions. It is important to resist extrinsic pressure from the athlete, family members, coaching staff, administrators, alumni, and the public. All of these may impact the decision making medical process. In *Gathers v. Loyola-Marymount University*,[11] the sudden cardiac death of an elite college basketball player likely owing to an inflammatory cardiomyopathy was alleged to have been influenced by a reduction in β-blocker dosage to nontherapeutic levels to allow him to compete without medication side effects. Although the case settled before judicial resolution, it illustrates that, in addition to appropriate disqualification (temporary and/or long term), one needs to be aware of competing interests and outside pressures that may influence proper medical judgment. Although often presented with this ethical dilemma, the role of the physician and associated sports medicine staff is to provide for the athlete's best medical interests and not succumb to any conflict with regard to performance expectations or competing interests. The legal responsibility for the return-to-play decision ultimately belongs to the licensed physician.[12]

LIMITING POTENTIAL EXPOSURES

There exists no road map that can guarantee professional health care providers will not find themselves involved in a professional claim brought by an athlete. However, there are certain considerations that may assist in limiting potential exposures. Key among these is careful, complete documentation. If there is one takeaway, it should be to document, document, document! Documentation should be performed consistently during all aspects of medical care, including histories, screenings, physical examinations (noting both the relevant positives and negatives), and the basis for any diagnosis and clinical recommendations including outside materials that may have been relied on or considered (eg, review of other medical records, consensus guidelines, published literature, including any consultations with others, such as other physicians, athletic trainers, players, or family when appropriate). When a claim is brought, clear documentation forming the basis for reasonable clinical judgment is the "bread and butter" in defending against such claims.

Obtaining a patient–athlete's informed consent when necessary under the circumstances should also be well-documented and is similar to the nonathlete population. All pertinent risks and benefits of procedures need to be discussed in detail and documented. Here again, however, there is a potential difference between the elite athlete and "normal patient." The "benefit" to the elite athlete is being able to compete in their respective sport at the highest level. They are going to want to hear what they want to hear. Hence, realistic goals need to be thoroughly discussed and well-documented.

Issues involving short-term and long-term restriction need to be well-documented. Of particular importance is careful documentation of any noncompliance with restriction recommendations. It should be documented that the patient–athlete understands the importance of the recommended restrictions and the medical risks potentially attendant to noncompliance.

PREPARTICIPATION PHYSICAL EXAMINATION

In 2014, The National Athletic Trainers' Association (NATA) published a position statement outlining prudent preparticipation physical examination standards and disqualifying conditions.[13] Among other recommendations, the authors note that, "A comprehensive medical and family history should be obtained from each participant. This is the cornerstone of the PPE and should take into account the areas of greatest concern for sport participation: specifically, the American Heart Association recommendations for pre-participation cardiovascular screening of competitive athletes." Under the heading "Cardiovascular Screening" the authors note, "Specific questions regarding risk factors should be asked during the history portion of the PPE. A positive response to any question should be confirmed and further evaluation conducted if necessary." Of note, The AHA has also recently updated their position statement and expanded their recommendations from 12 to 14 elements in the preparticipation history and physical.[6] The current NCAA Sports Medicine Handbook[9] does not address in detail the information contained in the NATA position statement, nor is there anything specific from the National Federation of State High School Associations[10] on this subject.

It is important to remember that the entire standard screening examination (PPE) and any additional diagnostic assessment must be completed before signing the official medical clearance form. Additionally, when a suspicion of cardiovascular disease is raised, standard practice requires a specialty consultation.[14] It is not appropriate to allow an athlete to compete (or even practice) if further cardiovascular assessment has been flagged as part of the standard PPE. This was illustrated by the case of *Izidor v. Knight*.[15] During the PPE of a community college basketball player, abnormal findings of a heart murmur and 2 prior episodes of syncope lead to performing an echocardiogram with a subsequent diagnosis of hypertrophic cardiomyopathy (HCM). However, the sports authorization clearance form was signed before the echocardiogram and diagnosis of HCM had been completed. The athlete died 6 weeks later after playing basketball. The allegation of inadequate screening was settled, but the case underscores that adherence to screening guidelines and prudence would suggest that final medical clearance be withheld pending the results of all diagnostic evaluations.

The literature has offered differing opinions on including routine ECG (or even an echocardiogram) screening as part of the PPE. Although there are proponents of both, the legal standard by which a physician offering such services either voluntarily or at reduced cost must adhere to is not well-established.

Professional sports represent a unique paradigm in terms of cardiovascular screening compared with high school and collegiate athletes. Among those factors is the relatively small cohort (around 4000) in comparison with high schools and colleges, the fact that they are largely of adult age with complex labor contracts being compensated for their services, and that professional teams possess greater financial resources to support more comprehensive screening initiatives with noninvasive testing.[16] As such, there is little to no judicial precedent related to screening and disqualification decisions in professional athletes with medicolegal guidelines generally directed toward high school and college participants.[14]

MEDICAL DISQUALIFICATION

At the collegiate level, the NCAA Sports Medicine Handbook[9] states the following under Guideline 2A: "*Withholding a student-athlete from activity*. The team physician has the final responsibility to determine when a student-athlete is removed or withheld from participation owing to an injury, an illness or pregnancy. In addition, clearance for that individual to return to activity is solely the responsibility of the team physician or that physician's designated representative."

The sentinel case on this at the collegiate level is the United States Court of Appeals for the Seventh Circuit decision in *Knapp v. Northwestern University*.[17] Knapp, while a student–athlete, suffered a sudden cardiac death during a pick-up basketball game during his senior year of high school and was successfully resuscitated by paramedics. Knapp subsequently had a defibrillator implanted. Northwestern University committed to honor his scholarship although the head team physician declared Knapp ineligible to participate. Knapp filed suit in federal district court asserting that the university's actions violated the Rehabilitation Act. Expert witnesses testified on both sides and the trial court found in favor of Knapp. The university appealed and the United States Court of Appeals reversed the decision, holding that the student was not "disabled" and not an "otherwise qualified individual" within the meaning of the

Rehabilitation Act. The Seventh Circuit language included, "Nicholas Knapp wants to play NCAA basketball for Northwestern University – so badly that he is willing to face an increased risk of death to do so…. In this case, the severity of the potential injury is as high as it could be – death."

The federal district court reasoned that, in the face of conflicting expert opinion and evidence regarding risk, and the fact that no scientific data existed to quantify that risk, the decision on whether Knapp should play falls in the lap of the court. The Seventh Circuit in reversing stated, "[w]e disagree with the district court's legal determination that such decisions are to be made by the courts and believe instead that medical determinations of this sort are best left to team doctors and universities as long as they are made with reason and rationality and with full regard to possible and reasonable accommodations. In cases such as ours, where Northwestern has examined both Knapp and his medical records, has considered his medical history and the relation between his prior sudden cardiac death and the possibility of future occurrences, has considered the severity of the potential injury, and has rationally and reasonably reviewed consensus medical opinions or recommendations in the pertinent field – regardless whether conflicting medical opinions exist – the university has the right to determine that an individual is not otherwise medically qualified to play without violating the Rehabilitation Act. The place of the court in such cases is to make sure that the decision-maker has reasonably considered and relied upon sufficient evidence specific to the individual and the potential injury, not to determine on its own which evidence it believes is more persuasive."

With regard to the consensus medical opinions, the court went on to reference the Bethesda Conferences: "Although the Bethesda Conferences were not convened by public health officials and such guidelines should not substitute for individualized assessment of an athlete's particular physical condition, the consensus recommendations of several physicians in a certain field do carry weight and support the Northwestern team doctors' individualized assessment of Knapp." The guidelines of the 26th Bethesda Conference [current at that time], which directly addressed this clinical situation, were offered by Northwestern's experts as substantiation, "For athletes with implantable defibrillators … all moderate and high intensity sports are contraindicated."

The Seventh Circuit concluded, "[w]e do not believe that, in cases where medical experts disagree in their assessment of the extent of a real risk of serious harm or death, Congress intended that the courts – neutral arbiters but generally less skilled in medicine than the experts involved – should make the final medical decision. Instead, in the midst of conflicting expert testimony regarding the degree of serious risk of harm or death, the court's place is to ensure that the exclusion or disqualification of an individual was individualized, reasonably made, and based upon competent medical evidence. So long as these factors exist, it will be the rare case regarding participation in athletics where a court may substitute its judgment for that of the school's team physicians."

Similar to the Knapp case involving a collegiate athlete, in the case of *Larkin v. Archdiocese of Cincinnati*,[18] a federal court held that a high school could exclude an athlete with HCM from its athletic football program without violating the Rehabilitation Act. Larkin claimed that the school's adherence to unanimous cardiologists' recommendations that playing posed an unacceptable risk of sudden death owing to heart disease violated the act. The federal court rejected Larkin's contention, reasoning that Larkin's inability to satisfy an Ohio High School Athletics Association bylaw requiring a "physician certification" before athletics participation was a "substantial justification" for the school's decision and that students do not have a compelling right to participate in extracurricular activities without medical clearance.

As stated previously, consideration for participation and disqualification of a professional athlete may in fact differ from those at the high school and collegiate level. This is illustrated in the 2013 case of *Mobley v. Madison Square Garden LP*.[19] Mobley, a former National Basketball Association (NBA) basketball player who was previously diagnosed with HCM, had been cleared to play from 1999 to 2008 (subject to signing a liability waiver), but was subsequently medically disqualified by 2 cardiologists during the 2008 and 2009 season when the New York Knicks acquired him. Mobley claimed 3 other cardiologists examined him, and there had been no material change in his heart condition and was fit to play as in the prior seasons. A New York federal district court judge ruled that Mobley might have a valid state law disability discrimination claim against the New York Knicks.

This article is not intended to discuss the myriad of cases dealing with disqualification of competitive athletes, but rather to raise an awareness of pertinent issues. Additional excellent resources on this subject is the article "Medical and Legal Issues in the Cardiovascular Evaluation of Competitive Athletes", by Paterick and colleagues,[14] and the numerous publications and articles authored by Matt Mitten,[20] Professor of Law, Director of the National Sports Law Institute, Marquette University Law School. Professor Mitten's papers can be accessed on the Social Science Research Network (SSRN) at http://ssrn.com/author=586273.

WAIVERS

Because of the desire of the elite athlete to compete under some particular set of medical conditions, the issue of "waivers" may arise. Such an issue needs to be examined in consultation with professionals knowledgeable on such issues within any particular state jurisdiction. As a generality, courts tend not to look favorably on waivers when presented in defense of a claim of professional negligence.

In both the *Knapp* and *Larkin* cases, the athlete was willing to sign a waiver of future claims after complete disclosure of the medical risks of sports competition. However, there is no good legal precedent that "forces" a school to accept signed waivers in these circumstances and the legal validity of such waivers (exculpatory agreements) are questionable.

A potential exception may be between an adult, professional athlete and a team physician. Courts may view this relationship differently than the typical physician–patient relationship and could potentially uphold liability waiver in certain circumstances.[20] This was illustrated previously in the case of *Mobley v. Madison Square Garden LP*, where courts may be willing to adopt "the athlete informed consent model for professional athletes, which would enable a professional athlete to choose to participate, despite medical disqualification by the team physician, if other competent medical authority clears him or her to play."[21] However, this does not negate a physician's legal responsibility to follow good medical standards and conform to accepted, customary, or reasonable medical practice. This issue has not yet been completely resolved within the legal system.

THE SECOND OPINION

The second opinion is often part of the evaluation of an athlete and has important legal and ethical implications. This could be driven by an athlete to either confirm/refute a diagnosis and/or provide return-to-play decisions, or if they do not "like" the clinical recommendation and advice. Alternatively, a physician may recommend an athlete obtain a second opinion when they are uncomfortable with providing a diagnosis that could impact return-to-play decisions.

The assessment of and clinical decision making for athletes can be a complex issue. Understanding the sport specific cardiac adaptions that are at play in any given sport ("exercise-induced cardiac remodeling" and the "athlete's heart") and how that may overlap with certain structural and acquired heart conditions is paramount when assessing an athlete and making appropriate return-to-play decisions. We do not want to place an athlete at risk by returning them to training and competition with a potentially lethal cardiac condition, but we must also be mindful of inappropriately restricting an athlete. As such, a second opinion provided by another physician with expertise in understanding both the physiology of the "athlete's heart" as well as the pathologic substrates that create the proverbial "gray zone" may prove to be the prudent course of action.

The athlete may also drive the second opinion, often to empower themselves with a better understanding to allow them to make a more informed decision about their own medical care. With all that is at stake in making not only return-to-play decisions (scholarships, finances, professional career, etc), but also lifelong management of a potentially lethal disease, an athlete may in fact seek confirmation from a nationally recognized expert. Alternatively, an athlete may pursue a behavior more consistent with "doctor shopping," simply looking for someone (expert or not) willing to provide clearance for return-to-play.[22] Care must be taken to avoid participating in "doctor shopping" behavior by an athlete that may place the athlete at harm and increase medical costs.

When providing a second opinion, it is important to assure to the athlete that a complete and nonerroneous evaluation, diagnosis, or medical recommendation has been made from another point of view. Ensuring the athlete has all of the information explained thoroughly so that they can make an autonomous decision about proceeding with their own health care is important. A second opinion should not be used as an alternative to not providing an honest and meaningful evaluation for the athlete.[23]

A second opinion does not need to alter the clinical assessment from the primary health care provider. Just because a second opinion may disagree with the initial opinion, the first provider does not necessarily need to acquiesce to the second opinion and the initial provider is not bound by the second opinion. Rather, the second opinion presents an additional factor for consideration by the primary health care provider. The clinical judgment of the primary health care provider, considering all of the pertinent medical information, provides the basis for defending against claims of professional negligence if such judgment is consistent with accepted, reasonable medical practice. Reasonable medical decisions and clinical judgment may differ among medical practitioners yet fall within acceptable medical practice.

ENERGY DRINKS

The use of energy drinks in the youth population has been increasing rapidly. It is estimated that approximately 35% of teenagers (adolescents to college students) regularly consume energy drinks and that the "jock identity" was associated with increased consumption.[24] Pharmaceutical-grade caffeine as well as additional caffeine from natural sources can often be found in energy drinks with multiple caffeine sources tied to a higher rates of adverse effects.[25] Clinicians need to aware of potential adverse cardiovascular effects from energy drinks, including tachycardia, hypertension, obesity, and other medical problems, particularly when assessing the symptomatic athlete.

SUMMARY

The legal and ethical issues in the cardiovascular care of elite athletes continue to expand, not only with questions of screening and disqualification, but also from public pressure. It is important to recognize that SCA/SCD in an elite athlete is rare, yet they are a tragic and devastating outcome to the family and community. Remember that when the suspicion of cardiovascular disease is raised, standard practice requires specialty consultation and temporary restriction from participation is warranted. Be cognizant of competing interests and outside pressures and be clear that as the medical provider your primary responsibility is to protect the health and well-being of the athlete.

Although there is no national standard of care in providing services to athletes, the medical provider needs to understand the legal standards at play and conform to what is generally accepted, customary, or reasonable medical practice. Knowledge and documentation of adherence to national guidelines, such as the AHA PPE, 14th edition, and the 36th Bethesda Guidelines, do provide some evidence of good medical practice, but are not conclusive evidence of the medical or legal standard of care.

REFERENCES

1. Roberts WO, Stovitz SD. Incidence of sudden cardiac death in Minnesota high school athletes 1993–2012 screened with a standardized pre-participation evaluation. J Am Coll Cardiol 2013;62:1298–301.
2. Maron BJ, Doerer JJ, Haas TS, et al. Sudden deaths in young competitive athletes: analysis of 1866 deaths in the United States, 1980–2006. Circulation 2006;119:1085–92.
3. Maron B, Haas TS, Doerer JJ, et al. Comparison of U.S. and Italian experiences with sudden cardiac deaths in young competitive athletes and implications for preparticipation screening strategies. Am J Cardiol 2009;104:276–80.
4. Harmon KG, Asif IM, Klossner D, et al. Incidence of sudden cardiac death in national collegiate athletic association athletes. Circulation 2011;123:1594–600.
5. Thompson PD. The cardiovascular complications of vigorous physical activity. Arch Intern Med 1996;156:2297–302.
6. Maron BJ, Friedman RA, Kligfield P, et al. Assessment of the 12-lead electrocardiogram as a screening test for detection of cardiovascular disease in healthy general populations of young people (12–25 years of age). J Am Coll Cardiol 2014;64:1479–514.
7. American Academy of Family Physicians, American Academy of Pediatrics, American College of Sports Medicine, American Medical Society for Sports Medicine, American Orthopaedic Society for Sports Medicine, American Osteopathic Academy of Sports Medicine. In: Bernhardt DT, Roberts WO, editors. Preparticipation physical evaluation. 4th edition. Elk Grove Village (IL): American Academy of Pediatrics; 2012.
8. Maron BJ, Zipes DP. Eligibility recommendations for competitive athletes with cardiovascular abnormalities: Bethesda conference 36. J Am Coll Cardiol 2005;45:1318–73.
9. Parsons JT, editor. 2014–2015 NCAA sports medicine handbook. Indianapolis (IN): National Collegiate Athletic Association; 2014.
10. Koester MC, editor. NFHS sports medicine handbook. Indianapolis (IN): National Federation of State High School Associations; 2014.
11. Gathers v Loyola-Marymount, No. C795027 (LA Sup Ct April 20, 1990).

12. Courson R, Goldenberg M, Adams KG, et al. Inter-association consensus statement on best practices for sports medicine management for secondary schools and colleges. J Athl Train 2014;49:128–37.

13. Conley KM, Bolin DJ, Carek PJ, et al. National Athletic Trainers Association position statement: preparticipation physical examinations and disqualifying conditions. J Athl Train 2014;49:102–20.

14. Paterick TE, Paterick TJ, Fletcher GF, et al. Medical and legal issues in the cardiovascular evaluation of competitive athletes. JAMA 2005;294:3011–8.

15. Izidor v Knight, 2003 WL 21689978 (Wash App).

16. Maron BJ, Thompson PD, Ackerman MJ, et al. Recommendations and considerations related to preparticipation screening for cardiovascular abnormalities in competitive athletes: 2007 update: a scientific statement from the American Heart Association Council on nutrition, physical activity, and metabolism. Circulation 2007;115:1643–55.

17. Knapp v Northwestern University, 101 F3d 473 (7th Cir 1996).

18. Larkin v Archdiocese of Cincinnati, No. C-90–619 (SD Ohio August 31, 1990).

19. Mobley v. Madison Square Garden LP, 2013 U.S. Dist. LEXIS 46341.

20. Mitten MJ. Emerging legal issues in sports medicine: a synthesis, summary, and analysis. Saint John's Law Review 2002;76:5–86.

21. Mitten MJ. Enhanced risk of harm to one's self as justification for exclusion from athletics. Marquette Sports Law Journal 1998;8:189–223.

22. Sasone RA, Sasone LA. Doctor shopping: a phenomenon of many themes. Innov Clin Neurosci 2012;9:42–6.

23. Axon A, Hassan M, Niv Y, et al. Ethical and legal implications in seeking and providing a second medical opinion. Dig Dis 2008;26:11–7.

24. Blankson KL, Thompson AM, Ahrendt DM, et al. Energy drinks: what teenagers (and their doctors) should know. Pediatr Rev 2013;34:55–62.

25. American Heart Association. Poison control data show energy drinks and young kids don't mix. In: blog.heart.org. 2014. Available at: http://blog.heart.org/poison-control-data-show-energy-drinks-young-kids-dont-mix/. Accessed February 2, 2015.

Something Old, Something New

Using Family History and Genetic Testing to Diagnose and Manage Athletes with Inherited Cardiovascular Disease

Matthew J. Thomas, ScM, CGC[a],*, Robert W. Battle, MD[b,c,d]

KEYWORDS

- Athletes • Cardiovascular diseases/genetics • Genetic counseling
- Medical history taking • Pedigree • Genetic testing
- Genetic predisposition to disease • Sudden cardiac arrest

KEY POINTS

- Family history obtained during preparticipation screening may provide valuable information about an athlete's risk of an inherited cardiovascular disease.
- Cardiovascular genetic testing has the potential to distinguish athletes predisposed to develop life-threatening inherited cardiovascular diseases from athletes at low risk.
- As the access and use of genetic testing grow, the challenge of managing genotype-positive/phenotype-negative athletes will become more prevalent.
- Even in the absence of an abnormal genetic test result, disease-specific cardiovascular screening protocols are designed to detect disease in at-risk athletes who have concerning family histories and/or subtle clinical signs.

INTRODUCTION

Unrecognized inherited cardiovascular diseases are responsible for the majority of sudden cardiac arrest (SCA) events in young athletes during exertion.[1,2] National and

Funding Sources: University of Virginia Health System.
Conflict of Interest: None.
[a] Division of Genetics, Department of Pediatrics, University of Virginia Health System, Box 800386, Charlottesville, VA 22908, USA; [b] Division of Cardiology, Department of Medicine, University of Virginia Health System, Box 800158, Charlottesville, VA 22908, USA; [c] Division of Cardiology, Department of Pediatrics, University of Virginia Health System, Box 800386, Charlottesville, VA 22908, USA; [d] Department of Athletics, University of Virginia, Sports Medicine, McCue Center, PO Box 400834, Charlottesville, VA 22904, USA
* Corresponding author.
E-mail address: mjthomas@virginia.edu

international organizations recommend preparticipation screening for these diseases prior to competition, as the reduction of activity level may reduce the risk of life-threatening events in those deemed to be at high risk.[3–5] Although debate continues on the inclusion of certain cardiovascular screening modalities (eg electrocardiogram [EKG] or echocardiogram [TTE]), a targeted review of an athlete's history and physical examination prior to competition remain a consistent practice. Reviewing the family history may identify otherwise healthy athletes at risk for SCA simply based on the presence of disease or sudden death in one or more relatives. Genetic testing for cardiovascular disease has emerged as a valuable addition to the repertoire of cardiologists facing the decision of clearing athletes with concerning clinical signs or family histories.

For the purposes of this article, inherited cardiovascular diseases most relevant to the risk of SCA in young athletes fall within 3 overarching categories: (1) cardiomyopathies (eg, hypertrophic cardiomyopathy [HCM] or arrhythmogenic right ventricular dysplasia/cardiomyopathy [ARVD/C]), (2) primary arrhythmias (eg, long QT syndrome [LQTS], catecholaminergic polymorphic ventricular tachycardia [CPVT]), and (3) thoracic aortic diseases (eg, Marfan syndrome, familial thoracic aortic aneurysm, and dissection [FTAAD]). Recent publications offer comprehensive reviews on the clinical and genetic aspects of inherited cardiomyopathies,[6,7] primary arrhythmias,[8,9] and thoracic aortic diseases.[10,11] Rather than summarize individual inherited cardiovascular diseases pertinent to athletes, this article will address the overall approach to evaluate an athlete with an emphasis on: the role of the family history in identifying athletes at risk for SCA and scenarios in which genetic testing for inherited cardiovascular diseases may be considered in an athlete.

USING FAMILY HISTORY TO IDENTIFY ATHLETES AT RISK FOR SUDDEN DEATH

An athlete who dies suddenly and unexpectedly during activity frequently has one or more clues in his or her family history. Retrospective reviews performed following an athlete's sudden death found that between 10% and 53% of victims had a possibly related cardiovascular disease or early death in their family.[12] The autosomal-dominant pattern of inheritance of most hereditary heart diseases may explain this observation, because these disorders are often inherited from a parent and may have been present in a family for generations.[13] However, even following the most comprehensive review of an athlete's family history, certain features of inherited cardiovascular diseases preclude a clinician from easily recognizing the risk of disease, even if it truly exists in the family (**Box 1**).

Box 1
Challenging clinical features of inherited cardiovascular diseases when reviewing an athlete's family history

1. Most diseases are autosomal dominant, but some happen via new (ie, de novo) mutations that were not passed down by either parent

2. The age of disease onset may range from the perinatal period to the elderly, even within the same affected family members

3. Variable expressivity—the type of complications and disease severity often vary, even within the same affected family members

4. Reduced penetrance—patients with a genetic predisposition to disease may never develop the disease and die at an old age of unrelated complications

5. Many diseases have extended subclinical phases in which they may not be detected for years or even decades

Guidelines for Reviewing an Athlete's Family History

The American Heart Association (AHA)[14] and European Society of Cardiology (ESC)[15] dedicated elements of their preparticipation screening recommendations to the review of an athlete's family history for evidence of inherited cardiovascular disorders. Both groups recommend further clinical evaluation in athletes with a family history of (1) early sudden and unexpected death, (2) heart-related disability, or (3) specific inherited heart conditions (eg, HCM, LQTS, Marfan syndrome). Beyond these broad recommendations, additional aspects of the family history are particularly important to assess:[16,17]

- Certain circumstances at the time of a family member's death, including the drowning of a sober individual, an unexplained car accident where the relative was driving, and sudden infant death syndrome (SIDS)
- Certain signs of cardiac disease, such as unexplained seizures, recurrent syncope, syncope with exercise, and near drowning
- Medical procedures performed at a young age, including device placement (eg, implantable cardioverter defibrillator [ICD]) and heart surgery (eg, transplant, aneurysm repair)

Challenges of Obtaining a Meaningful Family History

In addition to the difficult features of inherited cardiovascular diseases (see **Box 1**), limitations of patient knowledge, a deliberate lack of truthful disclosure, and provider time constraints compromise the value of an athlete's family history. Patients have difficulty distinguishing certain cardiovascular conditions in their families (eg, myocardial infarction vs stroke), and up to 15% to 20% of patients may be unaware of what led to a sudden death or hospitalization of their closest relatives.[16,18] Furthermore, the recall of accurate family history declines when patients are asked about more distantly related but still medically relevant family like grandparents, aunts, uncles, and cousins.[18,19] Finally, the most critical aspect of the athlete's family history, premature SCA, may be incorrectly attributed to myocardial infarction, as patients commonly describe any sudden death or heart-related hospitalization as being caused by a heart attack.[20]

In practice, the family history aspect of a typical preparticipation screening evaluation relies on athletes and/or their parents filling out questionnaires. Organizations like the American Academy of Pediatrics (AAP) provide forms (eg, Preparticipation Physical Evaluation) typically asking the athlete yes-or-no questions such as "Has anyone died suddenly or unexpectedly before age 50?"[21] Rather than a few binary choice questions, systematically reviewing the family history relative by relative will likely increase the sensitivity of identifying relevant affected or deceased relatives.[22] However, documenting a 3-generation family history into a drawn pedigree takes time, which is not realistic during a preparticipation screening.

Acquiring a More Complete Family History of an Athlete

Improving the accuracy of the recorded family history while preserving limited clinician time may be possible if family members take the responsibility of gathering information from their relatives prior to the evaluation. Rather than filling out a questionnaire while sitting in an office waiting room, an athlete and/or parent may obtain much more valuable information by contacting the relatives who have the most knowledge of relevant family history. New information technologies may help facilitate this process as online family history tools allow patients to track their family histories and share them electronically with each other and their physicians (eg, My Family Health Portrait[23]).

Additional research may determine the aspects of the athlete's family history with the optimal balance of sensitivity and specificity in identifying an increased risk of SCA. One large population-based cohort study suggests that focusing on younger ages of death in the family (<35 years old) may reduce false-positives, because there is a higher likelihood that deaths closer to age 50 are attributable to multifactorial coronary artery disease rather than single-gene inherited cardiovascular disorders.[24,25]

Even the most knowledgeable patient historian makes mistakes in his or her recall or is unaware of important intricacies of family medical information. In the cardiovascular genetics clinic, family history reported by a patient is considered the starting point for additional investigation, particularly when there is a family history of sudden unexplained death.[16,17,26] As the investigation continues, clinicians work with families to retrieve medical records from those who are affected and postmortem reports from those who are deceased.

CARDIOVASCULAR GENETIC TESTING AND THE ATHLETE

Advances in technology, particularly the development of massively parallel sequencing (MPS) (also known as next-generation sequencing [NGS]), have led to discovery of and capability to test hundreds of genes associated with inherited cardiovascular diseases. As suggested by the name, MPS is a technique designed to simultaneously analyze multiple genes of interest. One of the greatest strengths of MPS is its adaptability, which allows laboratories to offer a variety of testing options: (1) disease-specific gene panels that look at anywhere from a few genes to hundreds of genes associated with a particular disorder or clinical presentation, (2) sequence all of the protein-coding genes (ie, exome sequencing), or (3) sequence the whole genome.

Multiple academic and commercial laboratories offer clinically available genetic testing panels for inherited cardiovascular diseases. The ability to find the disease-causing mutation responsible for a patient's diagnosis varies by disease (**Table 1**). For example, a patient with a clinical diagnosis of LQTS has up to an 80% chance of testing positive for a disease-causing mutation, whereas, someone with Brugada syndrome has up to 30% chance of carrying an identifiable mutation. Testing panels vary in size based on published gene–disease associations. **Tables 2–4** summarize clinically testable genes associated with inherited cardiomyopathies, primary arrhythmias, and thoracic aortic diseases, respectively.

Determining If a Gene Variant Causes Disease

Whether a laboratory analyzes a 14-gene thoracic aortic aneurysm panel or a 100-gene cardiomyopathy panel, they it often detect multiple variants in multiple genes in each analysis. After detecting differences between the normal reference sequence and the patient's sequence, careful curation and interpretation distinguish benign gene variants from those that cause or predispose to disease. The larger the gene panel, the larger the number of variants that will be detected during sequencing. Like the interpretation of other useful medical tests, the results of gene sequencing may not always be clearly positive or negative. The interpretation of gene variant traditionally occurs on a 5-tiered spectrum ranging from pathogenic (disease-causing) to benign (not disease-causing). In the middle of the spectrum rests the variant of unknown significance (VUS), which indicates the inability to determine whether a specific gene variant is benign or disease causing. Each of the 5 interpretations has different implications for the patient tested and the at-risk family members. Although the laboratory is responsible for detecting and interpreting individual gene variants, the ordering clinician has the critical role of understanding the results, explaining them to

Table 1
Likelihood of detecting a disease-causing mutation in a patient with a given cardiovascular disease

Inherited Cardiovascular Disease	Detection Rate (%)
Cardiomyopathies	
HCM with no family history	30–40
HCM with positive family history	60–70
Familial dilated cardiomyopathy	40
ARVD/C	60–65
Left ventricular noncompaction	35–40
Restrictive	35
Primary arrhythmias	
Long QT syndrome	75–80
Brugada syndrome	20–30
CPVT	60–70
Short QT syndrome	20
Thoracic aortic diseases	
Familial TAAD	23
Marfan syndrome	72–93
Ehlers-Danlos syndrome type 4	95
Early, autopsy-negative sudden death	25–35

Abbreviation: TAAD, thoracic aortic aneurysm and dissection.

the patient and family, and applying the results to the patient's management. **Table 5** demonstrates the spectrum of possible gene variants and their implications for affected patients and their at-risk family members.

The decision about how a laboratory interprets individual gene variants relies on assessing different types of evidence to determine where the variant falls on the tiered spectrum of pathogenicity (**Box 2**).[27,28] Genetic testing laboratories accumulate available evidence to determine whether each individual variant may be associated with the patient's disease or predicted to cause disease. Ideally, the laboratory will place data that support or refute the association between the variant and the disease in the laboratory report delivered to the ordering provider.

Variant interpretations are not static and may later be reclassified. One laboratory published its experience performing just under 5000 genetic tests on patients with HCM in whom 1472 gene variants were identified. Of those variants, 214 interpretations (15%) were changed.[29] Many clinical laboratories offer updates to the ordering provider if the classification has changed in a clinically relevant way. The ordering clinician may play a valuable role in reclassifying a VUS result by facilitating targeted gene variant testing in other family members to determine whether the variant segregates with disease.

Genetic Testing Scenarios for the Athlete

The healthy athlete with no concerning family history
Based on the low incidence of SCA in the athlete[1] and the low prevalence of inherited cardiovascular diseases in the general population,[30] most athletes are healthy without worrisome family histories. There are no recommendations to offer genetic testing for inherited cardiovascular diseases to these athletes. In fact, the AAP and the American

Table 2
Genes associated with inherited cardiomyopathies, other gene-specific clinical features, and inheritance patterns

Gene	Spectrum of Clinical Features						Inheritance
	HCM	DCM	ARVD/C	LVNC	RCM	Other Disorders[a]	
ABCC9		X					AD
ACTC1	X	X		X	X		AD
ACTN2	X	X					AD
ANKRD1	X	X					IU
CALR3	X						AD
CASQ2				X		CPVT	AR
CAV3	X	X				Myopathies, LQTS, hyperCKemia	AD, AR, IU
CTF1		X					IU
CTNNA3			X				AD
DES		X	X		X	Myofibrillar myopathy	AD
DMD		X				Duchenne and Becker muscular dystrophy	XL
DSC2		X	X				AD
DSG2		X	X				AD
DSP		X	X			Carvajal syndrome	AD, AR
DTNA				X			AD
EMD		X				Emery-Dreifuss muscular dystrophy	XL
GATAD1		X					AR
GLA	X[b]					Fabry disease[b]	XL
ILK		X					AD
JPH2	X						AD
JUP		X	X			Naxos disease	AD, AR
LAMA4		X					IU
LAMP2	X	X				Danon disease	XL
LDB3	X	X	X	X		Myofibrillar myopathy	AD
LMNA		X		X		Myopathies, muscular dystrophy, lipodystropy	AD
MIB1				X			AD
MYBPC3	X	X		X			AD
MYH6	X	X				CHD	AD
MYH7	X	X		X	X	Myopathies	AD
MYL2	X				X		AD
MYL3	X				X		AD
MYLK2	X						IU
MYOM1	X						AD
MYOZ2	X						AD
MYPN	X	X		X	X		AD
NEBL		X				Endocardial fibroelastosis	IU

(continued on next page)

Table 2 *(continued)*							
			Spectrum of Clinical Features				
Gene	HCM	DCM	ARVD/C	LVNC	RCM	Other Disorders[a]	Inheritance
NEXN	X	X					AD
PDLIM3	X	X					IU
PKP2		X	X				AD
PLN	X	X	X				AD
PRKAG2	X[b]					WPW, glycogen storage disease[b]	AD
RBM20		X					AD
RYR2	X		X			CPVT	AD
SCN5A		X				Brugada syndrome, LQTS	AD
TAZ		X[b]		X[b]		Barth syndrome[b]	XL
TGFB3			X				AD
TMEM43			X				AD
TMPO		X					IU
TNNC1	X	X					AD
TNNI3	X	X			X		AD
TNNT2	X	X		X	X		AD
TPM1	X	X		X	X		AD
TRIM63	X						AD
TTN	X	X	X			Myopathies	AD
TTR	X[b]	X[b]				Amyloidosis[b]	AD
VCL	X	X		X			AD

Abbreviations: AD, autosomal dominant; AR, autosomal recessive; CHD, congenital heart defect; IU, inheritance unknown; LVNC, left ventricular noncompaction; RCM, restrictive cardiomyopathy; WPW, Wolff-Parkinson-White syndrome; X, disease/gene association; XL, X-linked.
[a] Other conditions with or without cardiomyopathy associated with the given gene.
[b] Cardiomyopathy seen as part of a larger disease spectrum (disease noted).
Adapted from Teekakirikul P, Kelly MA, Rehm HL, et al. Inherited cardiomyopathies: molecular genetics and clinical genetic testing in the postgenomic era. J Mol Diagn 2013;15:160; with permission.

College of Medical Genetics and Genetics (ACMG) explicitly discourage school-based genetic testing,[31] and the American College of Preventative Medicine (ACPM) recommends against performing genetic testing for conditions that predispose to SCA in individuals without appropriate risk factors.[32]

Offering genetic testing for cardiovascular disease in low-risk athletes is fraught with challenges. Even with the increased affordability of testing due to technology advances, the yield and associated cost-effectiveness are likely to be low.[14] The diagnostic yield of genetic testing is not 100% unless a pathogenic variant has been previously identified in the family, so a negative genetic test result may offer false reassurance to an athlete. There is also the danger of misinterpreting a VUS result as being disease-causing when it may have no clinical relevance, which may lead to inappropriate disqualification, unnecessary treatment, or both.[14] Finally, in the unlikely event that a truly disease-causing mutation is found in a healthy athlete who received genetic testing without any indication, there is little to no evidence supporting his/her disqualification based solely on the genetic test result alone.

Even though performing genetic testing in healthy athletes with healthy families is not the current practice, there are some reasons to believe this may change. In the not-too-distant future, athletes may bring copies of their whole-genome sequencing results to a sports physical. These results could include variants found in heart-related genes. Since 2013, all patients undergoing clinical exome or genome sequencing for any reason in the United States are recommended to be tested for 56 genes associated with actionable medical conditions, which have been deemed incidental or secondary findings, since those conditions are most often not the primary reason for the testing.[33] Eleven of the 56 genes on the ACMG list are inherited cardiovascular disorders, all of which impact an athlete's risk of SCA. Furthermore, genome

Table 3
Genes associated with inherited primary arrhythmias, other gene-related disorders, and inheritance patterns

Gene	LQTS[a]	BrS[a]	CPVT[a]	SQTS[a]	Other Disorders[b]	Inheritance
AKAP9	LQT11					AD
ANK2	LQT4					AD
CACNA1C	LQT8	BrS3			Timothy syndrome	AD
CACNA2D1		BrS13		SQT6	Early repolarization, malignant hyperthermia	AD
CACNB2	LQT?	BrS4			Lambert-Eaton myasthenic syndrome	AD
CALM1			CPVT4		QT prolongation, epilepsy, developmental delay, osteoarthritis	AD
CASQ2			CPVT2			AR
CAV3	LQT9				HCM, DCM, myopathies, hyperCKemia, rippling muscle disease	AD
GPD1L		BrS2				AD
HCN4		BrS9			Sick sinus syndrome	AD
KCND3	LQT?	BrS12			Spinocerebellar ataxia	AD
KCNE1	LQT5				Jervell and Lange-Nielsen syndrome	AD
KCNE1L	LQT?	BrS11			AF	AD
KCNE2	LQT6	BrS?				AD
KCNE3		BrS6			Hyperkalemic periodic paralysis	AD
KCNH2	LQT2			SQT1		AD
KCNJ2				SQT3	Andersen-Tawil syndrome, familial AF	AD
KCNJ5	LQT13				Familial hyperaldosteronism	AD
KCNJ8		BrS8			Idiopathic ventricular fibrillation	AD
KCNQ1	LQT1			SQT2	Jervell and Lange-Nielsen syndrome, familial AF	AD
RANGRF		BrS10				AD
RYR2			CPVT1		ARVD/C, HCM	AD

(continued on next page)

Table 3 (continued)						
				Spectrum of Clinical Features		
Gene	LQTS[a]	BrS[a]	CPVT[a]	SQTS[a]	Other Disorders[b]	Inheritance
SCN1B		BrS5			Familial AF, cardiac conduction defect, generalized epilepsy	AD
SCN2B		BrS16			Familial AF, epilepsy	AD
SCN3B		BrS7			Familial AF	AD
SCN4B	LQT10				Familial AF	AD
SCN5A	LQT3	BrS1			DCM, familial AF, sick sinus syndrome, heart block, progressive conduction system disease	AD
SLMAP		BrS14			Muscular dystrophy	AD
SNTA1	LQT12					AD
TRDN			CPVT5		Muscle weakness	AR
TRPM4		BrS15			Progressive familial heart block	AD

Abbreviations: BrS#, Brugada syndrome type #; BrS?, Brugada syndrome type undesignated; CPVT#, catecholaminergic polymorphic ventricular tachycardia type #; CPVT, catecholaminergic polymorphic ventricular tachycardia; LQT#, Long QT type #; LQT?, long QT syndrome type undesignated; LQTS, long QT syndrome; SQT#, short QT type #; SQTS, short QT syndrome; SR, sarcoplasmic reticulum.
[a] The specific type of inherited primarily arrhythmia associated with the given gene.
[b] Other conditions with or without primary arrhythmia associated with the given gene.

and exome sequencing may now be initiated in healthy individuals as early as when they arrive in the newborn nursery. The National Institutes of Health (NIH) recently funded 4 clinical research studies offering genome and/or exome sequencing to newborns, some of whom have no medical indication.[34] Even though the prevalence of HCM has traditionally been reported as 1 case in every 500 people, as many as 3 of 500 individuals in the Framingham Heart Study (FHS) and Jackson Heart Study (JHS) cohorts from the general population tested positive for a disease-causing or likely disease-causing gene variant associated with HCM.[35,36] Therefore, any adoption of population-based genomic testing will result in genotype-first diagnoses, which pose a challenge for athletes who have no clinical evidence of the condition they are potentially predisposed to develop. This will be a complex challenge for the athletes' physicians, who need to integrate genetic test results into their care plan and make decisions about the participation.

The healthy athlete with a family history of an inherited cardiovascular disease
If an athlete reports a family history of a hereditary heart disease, a clinician should work with the athlete to obtain records to confirm the diagnosis in the affected family member(s). Obtaining relevant cardiology records will help determine whether the disease reported by the patient is accurate and the likelihood of the athlete being at risk for the disease based on the nature of its inheritance. If an athlete's family member truly has an inherited cardiovascular disease, then the affected relative is an ideal candidate for the initiation of genetic testing.

Finding a definitively disease-causing gene variant in an affected family member allows the opportunity to offer a gold standard predictive test to a healthy athlete.[37] When testing an athlete for a familial disease-causing variant, there are 2 possible genetic test results: positive and negative.

Table 4
Genes associated with inherited thoracic aortic diseases, disorder-specific features, and inheritance patterns

Gene	Disorder(s)	Select Extra-aortic Features	Inheritance
ACTA2	FTAAD	CV: PDA, coronary artery disease, premature stroke, moyomoya disease Skin: livedo reticularis Ocular: iris flocuuli	AD
COL3A1	EDS4	Tissue fragility: aterial, intestinal, or uterine rupture Skin: extensive brusing, thin/translucent skin Facial features: thin nose and lips, small chin, prominent eyes Ocular: ectopia lentis, myopia	AD
FBN1	Marfan syndrome	Skeletal: pectus deformity, scoliosis, long fingers, dolichostenomelia Other: MVP, pneumothorax, striae, dural ectasia	AD
FLNA	X-linked periventricular nodular heterotopia	Neurological: heterotopia on brain MRI, focal seizures	XL
MED12	Lujan-Fryns syndrome	Neurologial: developmental delay in males Other: characteristic facial features	XL
MYH11	FTAAD	CV: PDA	AD
MYLK	FTAAD	n/a	AD
NOTCH1	Aortic valve disease	Other: male preponderance	AD
PRKG1	FTAAD	n/a	AD
SLC2A10	Aterial tortuosity syndrome	CV: severe arterial tortuosity; stenosis of pulmonary arteries Skin: soft, doughy Other: dysmorphic features	AR
SMAD3	LDS, AOS, FTAAD	CV: arterial tortuosity, cerebral aneurysm Skeletal: osteoarthritis, pectus deformity Skin: tranluscent, easy brusing, abnormal scarring	AD
TGFB2	LDS, FTAAD	CV: arterial tortuosity, MVP	AD
TGFBR1	LDS, FTAAD	Skeletal: pectus deformity, club foot, tall stature	AD
TGFBR2	LDS, FTAAD	Other: craniofacial features, bifid uvula, cleft palate	AD

Abbreviations: AOS, aneurysms-osteoarthritis syndrome; EDS4, Ehlers-Danlos syndrome type 4; FTAAD, familial thoracic aortic aneurysm and dissection; LDS, Loeys-Dietz syndrome; MV, mitral valve; N/A, none applicable; PDA, patent ductus arteriosus; TGF, transforming growth factor; vSMC, vascular smooth muscle cell; X, disease/gene association.

Positive An asymptomatic athlete who tests positive for a familial pathogenic variant will need to undergo extensive disease-specific clinical screening. If the athlete subsequently has no clinical evidence of disease, he or she is considered genotype-positive/phenotype-negative and needs to receive ongoing surveillance based on disease-specific guidelines. The clearance of genotype-positive/phenotype-negative athlete will be reviewed.

Table 5
The spectrum of possible gene variants and their implications for affected patients and their at-risk family members

Variant Classification:	Benign	Likely Benign	Unknown Significance	Likely Pathogenic	Pathogenic
Interpretation:	Variant is not disease-causing	Variant is likely not disease-causing	Unknown whether variant is benign or disease-causing	Variant is likely disease-causing	Variant is disease- causing
Implications for affected patient:	Rely on clinical diagnosis No change in management	Rely on clinical diagnosis No change in management	Rely on clinical diagnosis Consider gene- guided investigation[a] No change in management	Diagnosis likely made or confirmed Apply genotype-phenotype correlation[b] with caution	Diagnosis made or confirmed Apply genotype-phenotype correlation[b]
Implications for at-risk family:	Continue family CV screening	Continue family CV screening	Continue family CV screening Offer segregation analysis[c]	Offer targeted testing w/some continued CV screening if (-) Offer segregation analysis[c]	Offer targeted testing If (-) low risk, no CV screening If (+) initiate surveillance and management

Abbreviations: (+), positive; (-), negative; CV, cardiovascular.

[a] Gene-guided investigation = consider clinical testing based on the variant found. For example, if a variant of unknown significance was found in a gene associated with arrhythmogenic right ventricular dysplasia/cardiomyopathy, consider a cardiac MRI and/or a signal-averaged electrocardiogram.

[b] Genotype–phenotype correlation = determine whether a specific affected gene or gene variant is associated with certain clinical features and differences in medical management.

[c] Segregation analysis = Test other affected patients in the family to determine if the variant is present in people in the family with clinical disease. Test the patient's parents to determine if the variant is *de novo*, which increases the likelihood of its pathogenicity.

Box 2
Methods laboratories use to classify a gene variant across the spectrum of disease-causing mutation to benign variants

1. Find and assess previous publications that establish a relationship between the gene variant and the disease

2. Establish segregation between the gene variant and the disease. Do people in a family who carry the gene variant develop the disease, and people who do not carry the variant remain disease-free?

3. The frequency of the variant in a large sample of the healthy general population should be very low or absent. Laboratories and clinicians can assess variant frequency using publically available databases of reportedly healthy individuals (eg, Exome Variant Server, http://evs.gs.washington.edu/EVS/)

4. Assess informatic evidence using in-silico computer models to determine how evolutionarily conserved the location of the variant is across other species and the predicted functional effect on the protein

5. Experimental support performed on affected tissues from patients with the disease or validated in-vitro animal or artificial cell models

Negative A healthy athlete who tests negative for a familial pathogenic variant did not inherit the predisposition for the disease in the family and can be considered unaffected and at population-risk of disease. This is the best-case scenario for the athlete who can now compete with the highest level of reassurance and avoid unnecessary cardiovascular surveillance and treatment.

If an athlete's family member does not pursue genetic testing or if the genetic test results are negative or inconclusive (ie, the laboratory finds a VUS), then there is no predictive or diagnostic genetic testing to offer the athlete. Therefore, the cardiologist must rely on disease-specific cardiovascular screening in the athlete. Fortunately, published recommendations and consensus statements detail specific surveillance plans for at-risk family members (**Table 6**). The screening modality (eg, EKG, TTE, or cardiac magnetic resonance [CMR]) and frequency of screening vary based on the nature of the disease and the typical age of onset.

Even though clinical cardiovascular screening offers an athlete reassurance, genetic testing in the affected family member remains the ideal approach when possible. First,

Table 6
Guidelines for the diagnosis and management of and family cardiovasclar screening recommendations for patients with inherited cardiovascular diseases

Inherited Cardiovascular Disease	United States	Europe
Cardiomyopathies (HCM, DCM, ARVD/C, LVNC, RCM)	Hershberger et al,[20] 2009	Charron et al,[38] 2010
HCM-specific	Gersh et al,[39] 2011	Elliott et al,[60] 2014
Primary arrhythmias (LQTS, Brugada, CPVT, SQTS, SCA victims)	Priori et al,[45] 2013	Priori et al,[45] 2013
Thoracic aortopathies (Marfan, FTAAD, LDS, EDS4)	Hiratzka et al,[64] 2010	Erbel et al,[62] 2014
Marfan-specific	Tinkle et al,[40] 2013	N/A

Abbreviations: EDS4, Ehlers-Danlos syndrome type 4; LDS, Loeys-Dietz syndrome; LVNC, left ventricular noncompaction; n/a, none applicable; N/A, none available; RCM, restrictive cardiomyopathy.

clinical screening may be an unnecessary use of resources for an athlete who did not inherit the predisposition to the heart disease in the family. Evidence suggests genetic testing is cost-effective versus clinical screening for conditions like HCM.[41,42] Second, if the athlete truly did inherit a yet-to-be-identified disease-causing mutation, then a normal cardiovascular screen does not eliminate the athlete's risk of disease based on the often delayed age of onset of some inherited diseases. Finally, the first sign of an inherited cardiovascular disease may be SCA, even in an athlete with no clinical features on cardiovascular examination.[43,44]

The asymptomatic athlete with a positive family history of sudden death
Even if the athlete's first-degree relative is deceased, the option of genetic testing may be possible if care was taken to store a sample from the deceased relative. The option of postmortem genetic testing will be summarized in greater detail, but this is traditionally not available to an athlete's family unless the death occurred recently or unless the specific medical examiner's office preserved proper samples for an extended period of time.

For most athletes who have family history of sudden death, a cardiologist must rely on clinical cardiovascular screening. The Heart Rhythm Society and the ESC developed an algorithm for the clinical workup of an otherwise healthy individual who has lost a family member to a premature sudden and unexplained death.[45] First, a high-quality autopsy may distinguish deaths that occurred due inherited disease from those that were unlikely to be familial (eg, anomalous coronary, myocarditis). The quality of postmortem examination varies dramatically across the developed world, which is evidenced by the frequency of a nondiagnostic autopsy in cases of sudden death in the young, which ranges from as low 3% to as high as 53%.[46] If the autopsy is normal, and the death in the family remains unexplained, the initial evaluation in first-degree relatives of the deceased should include a detailed medical and family history including a pedigree, a physical examination, resting EKG, exercise EKG, and a TTE. This level of evaluation is recommended, because a clinical diagnosis of an inherited disease is made in up to one-third of the surviving relatives of a victim of sudden unexplained death.[47] Although preliminary evidence suggests that 1 comprehensive cardiovascular evaluation by an expert inherited cardiovascular disease center offers a great amount of reassurance for surviving family members,[48] some level of follow-up is required due to the reduced penetrance and variable expressivity of inherited cardiovascular diseases.

The genotype-positive/phenotype-negative athlete
The decision to restrict athletes who carry disease-causing gene mutations without any clinical evidence of disease varies dramatically by condition and provider. The difficult nature of this decision is demonstrated in the dramatic difference of opinion between the United States' 36th Bethesda Conference[3] and ESC (**Table 7**).[4] With few exceptions, the US group opted to not restrict clinically healthy athletes due to a lack of compelling evidence, whereas the European group reviewed the same data and came to far more conservative conclusions.

The dilemma of clearing athletes with disease-causing or likely disease-causing gene variants who are otherwise healthy has been discussed in detail.[49–52] Richard and colleagues[50] suggest taking a case-by-case approach based upon the following factors: (1) the specific gene mutation identified, (2) the athlete's family history of sudden and early death, (3) the sport under consideration, and (4) the presence of risk factors detected in the clinical evaluation of the athlete. The practice of 1 high-volume HCM clinic is to engage athletes and their families in a transparent

Table 7
Guidelines for competitive sports participation of genotype-positive/phenotype-negative athletes

Condition	36th Bethesda Conference	European Society of Cardiology
Cardiomyopathies (HCM, DCM, ARVD/C)	No restriction	No competitive sports, only noncompetitive & leisure activities permitted
LQTS	No restriction, except LQT1 & swimming	No competitive sports, only noncompetitive & leisure activities permitted
CPVT	No restriction	No competitive sports
Brugada syndrome	No restriction	No restriction
Marfan syndrome	Only low-to-moderate allowed without aortic dilatation, moderate-to-severe mitral regurgitation or family history of aortic dissection or sudden death	No competitive sports

Abbreviation: LQT1, long QT syndrome type 1.

conversation about what is known and largely unknown about the risk of SCA while keeping the discussion grounded in patient autonomy.[51] Ultimately, the conversation depends on the athlete and his or her family's comfort level with an uncertain, but likely low-level risk or risk framed within the importance of the sport to the athlete.

Some empiric evidence regarding the safety of genotype-positive/phenotype-negative athletes has been provided by cardiovascular genetics programs. A group of 67 of 70 genotype-positive/phenotype-negative athletes with LQTS was followed for an average of 5.1 years, and none experienced a sport-related event.[53] No adverse events were observed in 2 groups of genotype-positive/phenotype-negative patients at risk for HCM with low conversion-to-disease rates of 0% for 32 patients over an average 4 years of follow-up and 6% for 36 patients over 12 years.[54,55] Unfortunately, there is a paucity of this type of valuable evidence for other inherited cardiovascular diseases. As the frequency of these difficult clinical scenarios grows due to increased access and use of genetic testing, this gap in knowledge becomes even more critical to fill.

It is important to emphasize the role advanced clinical screening may play in distinguishing a truly phenotype-negative athlete from one with subtle evidence of disease. For example, CMR may detect abnormal morphology (eg, myocardial crypts, elongated mitral valve leaflets, fibrosis, diastolic dysfunction) in genotype-positive HCM patients with no left-ventricular hypertrophy.[56–58] For LQTS and other primary arrhythmias, exercise or drug challenge testing may have greater sensitivity in identifying affected individuals than resting EKGs alone.[45]

The athlete with borderline clinical evidence of disease

The effects of cardiovascular remodeling associated with intense training may mimic the appearance of known inherited cardiovascular diseases (eg, HCM, dilated cardiomyopathy [DCM], and ARVD/C).[59] Therefore, an athlete who undergoes a screening EKG, TTE, or other clinical test may have potentially false-positive results due to extensive training rather than an inherited disease. An added benefit of genetic testing for these athletes is the potential to identify inherited cardiovascular disease when the clinical diagnosis is uncertain.[37] In these scenarios, genetic testing may provide an independent line of evidence that a cardiologist can use to assess the athlete's likelihood of having an inherited heart disease. For example, an elite basketball player with borderline left ventricular hypertrophy who undergoes genetic testing and is found to carry an established disease-causing variant in a sarcomere protein gene will have a high level of suspicion of being affected by HCM.[60] Similarly, a competitive swimmer with borderline QT prolongation who tests positive for a definitive potassium channel gene variant would subsequently receive the diagnosis of LQTS.[45] Although the decision to restrict these athletes from competition may not be as clear as it is for the symptomatic athlete with obvious evidence on imaging, the cardiologist at least has all of the available data to discuss the management plan with the athlete and his or her family.

The current sensitivity of genetic testing for inherited cardiovascular disorders is not 100% (see **Table 3**), so a negative result in a patient with possible/borderline disease does not rule out an inherited disorder. Therefore, in situations in which a patient has a borderline phenotype and a negative or inconclusive genetic test result, continued clinical surveillance is necessary. This is another scenario in which clinical screening of the athlete's family members may provide valuable information. If the athlete's blood relatives do not have evidence of disease, this offers some reassurance. If a relative has obvious disease or history of sudden death, then this may suggest the athlete is in the early stages of being affected.

The athlete with a clinical diagnosis of an inherited cardiovascular disease

After an athlete receives a clinical diagnosis of an inherited cardiovascular disorder, guidelines and consensus statements generally recommend offering genetic testing.[61,62] The major justification for performing genetic testing in an athlete who has already received a clinical diagnosis is for the benefit of the at-risk family members, many of whom may also participate in sports that place them at risk.

Even though the ability to predict disease onset and severity based on genetic test results (ie, genotype–phenotype correlation) is not high for most conditions, there are there are some situations in which the results of genetic testing can be used to directly modify medical management:

- Cardiomyopathies. Genetic testing can distinguish isolated cardiomyopathies from disorders that cause disease beyond the heart. For example, a patient with left ventricular hypertrophy due to Fabry disease is at risk for other medical complications (eg, kidney disease), and enzyme replacement therapy is clinically available.[63] Mutations in the LMNA gene are associated with familial DCM that predisposes to a high risk of conductive defects and arrhythmia, so pacemaker and ICD placement may be indicated sooner than for traditional DCM patients.[20]
- Primary arrhythmias. Genetic testing can determine the subtype of LQTS, which helps identify triggering events and stratify the risk of SCA.[45,61]
- Thoracic aortic diseases. Patients with diseases of the aorta may be candidates for earlier prophylactic aortic root repair based on the mutation identified, as the presence of some gene mutations predispose to dissection at smaller sizes (eg, aortic root repair recommended at a diameter of $\geq$4.2 cm for TGFBR1/2 mutation carriers).[64] Some gene mutations, such those in ACTA2, predispose to vascular disease beyond the aorta, so additional surveillance from the head to the pelvis is recommended.[62]

Fortunately, ongoing clinical research is attempting to identify treatments for a variety of inherited cardiovascular diseases. Some researchers investigate the utility of widely available and US Food and Drug Administration (FDA) approved medications (eg, Marfan syndrome and losartan,[65] HCM and diltiazem[66]), while others are developing novel therapeutics, such as small molecules designed to mitigate the effect of specific disease-causing mutations for patients with hypertrophic and dilated cardiomyopaties.[67]

After the sudden cardiac arrest of an athlete

If an athlete experiences an SCA, measures must be taken to protect the surviving family members and the athlete who is fortunate enough to survive. Genetic testing performed on an SCA survivor or victim of a sudden and unexplained death has a diagnostic yield up to 30%.[47,68] If the cause of death is identified on autopsy (eg, HCM), then the yield of testing is expected to be higher.[68]

The National Association of Medical Examiners (NAME) recommends saving blood samples from the victims of sudden and unexpected deaths who are less than 40 years old for the purpose of potential genetic testing and DNA banking for future genetic testing.[69] If a sample is properly stored, genetic testing panels can be performed based on the diagnosis at autopsy or if the cause of death is unexplained.

If a mutation is identified in the decedent or the athlete surviving SCA, then familial mutation testing can be performed in the surviving family to determine who is at risk. For these reasons, multiple international consensus statements recommend offering post-SCA genetic testing as an option to the affected and the surviving family members.[45,61]

Ethical, Legal, Social, and Financial Implications of Genetic Testing in Athletes

Access to genetic testing has improved dramatically over the last 10 years for a variety of reasons. Clinical genetic testing has become more affordable for the average patient with a personal or family history of inherited cardiovascular conditions. The adoption and advancement of MPS have dramatically reduced the per-gene cost of sequencing. Subsequently, the marketplace of genetic testing laboratories has grown significantly. In 2003, there was 1 laboratory offering clinical genetic testing for HCM in the United States,[70] and there are now 17 laboratories according to the NIH Genetic Testing Registry (www.ncbi.nlm.nih.gov/gtr/). Competition between genetic testing laboratories has created patient-friendly billing policies that commonly limit the patient's out-of-pocket expense to $100 for many cardiovascular-related genetic testing panels.[70] Fortunately, clinicians and testing laboratories can make far more compelling arguments to insurers regarding the cost-effectiveness of genetic testing versus repeated clinical screening of at-risk family members and improvements in medical management.[41,42,61]

The Genetic Information and Nondiscrimination Act (GINA) of 2008 prevents healthy individuals from being discriminated by their health insurance company and employers based on genetic test results and family history. There are some exceptions to this law (eg, the military), and GINA does not protect patients from discrimination from life, disability, and long-term care insurance coverage. Only a few states (eg, California) offer protections for these types of insurance.

After a disease or disease-predisposing mutation has been identified in an athlete, and his or her care has been modified, the clinician's next responsibility is to educate the athlete about the risk of disease to other family members. In some scenarios, relationships among family members may be strained, and there may not be a willingness to share potentially life-saving information with relatives. This scenario, commonly referred to as the clinician's duty to warn, is a common ethical dilemma in genetics practice.[71] The clinician's ethical and legal obligations to respect his or her patient's privacy conflict with the possible harm an un-notified and subsequently untreated relative may experience. The consensus from most experts is to hold patient privacy paramount (and respect laws like Health Insurance Portability and Accountability Act of 1996), while encouraging patients to share relevant health information with their families and providing them with an effective means of doing so.[72] Merely providing written letters for a diagnosed patient to share with his or her at-risk family has proven to be successful in a variety of cardiology settings, leading to the identification of asymptomatic patients who have underlying and treatable disease.[73,74]

SUMMARY

Genetic testing for inherited cardiovascular diseases has emerged as a valuable resource in the medical evaluation of athletes at increased risk for SCA. Genetic testing has the potential to offer an athlete reassurance, confirm a diagnosis in those with borderline clinical features, or identify disease predisposition prior to the onset of clinical signs. Obtaining a comprehensive family history is essential to properly interpreting genetic test results and applying them to an athlete's management. Based on the complexity of ordering appropriate genetic tests and the potentially life-altering implications of the results, referrals to cardiovascular genetics clinics should be considered in athletes who are at risk based on personal or family history. These clinics provide team-based, multidisciplinary care that includes cardiologists, nurses, medical geneticists, genetic counselors, and other specialists dedicated to the care of patients with inherited cardiovascular diseases and their families.

REFERENCES

1. Harmon KG, Drezner JA, Wilson MG, et al. Incidence of sudden cardiac death in athletes: a state-of-the-art review. Heart 2014;100:1227–34.
2. Vaartjes I, Hendrix A, Hertogh EM, et al. Sudden death in persons younger than 40 years of age: incidence and causes. Eur J Cardiovasc Prev Rehabil 2009;16:592–6.
3. Maron B, Zipes D. 36th Bethesda Conference eligibility recommendations for competitive athletes with cardiovascular abnormalities. J Am Coll Cardiol 2005; 45:1312.
4. Pelliccia A, Fagard R, Bjørnstad HH, et al. Recommendations for competitive sports participation in athletes with cardiovascular disease. Eur Heart J 2005; 26:1422–45.
5. Ljungqvist A, Jenoure P, Engebretsen L, et al. The International Olympic Committee (IOC) consensus statement on periodic health evaluation of elite athletes. Br J Sports Med 2009;2009(43):631–43.
6. Sturm AC. Genetic testing in the contemporary diagnosis of cardiomyopathy. Curr Heart Fail Rep 2013;10:63–72.
7. Teekakirikul P, Kelly MA, Rehm HL, et al. Inherited cardiomyopathies: molecular genetics and clinical genetic testing in the postgenomic era. J Mol Diagn 2013; 15:158–70.
8. Webster G, Berul CI. An update on channelopathies from mechanisms to management. Circulation 2013;127:126–40.
9. Schwartz PJ, Ackerman MJ, George AL Jr, et al. Impact of genetics on the clinical management of channelopathies. J Am Coll Cardiol 2013;62:169–80.
10. Pyeritz R. Heritable thoracic aortic disorders. Curr Opin Cardiol 2014;2014(29): 97–102.
11. Pomianowski P, Elefteriades JA. The genetics and genomics of thoracic aortic disease. Ann Cardiothorac Surg 2013;2:271–9.

12. Campbell RM, Berger S, Drezner J. Sudden cardiac arrest in children and young athletes: the importance of a detailed personal and family history in the pre-participation evaluation. Br J Sports Med 2009;43:336–41.
13. Lebo MS, Baxter SM. New molecular genetic tests in the diagnosis of heart disease. Clin Lab Med 2014;34:137–56.
14. Maron BJ, Thompson PD, Ackerman MJ, et al. Recommendations and considerations related to preparticipation screening for cardiovascular abnormalities in competitive athletes: 2007 update. Circulation 2007;115:1643–55.
15. Corrado D, Pelliccia A, Bjørnstad HH, et al. Cardiovascular pre-participation screening of young competitive athletes for prevention of sudden death: proposal for a common European protocol. Eur Heart J 2005;26:516–24.
16. Dunn KE, Caleshu C, Cirino AL, et al. A clinical approach to inherited hypertrophy the use of family history in diagnosis, risk assessment, and management. Circ Cardiovasc Genet 2013;6:118–31.
17. Morales A, Cowan J, Dagua J, et al. Family history: an essential tool for cardiovascular genetic medicine. Congest Heart Fail 2008;14:37–45.
18. Facio FM, Feero WG, Linn A, et al. Validation of my family health portrait for six common heritable conditions. Genet Med 2010;12:370–5.
19. Hastrup JL, Hotchkiss AP, Johnson CA. Accuracy of knowledge of family history of cardiovascular disorders. Health Psychol 1985;4:291–306.
20. Hershberger RE, Lindenfeld J, Mestroni L, et al. Genetic evaluation of cardiomyopathy—a Heart Failure Society of America Practice Guideline. J Card Fail 2009; 15:83–97.
21. Bernhardt DT, Roberts WO. PPE: preparticipation physical evaluation. Elk Grove Village, IL: American Academy of Pediatrics; 2010.
22. Bennett RL. Practical guide to the genetic family history. 2nd edition. Hoboken (NJ): Wiley-Blackwell; 2010.
23. Health and Human Services. My family health portrait 2005. Available at: https://familyhistory.hhs.gov/. Accessed December 12, 2014.
24. Ranthe MF, Winkel BG, Andersen EW, et al. Risk of cardiovascular disease in family members of young sudden cardiac death victims. Eur Heart J 2013;34: 503–11.
25. Asif IM, Drezner JA. Detecting occult cardiac disease in athletes: history that makes a difference. Br J Sports Med 2013;47:669.
26. Miller EM, Hinton RB. A pediatric approach to family history of cardiovascular disease: diagnosis, risk assessment, and management. Pediatr Clin North Am 2014; 61:187–205.
27. Richards CS, Bale S, Bellissimo DB, et al. ACMG recommendations for standards for interpretation and reporting of sequence variations: revisions 2007. Genet Med 2008;10:294–300.
28. MacArthur DG, Manolio TA, Dimmock DP, et al. Guidelines for investigating causality of sequence variants in human disease. Nature 2014;508:469–76.
29. Aronson SJ, Clark EH, Varugheese M, et al. Communicating new knowledge on previously reported genetic variants. Genet Med 2012;14:713–9.
30. Burton H, Alberg C, Stewart A. PHG Foundation | Heart to Heart: inherited cardiovascular conditions services 2009. Available at: http://www.phgfoundation.org/reports/4986/. Accessed October 3, 2013.
31. Ross LF, Saal HM, David KL, et al, American Academy of Pediatrics, American College of Medical Genetics and Genomics. Technical report: ethical and policy issues in genetic testing and screening of children. Genet Med 2013;15: 234–45.

32. Mahmood S, Lim L, Akram Y, et al. Screening for sudden cardiac death before participation in high school and collegiate sports: American college of preventive medicine position statement on preventive practice. Am J Prev Med 2013;45: 130–3.
33. Green RC, Berg JS, Grody WW, et al. ACMG recommendations for reporting of incidental findings in clinical exome and genome sequencing. Genet Med 2013;15:565–74.
34. National Institutes of Health. NIH program explores the use of genomic sequencing in newborn healthcare 2013. Available at: http://www.nih.gov/news/health/sep2013/nhgri-04.htm. Accessed November 23, 2014.
35. Maron BJ, Gardin JM, Flack JM, et al. Prevalence of hypertrophic cardiomyopathy in a general population of young adults echocardiographic analysis of 4111 subjects in the CARDIA study. Circulation 1995;92:785–9.
36. Bick AG, Flannick J, Ito K, et al. Burden of rare sarcomere gene variants in the Framingham and Jackson heart study cohorts. Am J Hum Genet 2012;91:513–9.
37. Landstrom AP, Tester DJ, Ackerman MJ. Role of genetic testing for sudden death predisposing heart conditions in athletes. In: Lawless CE, editor. Sports cardiology essentials. New York: Springer; 2011. p. 85–100.
38. Charron P, Arad M, Arbustini E, et al. Genetic counselling and testing in cardiomyopathies: a position statement of the European Society of Cardiology Working Group on Myocardial and Pericardial Diseases. Eur Heart J 2010;31:2715–26.
39. Gersh BJ, Maron BJ, Bonow RO, et al. ACCF/AHA guideline for the diagnosis and treatment of hypertrophic cardiomyopathy: a report of the American College of Cardiology Foundation/American Heart Association Task Force on Practice Guidelines. Circulation 2011;124:e783–831.
40. Tinkle BT, Saal HM, The Committee on Genetics. Health Supervision for Children With Marfan Syndrome. Pediatrics 2013;132:e1059–72.
41. Ingles J, McGaughran J, Scuffham PA, et al. A cost-effectiveness model of genetic testing for the evaluation of families with hypertrophic cardiomyopathy. Heart 2012;98:625–30.
42. Wordsworth S, Leal J, Blair E, et al. DNA testing for hypertrophic cardiomyopathy: a cost-effectiveness model. Eur Heart J 2010;31:926–35.
43. Christiaans I, Lekanne dit Deprez RH, van Langen IM, et al. Ventricular fibrillation in MYH7-related hypertrophic cardiomyopathy before onset of ventricular hypertrophy. Heart Rhythm 2009;6:1366–9.
44. Mellor G, Raju H, de Noronha SV, et al. Clinical characteristics and circumstances of death in the sudden arrhythmic death syndrome. Circ Arrhythm Electrophysiol 2014;7:1078–83.
45. Priori SG, Wilde AA, Horie M, et al. HRS/EHRA/APHRS expert consensus statement on the diagnosis and management of patients with inherited primary arrhythmia syndromes expert consensus statement on inherited primary arrhythmia syndromes. Heart Rhythm 2013;10:e75–106.
46. Tester DJ, Ackerman MJ. The molecular autopsy: should the evaluation continue after the funeral? Pediatr Cardiol 2012;33:461–70.
47. Raju H, Behr ER. Unexplained sudden death, focussing on genetics and family phenotyping. Curr Opin Cardiol 2013;28:19–25.
48. Van der Werf C, Stiekema L, Tan HL, et al. Low rate of cardiac events in first-degree relatives of diagnosis-negative young sudden unexplained death syndrome victims during follow-up. Heart Rhythm 2014;11:1728–32.
49. Sylvester J, Seidenberg P, Silvis M. The dilemma of genotype positive-phenotype negative hypertrophic cardiomyopathy. Curr Sports Med Rep 2014;13(2):94–9.

50. Richard P, Denjoy I, Fressart V, et al. Advising a cardiac disease gene positive yet phenotype negative or borderline abnormal athlete: is sporting disqualification really necessary? Br J Sports Med 2012;46:i59–68.
51. Maron BJ, Yeates L, Semsarian C. Clinical challenges of genotype positive (+)–phenotype negative (−) family members in hypertrophic cardiomyopathy. Am J Cardiol 2011;107:604–8.
52. Sweeting J, Ingles J, Ball K, et al. Challenges of exercise recommendations and sports participation in genetic heart disease patients. Circ Cardiovasc Genet 2015;8(1):178–86.
53. Gray B, Ingles J, Semsarian C. Natural history of genotype positive–phenotype negative patient with hypertrophic cardiomyopathy. Int J Cardiol 2011;152(2):258–9.
54. Jensen MK, Havndrup O, Christiansen M, et al. Penetrance of hypertrophic cardiomyopathy in children and adolescents a 12-year follow-up study of clinical screening and predictive genetic testing. Circulation 2013;127(1):48–54.
55. Johnson JN, Ackerman MJ. Return to play? Athletes with congenital long QT syndrome. Br J Sports Med 2013;47:28–33.
56. Strijack B, Ariyarajah V, Soni R, et al. Late gadolinium enhancement cardiovascular magnetic resonance in genotyped hypertrophic cardiomyopathy with normal phenotype. J Cardiovasc Magn Reson 2008;10:58.
57. Rowin EJ, Maron MS, Lesser JR, et al. CMR with late gadolinium enhancement in genotype positive–phenotype negative hypertrophic cardiomyopathy. JACC Cardiovasc Imaging 2012;5:119–22.
58. Captur G, Lopes LR, Mohun TJ, et al. Prediction of sarcomere mutations in subclinical hypertrophic cardiomyopathy. Circ Cardiovasc Imaging 2014;7:863–71.
59. Battle RW, Mistry DJ, Malhotra R, et al. Cardiovascular screening and the elite athlete: advances, concepts, controversies, and a view of the future. Clin Sports Med 2011;30:503–24.
60. Elliott PM, Anastasakis A, Borger MA, et al. 2014 ESC guidelines on diagnosis and management of hypertrophic cardiomyopathy. Eur Heart J 2014;14:ehu284.
61. Ackerman MJ, Priori SG, Willems S, et al. HRS/EHRA expert consensus statement on the state of genetic testing for the channelopathies and cardiomyopathies. Heart Rhythm 2011;8:1308–39.
62. Erbel R, Aboyans V, Boileau C, et al. 2014 ESC guidelines on the diagnosis and treatment of aortic diseases document covering acute and chronic aortic diseases of the thoracic and abdominal aorta of the adult. Eur Heart J 2014; 35(41):2873–926.
63. Palecek T, Honzikova J, Poupetova H, et al. Prevalence of Fabry disease in male patients with unexplained left ventricular hypertrophy in primary cardiology practice: prospective Fabry cardiomyopathy screening study (FACSS). J Inherit Metab Dis 2014;37:455–60.
64. Hiratzka LF, Bakris GL, Beckman JA, et al. 2010 ACCF/AHA/AATS/ACR/ASA/ SCA/SCAI/SIR/STS/SVM guidelines for the diagnosis and management of patients with thoracic aortic disease. J Am Coll Cardiol 2010;55:e27–129.
65. Lacro RV, Dietz HC, Sleeper LA, et al. Atenolol versus Losartan in children and young adults with Marfan's syndrome. N Engl J Med 2014;371:2061–71.
66. Ho CY, Lakdawala NK, Cirino AL, et al. Diltiazem treatment for pre-clinical hypertrophic cardiomyopathy sarcomere mutation carriers: a pilot randomized trial to modify disease expression. JACC Heart Fail 2015;3(2):180–8.
67. Spudich JA. Hypertrophic and dilated cardiomyopathy: four decades of basic research on muscle lead to potential therapeutic approaches to these devastating genetic diseases. Biophys J 2014;106:1236–49.

68. Hertz CL, Ferrero-Miliani L, Frank-Hansen R, et al. A comparison of genetic findings in sudden cardiac death victims and cardiac patients: the importance of phenotypic classification. Europace 2015;17(3):350–7.
69. Middleton O, Baxter S, Demo E, et al. NAME position paper: retaining postmortem samples for genetic testing. Acad Forensic Pathol 2013;3:191–4.
70. Maron BJ, Maron MS, Semsarian C. Genetics of hypertrophic cardiomyopathy after 20 years: clinical perspectives. J Am Coll Cardiol 2012;60:705–15.
71. Godard B, Hurlimann T, Letendre M, et al. Guidelines for disclosing genetic information to family members: from development to use. Fam Cancer 2006;5:103–16.
72. Offit K, Groeger E, Turner S, et al. The "duty to warn" a patient's family members about hereditary disease risks. JAMA 2004;292:1469–73.
73. Miller EM, Wang Y, Ware SM. Uptake of cardiac screening and genetic testing among hypertrophic and dilated cardiomyopathy families. J Genet Couns 2012;22:258–67.
74. Van der Roest WP, Pennings JM, Bakker M, et al. Family letters are an effective way to inform relatives about inherited cardiac disease. Am J Med Genet A 2009;149A:357–63.

How to Practice Sports Cardiology

A Cardiology Perspective

Christine E. Lawless, MD, MBA[a,b],*

KEYWORDS

- Athlete • Cardiac adaptation • Sports medicine • Sudden cardiac death
- Sports cardiology • Cardiac testing

KEY POINTS

- Sports cardiology is a quintessential "patient-centered" discipline.
- Athletes are unique cardiovascular (CV) patients, distinct from the general population from physiologic and medical perspectives.
- Multiple athlete "gray zones" exist, beyond the usual echocardiographic chamber size and wall thickness.
- There exist overlaps between sports cardiology care rendered by a primary care sports physician and a sports cardiologist. Each provider must recognize their unique roles in athlete CV care, and be mindful of the boundaries of their scope of practice.
- Systematic approach to evaluation of athletes is recommended, taking into consideration sports-specific CV demands, CV adaptations and their appearance on cardiac testing, any existing or potential interaction of the heart with the internal and external sports environment, CV risks, and prevalence of use of performance-enhancing agents and rules for drug testing.

INTRODUCTION

When the legendary courier Pheidippides (530–490 BC) collapsed and died after running 25 miles from Marathon to Athens to announce a Greek victory over Persia,[1] bystanders were unaware they had witnessed the first recorded incident of exercise-associated sudden cardiac death (SCD). Clinician fascination with such events began that day, and persists to this day. Thus, it can be said that the practice of sports cardiology began with that first collapse. However, it has not been until the past 10 to 15 years that sports cardiology has come into its own as a discipline. Recently, the

a Sports Cardiology Consultants LLC, 360 West Illinois Street, #7D, Chicago, IL 60654, USA;
b Department of Nutrition and Health Sciences, University of Nebraska, Lincoln, 110 Ruth Leverton Hall, Lincoln, NE 68583-0806, USA
* Sports Cardiology Consultants LLC, 360 West Illinois Street, #7D, Chicago, IL 60654.
E-mail address: drlawless1221@gmail.com

Clin Sports Med 34 (2015) 539–549
http://dx.doi.org/10.1016/j.csm.2015.03.009   **sportsmed.theclinics.com**
0278-5919/15/$ – see front matter © 2015 Elsevier Inc. All rights reserved.

American College of Cardiology[2] and the European Society of Cardiology[3] have provided a rationale for the specialty of sports cardiology, described what team physicians and cardiologists "need to know" to practice it, and laid the foundation for its development throughout the United States and Europe. Although the European Society of Cardiology has proposed a core curriculum in sports cardiology for sports physicians and cardiologists (**Fig. 1**),[3] the American College of Cardiology has focused on cardiologists, noting that unique sports cardiology competencies overlap with existing cardiology learning pathways (**Fig. 2**).[2] When asymptomatic athletes present for CV screening, primary care sports medicine physicians and cardiologists use distinct sports cardiology competencies (see **Fig. 2**, *left side*). After an underlying disease is suspected or detected, competencies in cardiac disease and technology become operational (see **Fig. 2**, *center* and *right side*). Any cardiologist, either general or subspecialist, may be called on to evaluate athletes. Thus, it is essential that all cardiologists develop some basic proficiency in athlete CV care. This article outlines a systematic approach to the sports-specific CV care of any athlete (using soccer as an example), and reviews the knowledge base required to practice sports cardiology.

HOW TO PRACTICE SPORTS CARDIOLOGY: A PRACTICAL APPROACH TO THE SPORTS-SPECIFIC CARDIOVASCULAR CARE OF ANY ATHLETE

One of the challenges of sports cardiology is sifting through large amounts of published data on athletes, and organizing it in some fashion that allows comfortable

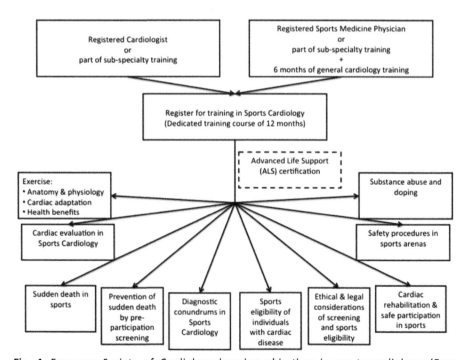

Fig. 1. European Society of Cardiology learning objectives in sports cardiology. (*From* Heidbuchel H, Papadakis M, Panhuyzen-Goedkoop N, et al. Position paper: proposal for a core curriculum for a European Sports Cardiology qualification. Eur J Prev Cardiol 2013;20:29; with permission.)

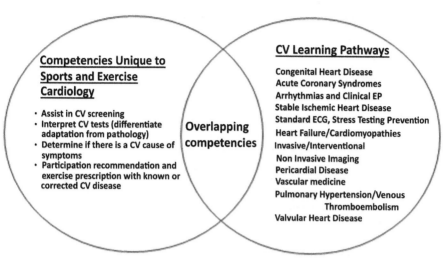

Fig. 2. Core competencies in sports and exercise cardiology overlap with existing competencies. CV, cardiovascular; ECG, electrocardiogram; EP, electrophysiology. (*Adapted from* Lawless CE, Olshansky B, Washington RL, et al. Sports and exercise cardiology in the United States: cardiovascular specialists as members of the athlete healthcare team. J Am Coll Cardiol 2014;63:1468; with permission.)

navigation through the sports' culture, assessment of sports-specific CV risk, and accurate interpretation of CV testing in any individual athlete. Challenge is posed by athlete heterogeneity. In the United States, athletes can be grouped according to high school, collegiate, professional, and older or masters athletes (>35 years) (**Table 1**).[2] Beyond that, they can be grouped according to sport, gender, size, ethnicity, and type of training. CV risk, cardiac adaptations, and appearance of cardiac tests all vary among individual groups of athletes based on these individual demographic characteristics.[2] Thus, we recommend an individualized, systematic, sports-specific, five-step approach to the CV care of any athlete (**Box 1**). This approach lends itself particularly well to professional and endurance athletes, where the most published data are available. Less information might be available in collegiate or high school age athletes or younger. These groups, although largest in terms of numbers of athletes, are probably the groups in most need of research and knowledge creation, especially in the United States.

Table 1 Number of athletes in the United States continues to increase		
Athlete Type	**2001**	**2011**
High school	3.3 million	7.7 million
Collegiate	~300,000	463,202
Masters (>35 y)		
Marathon finishers	353,000	>500,000
Triathlon memberships	21,431	>143,000

Data from Lawless CE, Olshansky B, Washington RL, et al. Sports and exercise cardiology in the United States: cardiovascular specialists as members of the athlete healthcare team. J Am Coll Cardiol 2014;63:1461–72.

Box 1
Systematic sports-specific approach to cardiovascular care of any athlete

1. Understand the sport and how it is governed

2. Define CV demands of the sport

3. Consider the internal and external sports environment

4. Identify range of normal CV adaptations for the sport

5. Evaluate CV risk, including risk of performance-enhancing agents

---

My personal introduction to sports cardiology was through the world of soccer. In 2006, I was asked to serve as Team Cardiologist to the Columbus Crew, an American professional soccer team based in Ohio. This led to 5 years of service as the Major League Soccer (MLS) Consulting Cardiologist, where I served at the recruitment combine, and wrote an extensive cardiac policy. My experiences inspired me to develop a systematic athlete-centered approach to the CV care of athletes, and to study and organize the essentials of the knowledge base required to provide CV care to athletes. This approach can be applied to any athlete, but here I demonstrate this method in a practical example that I am most familiar with: the professional soccer athlete.

FIVE-STEP APPROACH TO THE CARDIOVASCULAR CARE OF AN ATHLETE: EXAMPLE OF THE PROFESSIONAL SOCCER ATHLETE
Understand the Sport, How It Is Governed, and the Role of the Team Doctor and Cardiologist

Soccer is the world's most popular sport, with more than 200 million active players.[4] Founded in 1904, soccer's governing body the Fédération Internationale de Football Association (FIFA) is based in Zurich, Switzerland and is comprised of 209 member associations.[5] FIFA generates more than $1.386 billion in revenue, with 90% going back into the improvement of soccer.[5] Sanctioned by FIFA, the American professional football association, the MLS, is aligned with all of FIFA's policies and regulations. At the MLS player recruitment combine in Florida, local cardiologists partner with league medical staff to conduct and oversee athlete CV testing. Beyond the combine, each of the 20 MLS teams has designated a local "team cardiologist," who is available to provide immediate athlete CV care, allowing for efficient evaluation. Most team cardiologists assist in the interpretation of baseline electrocardiograms (ECG) and/or echocardiograms.

Define Cardiovascular Demands of the Sport

Soccer is a highly dynamic sport, categorized as IC (low static, high dynamic) per the 36th Bethesda Conference (**Fig. 3**).[6] During a 90-minute soccer match, field players cover 10 to 12 km (6.2–7.5 miles) and goalkeepers about 4 km (2.5 miles); players also sprint 2 to 4 seconds every 90 seconds.[7,8] Soccer has an underappreciated static component, because of "heading" or holding the ball against opponents.[7] During a soccer match, players average 80% to 90% of their heart rate maximum.[8] The highest mVo_2 recorded in soccer is about 80.9 mL/kg/min; most are in the 55 to 68 mL/kg/min range.[9,10]

Consider the Internal or External Sports Environment

During a 90-minute soccer match, catecholamines increase significantly compared with resting values.[11] Cortisol concentrations also increase.[11,12] Like marathoners,

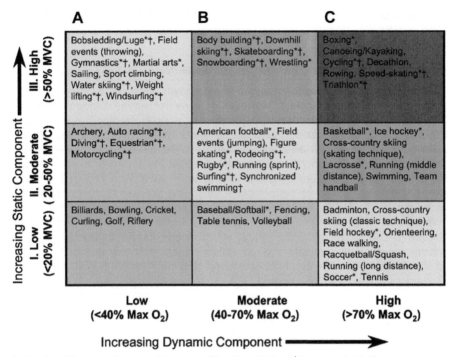

	A	**B**	**C**
III. High (>50% MVC)	Bobsledding/Luge*†, Field events (throwing), Gymnastics*†, Martial arts*, Sailing, Sport climbing, Water skiing*†, Weight lifting*†, Windsurfing*†	Body building*†, Downhill skiing*†, Skateboarding*†, Snowboarding*†, Wrestling*	Boxing*, Canoeing/Kayaking, Cycling*†, Decathlon, Rowing, Speed-skating*†, Triathlon*†
II. Moderate (20-50% MVC)	Archery, Auto racing*†, Diving*†, Equestrian*†, Motorcycling*†	American football*, Field events (jumping), Figure skating*, Rodeoing*†, Rugby*, Running (sprint), Surfing*†, Synchronized swimming†	Basketball*, Ice hockey*, Cross-country skiing (skating technique), Lacrosse*, Running (middle distance), Swimming, Team handball
I. Low (<20% MVC)	Billiards, Bowling, Cricket, Curling, Golf, Riflery	Baseball/Softball*, Fencing, Table tennis, Volleyball	Badminton, Cross-country skiing (classic technique), Field hockey*, Orienteering, Race walking, Racquetball/Squash, Running (long distance), Soccer*, Tennis
	Low (<40% Max O$_2$)	**Moderate (40-70% Max O$_2$)**	**High (>70% Max O$_2$)**

Increasing Static Component ↑

Increasing Dynamic Component ➡

Fig. 3. Classification of sports. * Danger of bodily collision. † Increased risk if syncope occurs. MVC, maximal voluntary contraction. (*From* Maron BJ, Zipes DP. 36th Bethesda Conference: eligibility recommendations for competitive athletes with cardiovascular abnormalities. J Am Coll Cardiol 2005;45:1366; with permission.)

troponin-I is elevated in 43% of soccer players after a match,[13] and may remain elevated for up to 48 hours.[14] Core temperature increases during play, starting at 20 minutes, and reaching 39°C at the end of a match.[15]

Identify Range of Normal Cardiovascular Adaptations for the Sport

MLS cardiac policy requires ECGs be done in all players at the combine and team level, followed by echocardiograms in any abnormal players. Team doctors and cardiologists must be well acquainted with the appearance of athletic adaptations on the soccer ECG/echocardiograms and develop proficiency in distinguishing these from cardiac pathology. Soccer poses a sustained volume load to the heart, resulting in four-chamber enlargement and increased stroke volume at rest and exercise.[16] Soccer-induced electrophysiologic adaptations appear on the ECG in the form of atrioventricular and interventricular blocks, ectopic beats, interval prolongations, increased voltage, and repolarization changes. In 582 professional soccer players undergoing cardiac assessment at the 2006 FIFA World Cup, 4.8% were found to have a potentially "pathologic" ECG, most commonly caused by T wave inversion.[17] Echocardiographic data in the same group suggest that ventricular enlargement is common: 30% of players demonstrate left ventricular end-diastolic dimension greater than 55 mm, whereas 10% show right ventricular end-diastolic dimension greater than 30 mm. Normal left ventricular ejection fraction ranges 45% to 85% in soccer players, whereas left atrial and aortic dimensions are 22 to 49 (mean, 36 ± 4) and 19 to 43 (mean, 31 ± 3) mm, respectively.[17] Three percent of players demonstrate left ventricular wall thickness greater than 13 mm.[17] Although MRI features of soccer have not been published, data on MRI in endurance athletes suggest that some normal players may demonstrate late gadolinium enhancement.[18] The clinical significance of this is not known.

Evaluate Cardiovascular Risk, Including that from Performance-Enhancing Agents

The exact risk of SCD in soccer players is not known, because occurrences have not been systematically tracked. However, in a recent survey conducted among 74.1% FIFA member organizations, 107 cases of sudden cardiac arrest (SCA) or SCD had been recalled over the past 10 years (mean age, 24.9 years), with 20.5% overall survival.[19] If an automated external defibrillator was placed on the pitch (field), survival was increased dramatically to 52.2%.[19] Similar to other endurance athletes, soccer players are prone to long-term risk of atrial fibrillation.[20] Adding to CV risk is the use of performance-enhancing agents. Professional soccer players may be tested for performance-enhancing agents in or out of competition, in compliance with FIFA antidoping regulations and the new World Anti-Doping Agency (WADA) Code of 2015.[21] Players have been known to test positive for performance-enhancing agents and recreational drugs, primarily anabolic steroids, and stimulants (ephedrine, amphetamines, and cocaine).[22] In 2011, WADA recorded 117 antidoping rule violations among FIFA-registered athletes, which is the highest number of positive tests in any of the professional sports committed to WADA regulations.[23]

This five-step approach to the CV care of an athlete can be adapted to fit any athlete, in any sport. Adolescent athletes demonstrate distinct training response,[24] echocardiographic adaptations,[25,26] and CV risk.[27,28] Older athletes are well represented in marathon athlete literature, where the CV demands, risks, and adaptations have been well-described.[29–31] Although the systematic approach allows for an organized thought process in approaching any athlete, equally important is a specialized sports cardiology knowledge base (**Box 2**).[2,3]

KNOWLEDGE BASE REQUIRED TO PROVIDE ATHLETE CARDIOVASCULAR CARE (SPORTS CARDIOLOGY)
Basic Exercise Physiology

Sports cardiology begins with an understanding of the basics of exercise physiology. Athletic adaptation occurs in response to training,[32] whereas certain physiologic reflexes may be triggered by the sports environment.[33]

Box 2
Knowledge base required to provide athletes CV care (sports cardiology)

1. Basic exercise physiology
2. CV screening
3. Choice of cardiac testing
4. Interpretation of CV testing: differentiating normal athletic adaptation from inherited diseases
5. Tailored management of CV conditions
6. Determine if CV cause of symptoms
7. Participation recommendation in those with known or suspected CV disease

Cardiovascular Screening

Although one of the most contentious areas of sports cardiology, the on-going debate in the United States regarding screening ECG has been one of the main drivers of the development of sports cardiology. The great screening debate and the interpretation of the athlete ECG are discussed in detail elsewhere in this issue. Regardless of the debate, sports physicians and cardiologists providing CV care to athletes are advised to be well-versed in athlete ECG and echocardiogram interpretation, and how to differentiate "normal" adaptation from pathology.

Choice of Cardiac Testing

Athletes frequently require ambulatory monitoring, but difficulty with lead adherence during physical activity, or contact with an opponent, can impede monitoring. In such instances, ALIVE-COR monitors (AliveCor, Inc, San Francisco, CA),[34] special water-resistant external devices,[35] implantable loop recorders,[36] commercial heart rate monitors,[37] or smart shirts[38] may be helpful. Bruce protocol stress testing, intended to diagnose coronary artery disease, may be insufficient to reproduce athlete symptoms. Clinicians are advised to either monitor during the sporting activity, or to recreate exercise load and conditions in the exercise laboratory.[2] Upright tilt table testing is considered unreliable in athletes, perhaps related to the interaction of high vagal tone with neurocardiogenic responses.[39]

Interpretation of Cardiovascular Testing

In differentiating normal athletic adaptation from inherited diseases, training-related adaptations mimic the phenotypic appearance of inherited diseases. These can place athletes into a unique category known as the "grey-zone."[16] Although most often applied to ventricular cavity dimensions and wall thickness, the "grey-zone" may also apply to the right ventricle, QT interval, and ST segment.[40–42] The clinician has access to a variety of specialized tools (cardiopulmonary exercise testing, advanced echocardiography, cardiac MRI, supervised detraining, pharmacologic infusion, genetic testing) to differentiate between normal and true pathology.[43] However, to successfully navigate this minefield, cardiologists must have a clear understanding of the "normal" limits to cardiac athletic adaptations, and the cardinal features of the inherited diseases that cause athlete SCA/SCD.[44]

Tailored Management of Cardiovascular Conditions

When making treatment recommendations, cardiologists must tailor therapies to the needs of the athlete. Some CV pharmacologic agents may be on the WADA prohibited list and thus not suitable for certain athletes. β-Blockade may not be the best choice because of negative effects on cardiac performance.[45] Need for anticoagulant therapy may influence choice of valve replacement versus repair in those wishing to resume contact sports after surgery. Ablation may be recommended earlier for athletes with reentrant arrhythmias or accessory pathways.[46] In athletes with pacemakers, upper rate limit behaviors can negatively impact athletic performance. In these cases, custom-made devices or custom programming can be helpful.[47]

Determine if Cardiovascular Cause of Symptoms

Although it has been shown that prodromal symptoms are common in those who succumb to SCA,[48] the predictive value of exertional and nonexertional chest pain, syncope, fatigue, palpitations, and shortness of breath in athletes is not known with certainty. Nonetheless, this is one of the more common reasons a cardiologist may be asked to see an athlete. Clearly, more study is necessary to define the predictive value of symptoms in this patient group.

Participation Recommendation in Those with Known or Suspected Cardiovascular Disease

In the United States, the 36th Bethesda Conference has been the gold standard for participation recommendation in athletes with established heart disease.[6] This document has been criticized for being too restrictive and lacking an evidence base.[2,49,50] Preliminary data in athletes and exercising individuals with implanted defibrillators,[51] and long QT,[52] suggest that the risk of exercise and/or sports may be acceptably low in certain individuals with these conditions. Further studies are planned, but outcome data like this will provide the Bethesda (participation recommendation) writers with information they need to allow the guideline to evolve.

SUMMARY/DISCUSSION

Sports cardiology may have had its beginnings more than 2000 years ago in ancient Greece with the sudden death of Pheidippides, but its contemporary practice is focused on the prevention of such instances, and requires that all primary care sports physicians and cardiologists develop basic competencies in athlete CV care. The systematic approach to individual athlete CV care, combined with an athlete-centered sports cardiology knowledge base, provides these clinicians with what is necessary to approach any athlete's cardiac risk assessment and evaluation. This dynamic field is developing quickly, and is likely to grow exponentially in years to come, based on the popularity of sports participation and the on-going screening debate.

REFERENCES

1. Sekunda N. Marathon 490 BC: the first Persian invasion of Greece. Oxford, United Kingdom: Osprey Publishing; 2002. ISBN 1841760005.
2. Lawless CE, Olshansky B, Washington RL, et al. Sports and exercise cardiology in the United States: cardiovascular specialists as members of the athlete health-care team. J Am Coll Cardiol 2014;63:1461–72.
3. Heidbuchel H, Papadakis M, Panhuyzen-Goedkoop N, et al. Position paper: proposal for a core curriculum for a European Sports Cardiology qualification. Eur J Prev Cardiol 2013;20:889–903.
4. Dvorak J. Football is the most popular sport worldwide. Am J Sports Med 2004; 32:3S–4S.
5. Available at: http://www.fifa.com/. Accessed March 7, 2015.
6. Maron BJ, Zipes DP. 36th Bethesda Conference: eligibility recommendations for competitive athletes with cardiovascular abnormalities. J Am Coll Cardiol 2005; 45:1313–75.
7. Stolen T, Chamari K, Castagna C, et al. Physiology of soccer: an update. Sports Med 2005;35:501–36.
8. Stroyer J, Hansen L, Klausen K. Physiological profile and activity pattern of young soccer players during match play. Med Sci Sports Exerc 2004;36:168–74.
9. Tumilty D. Physiological characteristics of elite soccer players. Sports Med 1993; 16(2):80–96.
10. Hoff J. Training and testing physical capacities for elite soccer players. J Sports Sci 2005;23(6):573–82.

11. Carli G, Bonifazi M, Lodi L, et al. Hormonal and metabolic effects following a football match. Int J Sports Med 1986;7:36–8.
12. Haneishi K, Fry AC, Moore CA, et al. Cortisol and stress responses during a game and practice in female collegiate soccer players. J Strength Cond Res 2007;21:583–8.
13. Löwbeer C, Seeberger A, Gustafsson SA, et al. Serum cardiac troponin T, troponin I, plasma BNP and left ventricular mass index in professional football players. J Sci Med Sport 2007;10(5):291–6.
14. Akyuz M. Changes in serum cardiac troponin T levels in professional football players before and after the game. African Journal of Pharmacy and Pharmacology 2011;5(11):1365–8. Available at: http://www.academicjournals.org/ajpp.
15. Ozgunen KT, Kurdak SS, Maughan RJ, et al. Effect of hot environmental conditions on physical activity patterns and temperature response of football players. Scand J Med Sci Sports 2010;20:140–7.
16. Maron BJ, Pelliccia A. The heart of trained athletes: cardiac remodeling and the risks of sports, including sudden death. Circulation 2006;114:1633–44.
17. Thunenkotter T, Schmied C, Dvorak J, et al. Benefits and limitations of cardiovascular pre-competition screening in international football. Clin Res Cardiol 2010; 99(1):29–35.
18. Breuckmann F, Möhlenkamp S, Nassenstein K, et al. Myocardial late gadolinium enhancement: prevalence, pattern, and prognostic relevance in marathon runners. Radiology 2009;251(1):50–7.
19. Schmied C, Drezner J, Kramer E, et al. Cardiac events in football and strategies for first-responder treatment on the field. Br J Sports Med 2013; 47(18):1175–8.
20. Abdulla J, Nielsen J. Is the risk of atrial fibrillation higher in athletes than in the general population? A systematic review and meta-analysis. Europace 2009; 11(9):1156–9.
21. Available at: http://fr.m.fifa.com/worldcup/news/y=2014/m=6/news=dvorak-le-profil-biologique-une-approche-completement-nouvelle-2354963.html. Accessed March 7, 2015.
22. Available at: http://www.nytimes.com/2014/06/21/sports/worldcup/no-doping-at-the-world-cup-thats-what-fifa-says.html?_r=0. Accessed March 7, 2015.
23. Available at: http://www.sportsonearth.com/article/67536920/soccer-doping-problem-shows-no-signs-of-stopping. Accessed March 7, 2015.
24. Baquet G, van Praagh E, Berthoin S. Endurance training and aerobic fitness in young people. Sports Med 2003;33:1127–43.
25. Makan J, Sharma S, Firoozi S, et al. Physiological upper limits of ventricular cavity size in highly trained adolescent athletes. Heart 2005;91(4):495–9.
26. Sharma S, Maron B, Whyte G, et al. Physiologic limits of left ventricular hypertrophy in elite junior athletes: relevance to differential diagnosis of athlete's heart and hypertrophic cardiomyopathy. J Am Coll Cardiol 2002;40:1431–6.
27. Maron BJ, Haas T, Ahluwalia A, et al. Incidence of cardiovascular sudden deaths in Minnesota high school athletes. Heart Rhythm 2013;10:374–7.
28. Roberts WO, Stovitz SD. Incidence of sudden cardiac death in Minnesota high school athletes 1993-2012 screened with a standardized pre-participation evaluation. J Am Coll Cardiol 2013;62:1298–301.
29. Predel HG. Marathon run: cardiovascular adaptation and cardiovascular risk. Eur Heart J 2014;35(44):3091–8.
30. Kim J, Malhotra R, Chiampas G, et al. Cardiac arrests during long-distance running races. N Engl J Med 2012;366:132–42.

31. Baggish AL, Yared K, Wang F, et al. The impact of endurance exercise training on left ventricular systolic mechanics. Am J Physiol Heart Circ Physiol 2008;295: H1109–16.
32. Baggish AL, Wood MJ. Athlete's heart and cardiovascular care of the athlete: scientific and clinical update. Circulation 2011;123:2723–35.
33. Gooden BA. Mechanism of the human diving response. Integr Physiol Behav Sci 1994;29:6–16.
34. Available at: http://www.alivecor.com/home. Accessed March 7, 2015.
35. Saxon LA, Tun H, Riva G, et al. Dynamic heart rate behavior of elite athletes during football. Paper presented at: Heart Rhythm 33rd Annual Scientific Sessions. Boston, May 10, 2012.
36. Rossano J, Bloemers B, Sreeram N, et al. Efficacy of implantable loop recorders in establishing symptom-rhythm correlation in young patients with syncope and palpitations. Pediatrics 2003;112:e228–33.
37. Müssigbrodt A, Richter S, Wetzel U, et al. Diagnosis of arrhythmias in athletes using leadless, ambulatory HR monitors. Med Sci Sports Exerc 2013;45:1431–5.
38. How to use the smart shirt. Available at: http://www.gtwm.gatech.edu/index/how_to_use.html. Accessed March 7, 2015.
39. Gopinathannair R, Olshansky B. Electrophysiological approach to syncope and near-syncope in the athlete. In: Lawless CE, editor. Sports cardiology essentials: evaluation, management and case studies. New York City: Springer-Verlag; 2011. p. 181–212.
40. Zaidi A, Ghani S, Sharma R, et al. Physiological right ventricular adaption in elite athletes of African and Afro-Caribbean origin. Circulation 2013;127:1783–92.
41. Basavarajaiah S, Wilson M, Whyte G, et al. Prevalence and significance of an isolated long QT interval in elite athletes. Eur Heart J 2007;28:2944–9.
42. Adler A, Rosso R, Viskin D, et al. What do we know about the "malignant form" of early repolarization? J Am Coll Cardiol 2013;62:863–8.
43. Maron BJ. Distinguishing hypertrophic cardiomyopathy from athlete's heart physiological remodelling: clinical significance, diagnostic strategies and implications for preparticipation screening. Heart 2005;91(11):1380–2.
44. Maron BJ, Doerer JJ, Haas TS, et al. Sudden deaths in young competitive athletes: analysis of 1866 deaths in the US, 1980–2006. Circulation 2009;119:1085–92.
45. Tesch PA. Exercise performance and beta-blockade. Sports Med 1985;2:389–412.
46. Blomström-Lundqvist C, Scheinman MM, Aliot EM, et al. ACC/AHA/ESC guidelines for the management of patients with supraventricular arrhythmias—executive summary: a report of the American College of Cardiology/American Heart Association Task Force on Practice Guidelines and the European Society of Cardiology Committee for Practice Guidelines (Writing Committee to Develop Guidelines for the Management of Patients With Supraventricular Arrhythmias). J Am Coll Cardiol 2003;42:1493–531.
47. Bennekers JH, van Mechelen R, Meijer A. Pacemaker safety and long-distance running. Neth Heart J 2004;12:450–4.
48. Tretter J, Kavey R. Distinguishing cardiac syncope from vasovagal syncope in a referral population. J Pediatr 2013;163:1618–23.
49. Lawless CE, Asplund C, Asif I, et al. Protecting the heart of the American athlete. J Am Coll Cardiol 2014;64(20):2146–71.
50. Longmuir PE, Brothers JA, de Ferranti SD, et al. Promotion of physical activity for children and adults with congenital heart disease. Circulation 2013;127:2147–59.

51. Lampert R, Olshansky B, Heidbuchel H, et al. Safety of sports for athletes with implantable cardioverter-defibrillators: results of a prospective, multinational registry. Circulation 2013;127:2021–30.
52. Johnson JN, Ackerman MJ. Competitive sports participation in athletes with congenital long QT syndrome. JAMA 2012;308:764–5.

The Management of Athletes with Congenital Heart Disease

Silvana Molossi, MD, PhD[a],*, Michelle Grenier, MD[b]

KEYWORDS

- Sudden cardiac death • Congenital heart disease • Congenital coronary anomalies
- Kawasaki disease • Sports cardiology

KEY POINTS

- Sudden cardiac death is a devastating event and efforts should be made to its prevention by careful evaluation of athletes, especially pertaining to underlying cardiovascular conditions.
- Congenital heart defects affect about 1% of the population and it is of utmost importance the basic knowledge of commons defects for the evaluation of athletes.
- Repaired congenital heart defects restoring normal physiology usually allow exercise activities and sports participation in most individuals.
- Unrepaired or palliated congenital heart defects usually pose at least some degree of limitations on the ability to participate in sports and athletics activities.
- Coronary anomalies, either congenital or acquired, are an important cause of sudden cardiac events during sports and exercise participation.

Gone are the days when we ran outside freely, climbed tress, rode bikes, and ran as long as humanly possible without having been prescreened by a health practitioner. The impact of sudden loss of basketball greats Reggie Lewis and Len Bias, volleyball Olympians such as Flo Hyman, countless world soccer players clipped of life mid-sprint, karate competitors heel-struck in the chest falling dramatically to their death is undeniable. Although rare, sudden cardiac death (SCD) is devastating to families and communities, and society dictates avoidance of any circumstances predisposing to the loss of human life during exertion.

SCD can only be "sudden" when there are no predictive factors, herein is the difficulty in prevention. Some of the more common risk factors for SCD have been described, although the true incidence and prevalence worldwide are difficult to ascertain given

[a] Section of Pediatric Cardiology, Department of Pediatrics, Texas Children's Hospital, Baylor College of Medicine, 6621 Fannin Street WT 19345-C, Houston, TX 77030, USA; [b] Pediatrix Cardiology Associates of New Mexico, 201 Cedar Street SE, Suite 700, Albuquerque, NM 87106, USA
* Corresponding author.
E-mail address: sxmoloss@texaschildrens.org

Clin Sports Med 34 (2015) 551–570
http://dx.doi.org/10.1016/j.csm.2015.04.001
0278-5919/15/$ – see front matter © 2015 Elsevier Inc. All rights reserved.

the complexity in defining the denominator (defined population in which SCD occurs). The most common final pathway leading to sudden cardiac arrest is ventricular tachycardia/fibrillation, which might be managed by the presence of an automated external defibrillator at all sports and exercise activities, along with trained experts in cardiopulmonary resuscitation. The exceptions are those with known connective tissue abnormalities (Marfan and Loeys-Dietz syndromes, for example) leading to sudden aortic dissection.

Screening of athletes before sports participation by trained professionals is useful in identifying individuals who carry the known risk factors for SCD. Overrestriction may be almost as harmful as underrestriction of athletes, however. For example, patients with congenital heart disease (CHD) have been and continue to be overrestricted in their activities because there remains a paucity of data as to the safety of exercise in this population. There is a burgeoning population of children and adult survivors with CHD that may be inappropriately restricted by health care providers who have no or few data to advise them, parents who fear for their vulnerable children, or patients who self-restrict themselves for lack of appropriate counseling and not knowing their true limitations (or lack of).

Sports medicine specialists are tasked with providing individual exercise prescriptions for exercising individuals with and without CHD, and these are currently outlined in the 36th Bethesda guidelines.[1] There is precedent in the Special Olympics and para-Olympians. Sports medicine specialists should be able to identify those at overwhelming risk for adverse events surrounding vigorous activity and direct appropriate evaluation by the specialist (ie, cardiologist). Equally importantly, they should be able to coach individuals to improve performance and quality of life with exercise.

EXERCISE AS MEDICINE

How does exercise figure into the mental and emotional well-being, quality of life, societal productivity, and general well-being of people with CHD? Can exercise attenuate the natural history of heart failure described in adolescents and adults after surgery for CHD[2]? Competitive and recreational sports participation may improve the quality of life and exercise capacity as well as lower body mass index in patients with mild, moderate, or severe CHD.[3] In one population of patients with a variety of complex congenital heart lesions, 50% participated in competitive sports, 25% were recreational athletes, and 29% of the severely affected congenital heart patients participated in competitive sports despite recommendations against such activities by the 36th Bethesda guidelines,[4] indicating the perceived benefits of exercise far outweighed the reported risks in the population studied. The job of sports medicine professionals is to help patients balance the risk:benefit ratio. The neurocognitive benefits of exercise are myriad and not to be underestimated in a population that is at risk for neurocognitive delays due to the effects of their disease, underlying genetics, or complexity of necessary interventions.

The positive effects of exercise on the myocardium, including enhanced myocardial contractility, improved diastolic filling due to improved myocardial relaxation, better compliance, decreased filling pressure, and improved atrial compliance, all contributing to increases in stroke volume and cardiac output, have been well documented,[5–7] although less well documented in the myocardium of patients with CHD that has been manipulated by surgical or catheter interventions or affected by residual lesions.

Despite the latest observation that there is an increase in coronary calcium scoring in elite runners, the cardioprotective effects of exercise are well demonstrated. Exercise acts directly on coronary blood flow by increasing myocardial oxygen demand, which then stimulates a compensatory increase in myocardial oxygen supply.[8] Endo-thelial factor (nitric oxide–mediated) improves coronary smooth muscle relaxation and enhanced coronary vasodilation, which thereby promotes vascular collateralization in previously ischemic areas.[8] In the case of children predisposed to coronary abnormal-ities (ie, patients after arterial switch operation for transposition of the great arteries and patients post-Kawasaki disease), an appropriate exercise regimen may provide the benefit of enhanced coronary flow. Exercise attenuates chemotherapy-induced myocardial damage and may be cardioprotective in those patients exposed to anthra-cycline therapy by inducing angiogenesis and improving myocardial energetics.[9] There are similar studies in patients with HIV infection who benefit from the increased myocardial insulin sensitivity induced by recurrent exercise.[10] Heart muscle adapta-tions are dictated by type and dose of sports, gender, genetics, race/ethnicity, and body mass index (further addressed in another article in this issue).

INCIDENCE AND PREVALENCE, BASIC ANATOMY, PHYSIOLOGY, AND NATURAL HISTORY OF COMMON CONGENITAL CARDIAC LESIONS

CHD is the most common congenital anomaly affecting 0.7% to 1% of live newborns, with 0.3% being critical lesions that require intervention in the first month of life.[11–13] The evolution in the treatment of CHD has led to very low mortality in large academic centers, nearing 1%, including all risk categories. Therefore, one is left nowadays to deal with the maintenance of health in this ever-growing population with repaired congenital lesions. It is estimated that more than 1 million adults live with CHD currently in the United States,[14] and the number of children with moderate and severe congenital defects equals the number of adults with such defects.[15] Standard exer-cise recommendations for these patients typically follow the 36th Bethesda guide-lines, however, with great variability in the cardiology outpatient setting. Data on exercise activities and participation are at best sparse in this population.

Sudden Death and Congenital Heart Disease

Congenital heart lesions that are not hemodynamically significant are very well toler-ated, cope well with the increased demands of exercise activity, and typically do not impact the athlete's performance. On the other hand, hemodynamically significant lesions pose an increased risk to exercise activities, especially those that course with intense dynamic or isometric activities. Normal adaptive changes to exercise, such as an increase in systemic output and myocardial oxygen demand with a concomitant increase in the systemic and arterial blood pressures, may decompensate a borderline hemodynamic status, leading to myocardial ischemia and arrhythmias with subse-quent sudden cardiac arrest or death. Specific conditions linked to SCD, many times without a known prior diagnosis, include aortopathy (discussed in detail in another article in this issue) and coronary anomalies (discussed in detail later in this article). Mitral valve prolapse is reportedly another cause of SCD given the only abnormality detected in autopsy cases,[16–18] although exceedingly rare, and also recently in survi-vors of "unexplained" out-of-hospital cardiac arrest.[19]

For the purposes of discussion, the common congenital cardiac lesions are divided into shunting lesions, pressure lesions, more complex lesions that may be associated with cyanosis, and coronary anomalies.

SHUNT VERSUS PRESSURE LESIONS

Dynamic and static/isometric exercises have differing direct effects on the myocar-dium, causing eccentric versus concentric left ventricular hypertrophy, as described by Baggish and Wood.[5] Long distance running (dynamic exercise) causes a sustained volume load to the heart for prolonged periods of time,[20] inducing increased stroke volume at rest and during exercise through an enlarged ventricular cavity.[5] Strength training (static/isometric exercise) induces a pressure load[20] in the heart leading to a disproportionate increase in wall thickness in relation to cavity size.[21–23] A combination of dynamic and isometric/static exercise causes a composite of these changes as the heart adapts to the exercise environment, and there is robust literature to support these observations.[5,20–23] Heart muscle adaptations are dictated by type and dosing sports, gender, genetics, race/ethnicity, and body mass index.

Shunt Lesions as Dynamic Exercise

Shunt lesions are typically septal defects between the atria (atrial septal defect or ASD), between the ventricles (ventricular septal defect or VSD), involving both atrial and ventricular septa, or persistence of congenital vessel connecting the high-pressure systemic circulation to the low-pressure pulmonary circulation (patent ductus arteriosus or PDA). These shunts lead to a volume overload system wherein blood is essentially "stolen" from the systemic system and directed into the pulmonary system. The effect is similar to that of chronic dynamic exercise (as in long-distance runners), where the myocardium is exposed to higher volume load given the presence of the shunt; this means the myocardium responds by enlarging the ventricular cavity, which handles the increased blood volume, also dealt with to a greater or lesser extent by the lungs.

Atrial Septal Defect

This defect between the low-pressure atrial chambers can remain silent for long periods of time, depending on its size. The so-called patent foramen ovale (PFO) is a very small defect in the atrial septum commonly found in about 20% to 25% of the adult population. It does not culminate with substantial shunting or lead to overload of the right heart. Long-term implications of PFO will not be discussed in this section, but typically these tiny defects do not impose any acute need for intervention and are not a cause for restriction from activity.

The size of the ASD determines how much load is placed on the right heart, and how audible the murmur is by increased flow across the pulmonary outflow tract. As blood returns from the lungs to the left atrium, it flows directly through the mitral valve into the left ventricle, where it is then pumped through the aorta to the rest of the body (systemic circulation). In the setting of an ASD, a portion of the blood coming to the left atrium will divert into the right atrium through the defect, where is goes through the tricuspid valve into the right ventricle and is pumped right back out into the lungs (the pulmonary circulation).

A chronic volume load on the right atrium and right ventricle causes enlargement of these chambers, and increased volume load to the lungs. Chronic exposure to an ASD may cause lung (vasculature) damage proportional to the size of the shunt, and the "stretching" of the right-sided cavities imposes strain on the conduction system and decreased exercise capacity. Many years with a sizable ASD, therefore, may result in rhythm and pulmonary complications. It is not uncommon to find athletes with ASDs during screening. Most of the time, these athletes may continue to compete, but should be referred to a pediatric cardiologist to be certain the prolonged pulmonary exposure to increased flow has not caused irreversible pulmonary damage (pulmonary hypertension, rarely occurring in this setting). Pulmonary hypertension carries a high risk of SCD and would be a cause for exclusion from competition. One should also consider that the volume load of endurance training can amplify the degree of right ventricular dilation beyond what would be expected with the left-to-right shunt alone.

Ventricular Septal Defect

Any defect in the thick wall between the pumping chambers, the ventricles, constitutes a VSD. The behavior of the defect and its effect on the heart are dependent on its size and location within the ventricular septum. This type of defect may occur high up along the base of the heart or they may occur farther down within the muscular septum. The pressure in the ventricular (pumping) chambers is higher than that of the atria, and the pressure in the left ventricle is typically 3 to 4 times higher than that in the right ventricle. Therefore, the VSD murmur is directly due to the defect, as opposed to the ASD, where the murmur is attributable to the increased flow through the pulmonary (lung) artery. Small VSDs in the muscular septum are extremely common with an estimated incidence of 5% in live newborns.[24]

Similar to the ASD, blood returns from the lungs to the left atrium and is directed through the mitral valve into the left ventricle, where it is directed out the aorta into the systemic circulation. If there is a VSD, a proportion of the blood directed out of the aorta is diverted to the right ventricle through the defect, which pumps this "extra blood" to the lungs, eventually returning a larger volume back to the left atrium. The result is larger left atrial and left ventricular cavities proportional to the size and location of the defect. In fact, most large VSDs are diagnosed in the United States during infancy.

The athlete presenting with a serendipitous finding of VSD should be referred to a pediatric cardiologist who will evaluate for any degree of pulmonary hypertension or associated defects. Once again, unless there are elevated pulmonary pressures (pulmonary hypertension) or other associated defects, there is no need to restrict the athlete from competitive sports. There are many individuals with tiny but loud VSDs of no hemodynamic significance who should not be restricted from competition!

Atrioventricular Septal Defect or Complete Atrioventricular Canal

The atrioventricular septal defect (AVSD) encompasses a defect involving both the atrial and the ventricular septa where the atrioventricular valves (mitral and tricuspid) maintain their apparatus. It is a defect in the crux of the heart, hence altering the normal structure of both mitral and tricuspid valves. Once again, there is volume overload as described in the previous 2 defects, which affects the myocardium much as chronic dynamic exercise, causing eccentric enlargement of the atrial and ventricular cavities. As in the ASD and VSDs, there may be right, left, or biventricular and biatrial enlargement dependent on the size and locations of the shunt. As these defects are largely recognized and repaired during early childhood, the size of the left-to-right shunt and its chronicity determine the extent of residual damage. The lungs usually sustain some degree of damage from increased pulmonary blood flow, which is proportional to the size of the defects, but can completely recover if repair is achieved early in the first year of life. Again, it is important for these individuals to be evaluated by a pediatric cardiologist, who may advise the sports medicine practitioner in regard to any elevation of pulmonary artery pressures or residual valvar lesions (narrowing/stenosis or leakage/regurgitation).

AVSDs are commonly associated with Down syndrome. Those individuals with Down syndrome will require evaluation of other systems extrinsic to the cardiovascular system before participation in exercise.

Patent Ductus Arteriosus

The PDA is a remnant of the fetal/neonatal period, when its purpose was to keep an open communication between the aorta and the pulmonary arteries. After birth and when the pulmonary pressure drops lower than the aortic pressure, the PDA offers a direct communication from the higher-pressure aorta into the lower-pressure pulmonary artery. The lung or pulmonary bed receives this increased volume of blood, which transmits back to the left atrium and left ventricle, a situation similar to chronic dynamic exercise, resulting in an enlarged left atrium and left ventricle in proportion to the size of the shunt. Just as there are tiny PFOs, tiny ASDs, and tiny VSDs, there may be tiny and even silent PDAs. Unless there is evidence of increased pulmonary pressures (pulmonary hypertension), these athletes should not be restricted from participation in exercise.

PRESSURE LESIONS AS STATIC EXERCISE

As previously stated, pressure lesions within the heart are equivalent to static or isometric exercise. They have similar effects on the myocardium, including thickening of the ventricular walls that correspond to the chamber upstream of the obstruction. That is, a ventricle must push blood through a tightened/stenotic passage or valve. How thick (hypertrophied) the ventricular walls become is often proportionate to how hard the ventricle must work to push blood through the narrowed passage.

Pulmonary Valve Stenosis

The right ventricle is attached to the pulmonary valve, which allows blood from the ventricular cavity into the lung or pulmonary arteries. In cases where the valve is not formed well or is extremely tight (critical pulmonic stenosis), blood cannot get to the pulmonary arteries and lungs, and the patient may appear visibly blue (cyanotic). These extreme defects typically present in infancy and are treated at that time (see the later section on therapeutic interventions).

The murmur of pulmonary stenosis is due to the valve abnormality and may vary with the degree of tightness or stenosis. Occasionally, when the pulmonary artery is enlarged above the stenotic valve, the murmur is disproportionately loud with clicks (vibration of the thickened valve leaflets). Therefore, the echocardiogram is the best for determining the degree of pulmonary stenosis.

In general, patients with untreated mild-to-moderate pulmonary valve stenosis may perform most physical activities without restraint. Those with a moderate degree of stenosis should be evaluated by a cardiologist for right ventricular hypertension to assure their safety in activities, although isolated pulmonic stenosis is not typically listed as a risk factor for SCD.

Aortic Valve Stenosis

The aortic valve allows blood to flow from the high-pressured left ventricle into the systemic aorta. Like the pulmonary valve, where critical stenosis may present at birth or in infancy and be addressed appropriately, aortic valve stenosis can also present in this fashion. However, not infrequently, it may occur insidiously. In the case of a bicuspid aortic valve (estimated prevalence 1%–2%), there may be progressive stenosis or leak (insufficiency) over time. In the case of stenosis, the left ventricle responds to the pressure stimulus much as it would to static/isometric/weight-lifting: it becomes concentrically thickened or hypertrophied. Aortic stenosis may be asymptomatic and its progress may be insidious. The athlete may not be aware of the defect until they manifest symptoms, which, on rare occasion, is that of SCD.[25,26] Concentric left ventricular hypertrophy, while not causing SCD in and of itself, may be part of the substrate that leads to the final common pathway, ventricular arrhythmia, which predisposes to SCD.[25]

The murmur of aortic valve stenosis may correlate with the degree of aortic pressure gradient from the left ventricle into the aorta. Once again, it is a dynamic change that occurs, with left ventricular thickness/hypertrophy, which may be proportional to the degree of valvar tightness or stenosis. These patients should be restricted from activities until a cardiologist can evaluate them. There are now surgical and nonsurgical aortic valve interventions, which may be life-saving (see section on therapy).

Coarctation of the Aorta—Covert Systemic Hypertension

A narrowing in the aorta may lie undiagnosed for a long period of time. Critical coarctation, or interruption of the aortic arch, presents in the newborn period, because oxygen/nutrient-rich blood cannot pass beyond the area of obstruction in the aorta to perfuse important organs, such as the brain, kidneys and gastrointestinal system. However, narrowing in the aorta need not always be critical, and they are not relegated to the level of the isthmus and descending aorta. Narrowing, or coarctation, may occur in the thoracoabdominal aorta, which makes it more occult and difficult to diagnose. This aortic narrowing may also be accompanied by growth of ancillary vessels "collaterals," which circumvent the narrowed aorta.

Although there may be a murmur, it may not be in the typical place. A murmur heard best in the upper or lower back, corresponding to where the blood flow is impeded in the aorta, is an expected finding. There may also be continuous murmurs through the ribs, where the collateral vessels have grown.

The heralding sign of coarctation is more commonly hypertension in an upper extremity with simultaneous lower extremity normal to lower blood pressures. Upon feeling the upper and lower extremity pulses simultaneously (which may be tricky in a basketball player), there is a "lag" or a delay in the pulses in the feet. A case may be made for obtaining an upper and lower (thigh) extremity blood pressure simultaneously when there is systemic hypertension. This condition is a common cause of secondary systemic hypertension in youngsters (second only to renal abnormalities) and should always be considered in the presence of high blood pressure levels.

Once again, this pressure overload is similar to a static/isometric load on the left ventricle. From that standpoint, there is concentric left ventricular hypertrophy, which is a risk factor for SCD in and of itself.[25] These individuals should be restricted from exercise until evaluated and treated by a cardiologist.

COMPLEX LESIONS WITH CYANOSIS

Complex lesions with cyanosis lead to the mixture of venous blood with arterial blood and result in decreased systemic oxygenation and consequent cyanosis. Some of these defects are amenable to surgical intervention and largely restoring the normal cardiac physiology with 2 functional ventricles (1 leading the blood to the pulmonary circulation and 1 leading the blood to the systemic circulation). Conversely, other defects that culminate with a smaller ventricular chamber (either right or left) result in a so-called univentricular heart. These lesions are repaired or palliated with surgical intervention. Given the presence of cyanosis from the newborn period, typically the diagnosis is made in very early life. The sports physician will encounter these athletes already in a postrepair stage and the implications on sports participation will depend on the presence of residual lesions, more commonly seen in some of these conditions.

Tetralogy of Fallot

Tetralogy of Fallot is the most common cyanotic CHD. It includes the presence of a VSD and various levels of obstruction to the pulmonary circulation (pulmonary stenosis at the valvar, subvalvar [below the valve], and supravalvar [above the valve] level). This leads to increased pressure in the right ventricle that works hard to impel the blood to the lungs (acting as an isometric exercise). The pressure usually increases above the pressure in the left side, leading to shunting of blood from the right to the left circulation (out to the aorta from the left ventricle). Conversely to what is seen in the shunt of lesions without cyanosis where there is increased blood to the lungs, here there is a decreased amount of blood to the lungs and resulting in cyanosis.

In developed countries, this lesion is readily diagnosed, and surgical intervention is performed in the first year of life. Therefore, these patients will participate in exercise activities in their repaired stage, and their eligibility will depend largely on the presence of residual lesions.

Dextrotransposition of the Great Arteries

Dextrotransposition of the great arteries leads to 2 parallel circulations with the aorta leaving the right ventricle and the pulmonary artery leaving the left ventricle. Therefore, venous blood (poor in oxygen content) coming from the body to the right ventricle returns to the systemic circulation, and arterial blood (rich in oxygen content) coming from the lungs to the left ventricle returns to the lungs. Therefore, it is absolutely necessary that a defect between the 2 parallel circulations exists for the mixing of venous and arterial blood. This parallel circulation usually occurs at the atrial level through an ASD. The maintenance of a PDA shortly after birth helps to some extent by means of shunting of blood from the pulmonary artery (in this situation, where blood is rich in oxygen) to the aorta (in this situation, where blood is poor in oxygen).

This lesion will not be present in athletes evaluated by a sports physician later in life, except in its repaired stage. Cyanosis will no longer be present and, as in tetralogy of Fallot, participation in exercise activities will depend on the repair performed and the presence of residual lesions.

Single Ventricle

The single ventricle defect is a complex heart defect with several forms and associated lesions, but all leading to a univentricular heart. In other words, there is only one meaningful ventricular chamber, with the other one being small or hypoplastic, and this can be of a right or left ventricular morphology. Commonly, it presents in the newborn period with various degrees of cyanosis caused by the mixture of venous and arterial blood in this main ventricular chamber and may be associated with obstruction to either the pulmonary or the systemic circulation. Palliative surgical procedures usually start in the newborn period and continue until early childhood years (typically 3 different procedures), culminating with the passive venous blood return to the lungs without the pumping action of a ventricular chamber. The single functional ventricle is eventually solely used to maintain the systemic circulation (pump oxygenated/arterial blood to the aorta).

These severe lesions, as with the others mentioned above, will be present in their repaired stage in patients or athletes being evaluated for sports participation. Most of these will have by then normal oxygen saturation, with the venous and arterial blood completely separated through the various surgical procedures performed. Their functional capacity will largely depend on the presence of normal ventricular function, little or no atrioventricular valve regurgitation, absence of significant rhythm abnormalities, and unobstructed blood flow to both the pulmonary and the systemic circulations.

CONGENITAL HEART DISEASE AFTER INTERVENTION
Atrial Septal Defect

Surgical repair of the ASD should be evident by a healed median sternotomy, although nowadays most defects are closed through catheter intervention. The examination should be consistent with the lack of a murmur. A chest radiograph would reveal sternal wires, and a 12-lead electrocardiogram (ECG) should reveal sinus rhythm. Most surgical complications of ASD would have been addressed within the first 6 weeks postoperatively.

Similarly, device occlusion of ASD would be associated with no median thoracotomy scar, but there would be evidence of the device and its placement by chest radiograph or echocardiography. Clearance for participation should be made in consultation with a cardiologist who will verify placement of the device by echocardiography. The likelihood of device embolization or erosion through the aorta is rare,[27] and most individuals are cleared for competitive sports within 6 weeks of intervention.

Ventricular Septal Defect

Although device occlusion of VSDs is a possibility, most of these defects are addressed surgically and will be evident by a well-healed median sternotomy. The examination should reveal no murmur, although there may be a fixed split S2 consistent with a residual right bundle branch block (RBBB) from repair. The ECG may be entirely normal, but may reveal the aforementioned RBBB, which does not preclude the safety of the athlete in exercising. Consultation with a cardiologist before sports clearance is advocated, but these "repaired" athletes are usually safe to compete even if there are small residual defects.

Atrioventricular Septal Defect

Athletes with ASD exhibit a well-healed sternotomy on presentation given previous surgical repair. There may be a characteristic murmur of mitral regurgitation, not uncommon because the atrioventricular valves structure is altered in this defect, or of residual ASD/VSD. The degree of residual defect after repair determines the athlete's limitations. The repaired AVSD in and of itself is not a risk factor for SCD during exercise. There may be actual physical limitation based on the degree of residual mitral regurgitation. Consultation with a cardiologist is advisable to understand any physiologic limitations the patient might experience.

Frequently, the AVSD is associated with Down syndrome, a factor that alters the course of presentation of these defects as well as the age of diagnosis and repair. When these defects are repaired within the first year of life, Down syndrome does not affect the long-term results of the repair. However, there may be factors in children with Down syndrome that are extrinsic to the heart, affecting their ability to exercise.

Patent Ductus Arteriosus

The ductus arteriosus may be ligated by a lateral thoracotomy (so patients may have a scar beneath their armpit extending to the back) or they may be occluded with catheter intervention (coil or device). Six weeks after surgical or catheter intervention, these patients should be ready for competition, without further concerns.

Pulmonary Valve Stenosis

This lesion has perhaps the most benign natural history, being very amenable to catheter intervention with percutaneous balloon dilation to open up the valve. Even moderate to severe levels of obstruction are well tolerated and these individuals may be able to perform a very rigorous exercise regimen without symptoms. However, this is not advisable given the possible significant decrease in the right ventricular output with the association of increased heart rate, increased contractility, and decreased blood volume going into the pulmonary circulation; this in turn impacts the return of oxygenated blood to the left ventricle, compromising systemic output/circulation. Once the obstruction is relieved, these athletes can perform at normal levels, especially in the absence of significant residual obstruction. Evaluation with a cardiologist to determine the functional status of the pulmonary valve and advice on sports participation are warranted.

Aortic Valve Stenosis

As with pulmonary valve stenosis, this valvar disease is amenable to catheter intervention with percutaneous balloon dilation to open up the valve. A mild or moderate degree of narrowing may be well tolerated and generate no symptoms during exertion or sports participation. However, moderate to severe degrees will impact the performance, leading to substantial increase in the left ventricular pressure, and these individuals may be at risk of sudden cardiac events. They typically have a loud murmur on examination and may have a click in the setting of a bicuspid aortic valve. Even with successful relief of the obstruction with balloon valvuloplasty, some individuals may be left with residual regurgitation/leakage of the valve. This residual regurgitation/leakage of the valve needs to be followed, and eventually, patients might need surgical intervention to repair or replace the valve.

Exercise and sports participation will depend largely on the functional status of the valve, the left ventricle (degree of hypertrophy and function), or previous surgery for valve replacement and choice of valve. In individuals that undergo the so-called Ross procedure (removal of the native pulmonary valve with placement in the aortic position and replacement of the native pulmonary valve with a homograft/donor valve), they usually can participate at all levels. These individuals may follow with progressive dilation of the aorta, because it may occur in the setting of a bicuspid aortic valve, and therefore, high static exercise activities are usually discouraged.

Coarctation of the Aorta

Similar to the PDA, the isolated coarctation may be addressed by lateral thoracotomy (a scar beneath the armpit extending to the back), or there may have been catheter intervention with either angioplasty or stent implantation, where the aorta is dilated ± stent placement. It is important for these patients to follow-up with a cardiologist, because many have residual narrowing that may require intervention before safely exercising or engaging in sports competition. The examination may be remarkable for a murmur and systemic hypertension, even in the absence of residual obstruction, given the predisposition these patients have to develop systemic hypertension, especially if diagnosed later in childhood or adolescence.[28–30] The degree of residual coarctation can be estimated by blood pressure measurement in the upper extremity combined with a blood pressure measurement in the lower extremity (thigh cuff).

A cardiologist will obtain an echocardiogram and also likely an exercise stress test to risk-stratify assessing blood pressure elevation and development of ischemic changes on the ECG. Often the individual requires antihypertensive medications, which should not be a contraindication for many dynamic activities. However, consultation with the cardiologist is advised before making recommendations to this subgroup of athletes.

Tetralogy of Fallot

Surgical intervention usually confers restoration of normal physiology, with closure of the VSD and opening of the narrowed passage to the lungs (right ventricular outflow tract and pulmonary valve), although residual lesions are not uncommon that may require further intervention later in life. The most common residual lesion is the presence of pulmonary regurgitation, inherent to the repair performed in the first year of life. This leads to progressive overload of the right ventricle because of blood returning to the ventricle after every ventricular contraction. Typically, these patients will need another procedure for placement of a competent pulmonary valve between the right ventricle and the pulmonary artery.

There is an evident sternotomy scar in the middle of the chest from the surgery. The presence of a murmur is common that is originating in the right ventricular outflow tract. There is normal oxygen saturation. Rhythm abnormalities may occur and need surveillance. Thus, these patients should always be evaluated by a cardiologist before participating in sports. Their exercise capacity might be diminished because of the right ventricular overload, but many patients can perform at higher levels, especially in the absence of significant residual lesions. In addition, the benefits of exercise activity and sports participation have been documented in patients with repaired tetralogy of Fallot, with lower neurohormone levels and no adverse cardiac remodeling.[31–33]

Imaging with echocardiography to assess right ventricular size and ventricular function, as well as degree of valvar regurgitation, is routinely performed, as are the stress exercise test and Holter monitor (monitoring of the heart rate for 24 hours) for surveillance of asymptomatic arrhythmias. Cardiac magnetic resonance (MR) is very useful to determine right ventricular volume and function and to define the optimal timing for placement of a new pulmonary valve, typically occurring in the late teenage years or early adult life.

D-Transposition of the Great Arteries

D-transposition of the great arteries is repaired by switching the great arteries through a surgical procedure that then restores normal physiology. In other words, the aorta and pulmonary arteries are switched, although the valves remain attached to their respective ventricles; this means that the coronary arteries need to be translocated to the valve in the left side (the neo-aortic valve). Individuals who have undergone the arterial switch procedure in infancy typically do quite well and are safe to participate in most activities, with a few exceptions. Long-term complications of the arterial switch operation include narrowing or kinking of the coronary arteries and aortic root dilation.[34]

The aortic valve, or neo-aortic valve, was designed to be the pulmonary valve. As such, it may not sustain systemic pressure as well and it has a tendency to dilate. The coronary arteries translocate as "coronary buttons" at the time of operation. Because they are stretched and moved when the switch occurs, there may be kinking or an abnormal course of the coronary arteries with growth. Consultation with a cardiologist is recommended before release to competitive sports. The cardiologist will measure the aorta by echocardiography, evaluate the left ventricular function, assess the 12-lead ECG for any evidence of ischemic changes, obtain an exercise stress test with or without nuclear scan, and may consider additional imaging of the coronaries with computed tomographic (CT) angiography or cardiac MR in some situations.[35–37]

Single Ventricle

These lesions, as mentioned above, will be palliated (not resuming normal cardiac physiology) with multiple surgical and catheter intervention procedures in early infancy and childhood. The aim is to eventually have all the venous blood returning from the body to reach the pulmonary circulation directly to the lungs passively (without a pumping chamber), the so-called Fontan operation (also known as Fontan physiology).

Patients with Fontan physiology typically cannot perform at normal levels of exercise capacity, especially at moderate or high levels of dynamic and static exercises, given the limitation in maintaining increased cardiac output. However, preadolescent children usually have normal or near normal exercise capacity and may well tolerate competitive sports that are appropriate for their age. As they reach adolescence, the level of performance is significantly different and they may lag behind and not be able to perform because of development of symptoms.[38] Careful evaluation and individual assessment are warranted, taking into consideration risk factors inherent to the specific patient/athlete. If they are able to participate, they should be allowed to hydrate frequently and rest as needed (in other words, participate to their tolerance level). It is unquestionable, however, the benefits of exercise activity not only from a cardiovascular standpoint, but also, perhaps equally or more importantly, from a quality-of-life and psychological perspective.[3]

CORONARY ANOMALIES—CONGENITAL AND ACQUIRED
Anomalous Aortic Origin of a Coronary Artery

Anomalous aortic origin of a coronary artery (AAOCA) is a congenital abnormality of the origin or course of a coronary artery that arises from the aorta. Anomalous coronary originating from the opposite sinus of Valsalva constitutes the second leading cause of SCD among young athletes,[24] occurring unexpectedly during or immediately after exercise.[24,39,40] Furthermore, an increasing number of children and young adults are being incidentally found to have AAOCA on imaging studies performed for other reasons or as part of screening campaigns with MRI.[41] The estimated prevalence of AAOCA varies according to the source of data, but it ranges from 0.06% to 0.9% for anomalous right coronary artery (ARCA) to 0.025% to 0.15% for anomalous left coronary artery (ALCA).[42–45] Recently, a screening program using limited cardiac MRI in 1839 middle school children has estimated a prevalence of 0.6% for ARCA and (0.1%) for ALCA.[41]

The precise mechanism leading to sudden cardiac arrest or death in this condition is yet to be defined, although it is postulated that occlusion or compression of the anomalous vessel during exercise leads to myocardial ischemia and consequent lethal ventricular arrhythmia (ventricular tachycardia and fibrillation). Factors thought to account for this include abnormal ostium of the anomalous coronary artery, course between the aorta and the pulmonary artery (interarterial), and course inside the aortic wall (intramural). Often the first manifestation is a sudden event, and it is unknown why an athlete can exercise intensely for several years with no symptoms until the sentinel event. Other clinical manifestations that are present in approximately half of the patients include the occurrence of chest pain, syncope or near syncope, dizziness, or palpitations during exertion.[39,40,46]

The workup of patients with AAOCA typically includes assessment of exercise performance (stress test), myocardial perfusion, and imaging. However, the stress test has limitations given that in published series it rarely is positive for ischemia, even in those who suffered sudden death.[39,47] Similarly, stress nuclear myocardial perfusion carries the same burden of false positive and false negative results. Imaging is crucial in determining details of ostial anatomy and course of the anomalous vessel. Cardiac MRI and CT angiogram (**Figs. 1** and **2**) are the preferred modes of imaging and the choice between the 2 varies among institutions. Cardiac catheterization is rarely

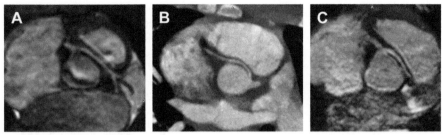

Fig. 1. CT angiogram of anomalous coronary arteries. Panel A depicts a single coronary artery arising from the right sinus of Valsalva. Panel B shows an anomalous right coronary artery arising from the left sinus of Valsalva with an interarterial course. Panel C shows an anomalous left coronary artery arising from the right sinus of Valsalva with an interarterial course.

used, except in some selected cases and usually only when additional information is sought, such as to determine coronary flow reserve and assess vessel compression throughout the cardiac cycle with intravascular ultrasound.

The management of these patients is challenging given the paucity of data in risk stratification and lack of longitudinal follow-up data. It varies significantly among different centers as recently published by the Congenital Heart Surgeons Society.[48] Strategies span from surgical approach to exercise restriction to doing nothing. In light of so many unknowns, in December 2012 the Coronary Anomalies Program was created at Texas Children's Hospital, aiming at a standardized approach to the diagnosis, management, and follow-up of these patients. A multidisciplinary team including a defined number of clinicians (cardiologists, surgeons, radiologists, and nurses), researchers, and outcomes program staff developed an algorithm (**Fig. 3**) that has been followed consistently.[49] Initial data analyzed in 90 patients seen and followed thus far and recently presented at the American College of Cardiology Scientific Session 2015 show that approximately 45% of patients are symptomatic on presentation, 4% present with either sudden cardiac arrest or shock, and 43% are asymptomatic. Of these, 35% underwent surgical intervention, and all have returned to exercise activities with no restrictions postoperatively.[50]

This area remains obscure where many questions are yet to be answered. However, efforts nationwide are ongoing to gather meaningful data with longitudinal follow-up of

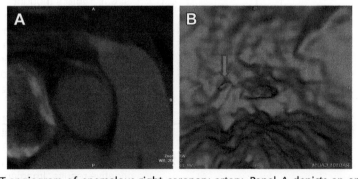

Fig. 2. CT angiogram of anomalous right coronary artery. Panel A depicts an anomalous right coronary artery arising from the left sinus of Valsalva with an interarterial course and narrowed course. Panel B shows virtual angioscopy with a normal, round left coronary ostium and a stenotic, slit-like ostium of the anomalous right coronary artery (*blue arrow*).

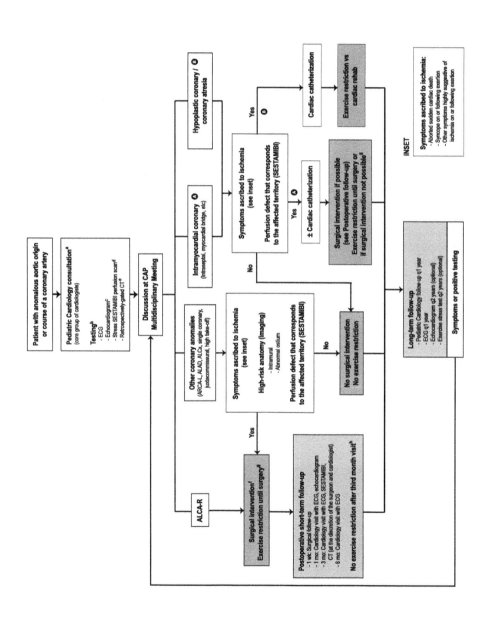

patients with AAOCA that will allow better risk stratification and, it is hoped, decrease the occurrence of SCD and unnecessary exercise restriction in these patients.

Kawasaki Disease

Kawasaki disease is an acquired inflammatory process that targets small vessels, particularly the coronary circulation, first described in 1967.[51] It has a robust clinical presentation with prolonged fever (>5 days), bilateral conjunctival injection, cervical lymphadenopathy (>1.5 cm), erythema of hands and feet with subsequent peeling, erythema, cracking of lips and tongue, and a polymorphous rash. Atypical (incomplete) presentation can occur in infants and older children and may go underdiagnosed. Without treatment in the acute phase, the occurrence of coronary involvement may reach one-fourth of all cases. With treatment, its incidence declines to less than 5% (statement Circ 2004). The changes in the coronary arteries vary from transient dilation/ectasia to substantial enlargement with aneurysm formation and later with areas of stenosis, leading to chest pain (angina), myocardial ischemia/infarction, ischemic cardiomyopathy, and sudden death.[52–54]

Here once again is the importance of the increased awareness to not only the occurrence of symptoms during exertion but also the past medical history of the athletes. Even those patients with no coronary artery involvement demonstrated in the acute phase may experience endothelial dysfunction (the inner layer of the vessel wall) and may be at increased risk of development of premature coronary artery disease in the future. It might be reasonable to ascertain that athletes with a history of Kawasaki disease in infancy or childhood have a cardiology evaluation performed to clear them for sports participation; in some instances, functional assessment may be indicated in selected cases.

THE PRACTICAL APPROACH
Athlete Versus Practitioner Preference and Choices

In general, athletes are strong willed and usually passionate about their given sport. There is physical, mental, and spiritual commitment, and any upset in this balance

---

Fig. 3. Clinical algorithm for evaluation and management of patients with anomalous aortic origin of a coronary artery developed by the Coronary Anomalies Program at Texas Children's Hospital. [a] Consent obtained for participation in prospective CHSS and TCH databases. [b] Additional studies (Holter, MRI, etc) may be performed depending on the clinical assessment. [c] External echocardiograms do not need to be repeated if the study is deemed appropriate. [d] SESTAMIBI perfusion scan not necessary on patients that present with aborted sudden cardiac death. [e] An external CT may be used if able to upload the images and the study provides all necessary information to make a decision. [f] Unroofing if significant intramural segment, neo-ostium creation or coronary translocation if intramural segment behind a commissure, coronary translocation or ostioplasty if no intramural segment. Surgical intervention will be offered for patients between 10 and 35 years of age. Other patients will be considered on a case-by-case basis. [g] Restriction from participation in all competitive sports and in exercise with moderate or high dynamic component (>40% maximal oxygen uptake - eg, soccer, tennis, swimming, basketball, American football).[20] [h] Postoperative patients will be cleared for exercise and competitive sports based on findings at the third month postoperative visit including results of SESTAMIBI and CT (if performed). ALAD, Anomalous left anterior descending artery; ALCA-R, Anomalous left coronary from the right sinus; ALCx, Anomalous left circumflex artery; ARCA-L, Anomalous right coronary from the left sinus; CAP, Coronary Anomalies Program. (Copyright © 2013 Texas Children's Hospital. Reprinted with permission.)

affects performance. The level of evidence concerning specific athletic activities in given congenital lesions is forthcoming in many areas, and it is important to advise the athlete that recommendations are based on the current level of evidence (36th Bethesda guidelines[4]). It is also important to remind the athlete that the practitioner is a part of the team advising them on their safety and risk, but the ultimate decision is theirs.

In some cases, the risk level is clear and there may be a preponderance of evidence advising against certain risky activities. For example, a patient with severe aortic stenosis and chest pain may be ill-advised to compete in a marathon until the aortic valve can be appropriately addressed. Although a patient with repaired tetralogy of Fallot with inherent severe aortic root dilation may be advised not to compete in body building based on the suspicion that elevated aortic pressures with weight-lifting may cause irreparable damage and even sudden death, there are no significant data to support the allegation. The athlete should, at all times, be educated by the practitioner with the best and most current data. In the absence of data, a frank discussion of the known physiology (a >300 mm Hg change in pressure in the aorta of the weight-lifting tetralogy of Fallot patient) must be put forth for the athlete's consideration. For instance, there is documentation of a significant pressure increase in the aorta during weight-lifting, in normal subjects, in excess of 200 mm Hg.[55] This extreme pressure in patients with tetralogy of Fallot is not known, but it is speculated as deleterious.

Medical-Legal Aspects

The first duty of the team physician is to protect the health and well-being of the athlete.

Many practitioners are adverse to mass sports screening because of the medical liability associated with false negative findings, or "missing" a lethal cardiac defect. Others are concerned with false positives, or overrestricting athletes, and the repercussions of preventing a talented athlete from achieving their ultimate goals, such as acquiring a college scholarship or pursuing a career in professional sports. An athlete prevented from participating in their sport of choice is subject to feelings of depression and defeat as well as potential loss of a lucrative career.

"Good clinical practice" is described as what is commonly done by physicians in the same specialty.[56] To that end, the American College of Cardiology developed the 36th Bethesda Guidelines[4] soon to be replaced by a set of guidelines, which have been updated with latest data affording the best level of evidence, as opposed to expert opinion. These guidelines are frequently cited in court as evidence of good medical practice. The inherent difficulty lies in the disagreement among experts in this field, where there may not be any level of evidence. Therefore, the best avoidance of liability is to keep up-to-date with the latest research, which will allow the practitioner "to act in a careful and diligent manner."[56] Some states have instituted laws demanding athlete screening before athletic participation; this continues to be a heated debate in various forums.

Awareness and Preparedness

The debate regarding the necessity and best methodology of pre-sports screening continues. What seems to be resolved, however, is the need for a backup plan. Automated defibrillators have become more affordable, and many public areas, schools, athletic clubs, and fields have access to these life-saving devices. The parents, coaches, and team members should all know the exact locations of these devices (which should be close!). In addition, basic life support skills should be mandated of each team member, high school graduate, and coach. There are several anecdotal cases and unsung heroes who have aborted SCD with automated external defibrillators and cardiopulmonary resuscitation. These methods are easy and cost-effective to save a life in any athlete, whether with known CHD or otherwise.

REFERENCES

1. Mitten MM, Maron BJ, Zipes DP. Task Force 12: legal aspects of the 36th Bethesda Conference recommendations. J Am Coll Cardiol 2005;45:1373–5.
2. Norozi K, Wessel A, Alpers V, et al. Incidence and risk distribution of heart failure in adolescents and adults with congenital heart disease after heart surgery. Am J Cardiol 2006;97:1238–43.
3. Dean PN, Gillespie CW, Greene EA, et al. Sports participation and quality of life in adolescents and young adults with congenital heart disease. Congenit Heart Dis 2015;10(2):169–79.
4. Maron BJ, Zipes DP. 36th Bethesda Conference: eligibility recommendations for competitive athletes with cardiovascular abnormalities. J Am Coll Cardiol 2005; 45:1313–75.
5. Baggish AL, Wood MJ. Athlete's heart and cardiovascular care of the athlete: scientific and clinical update. Circulation 2011;123:2723–35.
6. Keteyian SJ, Schairer JR. Exercise training and prescription. In: Lawless CE, editor. Sports cardiology essentials. Evaluation, management and case studies. 1st edition. New York: Springer Science + Business Media; 2010. p. 63–84.
7. Levine BD. Exercise and sports cardiology. New York: McGraw-Hill; 2001.
8. Bruning RS, Sturek M. Benefits of exercise training on coronary blood flow in coronary artery disease patients. Prog Cardiovasc Dis 2015;57:443–53.
9. Hahn VS, Lenihan DJ, Ky B. Cancer therapy-induced cardiotoxicity: basic mechanisms and potential cardioprotective therapies. J Am Heart Assoc 2014;3(21): e000665.
10. Cade WT, Reeds DN, Overton ET, et al. Pilot study of pioglitazone and exercise training effects on basal myocardial substrate metabolism and left ventricular function in HIV-positive individuals with metabolic complications. HIV Clin Trials 2013;14:303–12.
11. Egbe A, Uppu S, Lee S, et al. Temporal variation of birth prevalence of congenital heart disease in the Unoited States. Congenit Heart Dis 2015;10(1):43–50.
12. Hoffman JI, Kaplan S. The incidence of congenital heart disease. J Am Coll Cardiol 2002;39:1890–900.
13. Van der Linde D, Konings EE, Slager MA, et al. Birth prevalence of congenital heart disease worldwide: a systematic review and meta-analysis. J Am Coll Cardiol 2011;58:2241–7.
14. Sable C, Foster E, Uzark K, et al. Best practices in managing transition to adulthood for adolescents with congenital heart disease: the transition process and medical and psychological issues. A scientific statement from the American Heart Association. Circulation 2011;1454:1485.
15. Marelli AJ, Mackie AS, Ionescu-Ittu R, et al. Congenital heart disease in the general population. Changing prevalence and age distribution. Circulation 2007;115: 163–72.
16. Vohra J, Sathe S, Warren R, et al. Malignant ventricular arrhythmias in patients with mitral valve prolapse and mild mitral regurgitation. Pacing Clin Electrophysiol 1993;16:387–93.
17. Nishimura RA, McGoon MD, Shub C, et al. Echocardiographically documented mitral-valve prolapse. Long-term follow-up of 237 patients. N Engl J Med 1985; 313(21):1305–9.

18. Duren DR, Becker AE, Dunning AJ. Long-term follow-up of idiopathic mitral valve prolapse in 300 patients: a prospective study. J Am Coll Cardiol 1988;11:42–7.

19. Sriram CS, Syed FF, Ferguson E, et al. Malignant bileaflet mitral valve prolapse syndrome in patients with otherwise idiopathic out-of-hospital cardiac arrest. J Am Coll Cardiol 2013;62:222–30.

20. Mitchell JH, Haskell W, Snell P, et al. Task Force 8: classification of sports. J Am Coll Cardiol 2005;45:1364–7.

21. Maron BJ, Pellicia A. The heart of trained athletes: cardiac remodeling and the risk of sports, including sudden death. Circulation 2006;114:1633–44.

22. Longhurst JC, Kelly AR, Gonyea WJ, et al. Echocardiographic mass in distance runners and weight lifters. J Appl Physiol 1980;48:154–62.

23. Pellicia A, Spataro A, Caselli G, et al. Absence of left ventricular wall thickening in athletes participating in intense power training. Am J Cardiol 1993;72:1048–55.

24. Maron BJ, Doerer JJ, Haas TS, et al. Sudden death in young competitive athletes: analysis of 1866 deaths in the United States, 1980–2006. Circulation 2009;119: 1085–92.

25. Monin JL, Lancelloti P, Monchi M, et al. Risk score for predicting outcome in patients with asymptomatic aortic stenosis. Circulation 2009;120:69–75.

26. Verzelatti A. Medical malpractice and the professional legal responsibility of the sports physician. J Law Med 2013;21:179–86.

27. Amin Z, Hijazi ZM, Bass JL, et al. Erosion of Amplatzer septal occluder device after closure of secundum atrial septal defects: review of registry of complications and recommendations to minimize future risks. Catheter Cardiovasc Interv 2004;63(4):496–502.

28. Krieger EV, Clair M, Opotowsky AR, et al. Correlation of exercise response ion repaired coarctation of the aorta to left ventricular mass and geometry. Am J Cardiol 2013;111(3):406–11.

29. Morgan GJ, Lee KJ, Chaturvedi R, et al. Systemic blood pressure after stent management for arch coarctation implications for clinical care. JACC Cardiovasc Interv 2013;6(2):192–201.

30. Bocelli A, Favilli S, Pollini I, et al. Prevalence and long-term predictors of left ventricular hypertrophy, late hypertension, and hypertensive response to exercise after successful aortic coarctation repair. Pediatr Cardiol 2013;34(3):620–9.

31. Van der Bom T, Winter MM, Knaake JL, et al. Long-term benefits of exercise training in patients with a systemic right ventricle. J Cardiol 2015;179:105–11.

32. Dupen N, Kapusta L, de Rijke YB, et al. The effect of exercise training on cardiac remodeling in children and young adults with corrected tetralogy of Fallot or Fontan circulation: a randomized controlled trial. J Cardiol 2015;179:97–104.

33. Duppen N, Geerdink LM, Kuipers IM, et al. Regional ventricular performance and exercise training in children and young adults after repair of tetralogy of Fallot: randomized controlled pilot study. Circ Cardiovasc Imaging 2015;8(4) [pii: e002006].

34. Villafane J, Lantin-Hermoso MR, Bhatt AB, et al. D-transposition of the great arteries: the current era of the arterial switch operation. J Am Coll Cardiol 2014; 64(5):498–511.

35. Mahle WT, McBride MG, Paridon SM. Exercise performance after the arterial switch operation for D-transposition of the great arteries. Am J Cardiol 2001; 87(6):753–8.

36. Chen RH, Wong SJ, Wong WH, et al. Arterial mechanics at rest and during exercise in adolescents and young adults after arterial switch operation for complete transposition of the great arteries. Am J Cardiol 2014;113(4):713–8.

37. Harris DM, Schelbert EB, Wong TC, et al. Myocardial ischemia after arterial switch procedure detected by regadenoson stress cardiac magnetic resonance. Int J Cardiol 2014;174(1):e16–8.
38. Khiabani RH, Whitehead KK, Han D, et al. Exercise capacity in single-ventricle patients after Fontan correlates with haemodynamic energy loss in TCPC. Heart 2015;101(2):139–43.
39. Basso C, Maron BJ, Corrado D, et al. Clinical profile of congenital coronary artery anomalies with origin from the wrong aortic sinus leading to sudden death in young competitive athletes. J Am Coll Cardiol 2000;35:1493–501.
40. Taylor AJ, Rogan KM, Virmani R. Sudden cardiac death associated with isolated congenital coronary artery anomalies. J Am Coll Cardiol 1992;20:640–7.
41. Angelini P, Shah NR, Uribe CE, et al. Novel MRI-based screening protocol to identify adolescents at high risk of sudden cardiac death. J Am Coll Cardiol 2013;61:E1621.
42. Drory Y, Turetz Y, Hiss Y, et al. Sudden unexpected death in persons less than 40 years of age. Am J Cardiol 1991;68:1388–92.
43. Davis JA, Cecchin F, Jones TK, et al. Major coronary artery anomalies in a pediatric population: incidence and clinical importance. J Am Coll Cardiol 2001;37: 593–7.
44. Angelini P, Villason S, Chan AV, et al. Normal and anomalous coronary arteries in humans, in coronary artery anomalies. In: Angelini P, editor. Coronary artery anomalies. Philadelphia: Lippincott Williams & Wilkins; 1999. p. 27–150.
45. Prakken NH, Cramer MJ, Olimulder MA, et al. Screening for proximal coronary artery anomalies with 3-dimensional MR coronary angiography. Int J Cardiovasc Imaging 2010;26:701–10.
46. Eckart RE, Scoville SL, Campbell CL, et al. Sudden death in young adults: a 25-year review of autopsies in military recruits. Ann Intern Med 2004;141:829–34.
47. Brothers JA, McBride MG, Seliem MA, et al. Evaluation of myocardial ischemia after surgical repair of anomalous aortic origin of a coronary artery in a series of pediatric patients. J Am Coll Cardiol 2007;50:2078–82.
48. Brothers J, Gaynor JW, Paridon S, et al. Anomalous aortic origin of a coronary artery with an interarterial course: understanding current management strategies in children and young adults. Pediatr Cardiol 2009;30:911–21.
49. Mery CM, Lawrence SM, Krishnamurthy R, et al. Anomalous aortic origin of a coronary artery: toward a standardized approach. Semin Thorac Cardiovasc Surg 2014;26(2):110–22.
50. Molossi S, Mery CM, Krishnamurthy R, et al. Standardized approach to patients with anomalous aortic origin of a coronary artery: results from the coronary anomalies program at Texas Children's Hospital. J Am Coll Cardiol 2015;65(10):A501.
51. Kawasaki T. Acute febrile mucocutaneous lymph node syndrome: clinical observations of 50 cases. Japan J Allergology 1967;16:178.
52. Committee on Rheumatic Fever Endocarditis, Kawasaki Disease, Council on Cardiovascular Disease in the Young, American Heart Association, American Academy of Pediatrics, Newburger JW, Takahashi M, Gerber MA, et al. Diagnosis, treatment, and long-term management of Kawasaki disease: a statement for health professionals from the Committee on Rheumatic Fever, Endocarditis and Kawasaki Disease, Council on Cardiovascular Disease in the Young, American Heart Association. Circulation 2004;110(17):2747–71.
53. Harmon KG, Drezner JA, Maleszewski JJ, et al. Pathogenesis of sudden cardiac death in National Collegiate Athletic Association athletes. Circ Arrhythm Electrophysiol 2014;7:198–204.

54. Attili A, Hensley AK, Jones FD, et al. Echocardiography and coronary CT angiography imaging of variations in coronary anatomy and coronary abnormalities in athletic children: detection of coronary abnormalities that create a risk for sudden death. Echocardiography 2013;30:225–33.
55. Elefteriades JA, Hatzaras I, Tranquilli MA, et al. Weight lifting and rupture of silent aortic aneurysms. JAMA 2003;290(21):2803.
56. Panhuyzen-Goedkoop NM, Smeets JL. Legal responsibilities of physicians when making participation decisions in athletes with cardiac disorders: do guidelines provide a solid legal footing? Br J Sports Med 2014;48(15):1193–5.

The Historical Perspective of Athletic Sudden Death

Walter J. Hoyt Jr, MD[a],*, Peter N. Dean, MD[a], Robert W. Battle, MD[b]

KEYWORDS

• Sudden death • Athletes • Historical perspective • Sports cardiology

KEY POINTS

• From ancient Greece to modern elite-level sports, the athlete has been celebrated within small communities and at the international level.
• Athletic sudden death is a rare event, but the sudden death of an athlete, particularly in youth with the paradox of vitality and mortality, seems particularly tragic and often difficult to reconcile, increasing the magnitude of the tragedy.
• Screening athletes for conditions associated with sudden death varies by country, competition level, and physician opinion.

INTRODUCTION

Since antiquity, the athlete has been elevated to a heroic status both within small communities and at the international level. The paradox of heroic fitness and the shocking occurrence of an athlete's death increases the magnitude of the tragedy within and beyond the athlete's community. Although population studies reassure us that sudden death is rare for the athlete, sudden death of an athlete, particularly a youth, seems especially tragic and often difficult to reconcile. Death in the athlete as a written subject is reviewed in an effort to better appreciate the upsetting impact of an athlete's death. Over the past 2 centuries, initiatives have increasingly developed to protect the athlete, which have provided modern medicine with the perhaps impossible task of keeping athletes safe. In addition, the historical origin of sport, the athlete as a status, and sudden death are examined to understand their respective inputs to the calamity of athletic sudden death. In this article, athlete sudden death is analyzed from a historical and literary perspective and the development of modern initiatives to protect athletes from sudden death is reviewed.

[a] Department of Pediatric Cardiology, University of Virginia, PO Box 800386, Charlottesville, VA 22908, USA; [b] Department of Cardiology, University of Virginia, PO Box 800386, Charlottesville, VA 22908, USA
* Corresponding author. UVA Children's Hospital Heart Center, PO Box 800386, Charlottesville, VA 22908.
E-mail address: WH7D@hscmail.mcc.virginia.edu

Clin Sports Med 34 (2015) 571–585
http://dx.doi.org/10.1016/j.csm.2015.03.002
0278-5919/15/$ – see front matter © 2015 Elsevier Inc. All rights reserved.

sportsmed.theclinics.com

ATHLETICS AND THE ATHLETE
Definition and Origins of Ancient and Modern Sport

At one time or another, organized athletics have been used to worship deities, mourn at funerals, determine pay grade, train soldiers, celebrate rulers, entertain spectators, and as a means to fame and profit.[1–5] Athletic contests began in various ancient civilizations around the Mediterranean as early as 4000 BC.[1] Although the Phoenicians, Egyptians, Chinese, and Japanese practiced athletic competition, the Greeks provide the most famous example of elite athletics from antiquity.[1,6,7] In addition to numerous local festivals, there were 4 primary international games for elite athletes in ancient Greece: the Olympic games dedicated to Zeus at Olympia beginning around 776 BC; the Pythian games dedicated to Apollo at Delphi beginning around 586 BC; the Isthmian games dedicated to Poseidon at the Isthmus of Corinth beginning around 582 BC; and the Nemean games dedicated to Zeus at both Nemea and Argos beginning around 573 BC.[3] Dedicated spectators endured arduous travel to the festival camp not only from around the Peloponnese but as far as Cadiz and Egypt.[4] Athletes competed in 12 sports at Olympia over the course of 5 days, which included 2-horse and 4-horse chariot racing; Pentathlon, which combined discus, javelin, long-jumping, running, and wrestling; youth competitions; 200-m, 400-m, and 3600-m running races; wrestling; boxing; the pankration, a violent sport similar to modern mixed martial arts; and a race-in-armor.[4] Herodotus and Plutarch noted that victors of the preeminent games won relative fortunes in proportion to the athlete's fame, event popularity, and reputation of the festival.[2] The prodigious influence of athletics on ancient Greek culture is highlighted by the widespread use of the athlete, sport, and festivals as a common subject in Greek art, religion, literature, and mythology.[3,8–11]

Although the origins of specific sports are scattered throughout the world, the resurgence of modern athletics in the West is predominately attributed to the British, with increasing organization of sport in the nineteenth century.[1] The first national championship in athletics is attributed to the Amateur Athletic Club in 1866, and the first governing athletic association to the Amateur Athletics Association in 1880. This development was shortly followed in the United States by the National Association of the Amateur Athletes of America in 1879 and Amateur Athletic Union in 1888.[1] The Olympic games themselves remained on a 1502-year hiatus as a stage for international competition until their revival in 1896 by the French Baron Pierre de Coubertin.[1,4,12] The popularity of athletics exponentially increased over the following century, and the centennial Olympic games in Atlanta included 10,600 participants from 197 countries.[12] Participation has similarly increased at the national and local levels, with the National Collegiate Athletics Association (NCAA) noting that more than 470,000 athletes participated in varsity college athletics during the 2013–2014 season.[13]

Heroic Status of the Athlete

The elite athlete has enjoyed a celebrated status since antiquity.[2,4,14] Not only were Greek champions greatly admired but some also were heralded as gods among mortals.[2,12] In circa AD 170, Lucian, addressing Apollo in writing, wittily mocks the god that his shrines are no longer as popular as the statues of the athlete Polydamas for both worship and prayers of healing.[2] Pausanias melds the athlete with mythology in the story of Theagenes, a champion of both the pyx and pankration at Olympia and Delphi, by attributing Theagenenes's success to being a purported illegitimate son of Herakles rather than purely human.[2] Greek deities themselves were also portrayed as athletes; Herakles, the Greek patron of wrestling, is commonly depicted as a wrestler in sculpture and pottery.[2,8–11] Analogously, Greek images of some gods were likely modeled from real-life athlete heroes. The wide variation in age and likeness of Herakles' depiction in classical art, which generally matches Philostros's description of the ideal wrestler, support the likelihood that the mythological subject was modeled from a variety of successful athletes.[2,8–11] Modern elite athletes receive similar fanfare, with some among the highest paid celebrities. Although no longer viewed as a divine source of healing, sports teams frequently visit inpatient wards at children's hospitals to encourage the sick, particularly the chronically ill.

The understanding of the competing athlete is both so widespread and so striking that numerous writers have invoked the metaphor of an athlete hero to describe concepts and figures of far greater heroism from a much grander arena. Theodore Roosevelt famously described a struggling athlete during his speech "Citizenship in a Republic", delivered in Paris in 1910[15]:

It is not the critic who counts; not the man who points out how the strong man stumbles, or where the doer of deeds could have done them better. The credit belongs to the man who is actually in the arena, whose face is marred by dust and sweat and blood; who strives valiantly; who errs, who comes short again and again, because there is no effort without error and shortcoming; but who does actually strive to do the deeds; who knows great enthusiasms, the great devotions; who spends himself in a worthy cause; who at the best knows in the end the triumph of high achievement, and who at the worst, if he fails, at least fails while daring greatly, so that his place shall never be with those cold and timid souls who neither know victory nor defeat.

The Apostle Paul also used the analogy of athletic struggle in his letters to Timothy and the Corinthians. Interestingly, both epistles were sent to residents of Greek cities: Timothy at Ephesus and the fledgling Christian church at Corinth:

I have fought the good fight, I have finished the race, I have kept the faith. Now there is in store for me the [victor's] crown of righteousness.
—2 Timothy 4:7–8[16]

Do you not know that in a race all the runners run, but only one gets the prize? Run in a way as to get the prize. Everyone who competes in the games goes into strict training. They do it to get a crown that will not last, but we do it to get a crown that will last forever. Therefore I do not run like someone running aimlessly; I do not fight like a boxer beating the air. No, I strike a blow to my body and make it my slave so that after I have preached to others, I myself will not be disqualified for the prize.
—1 Corinthians 9:24–27[16]

Although that association remains familiar today, the veneration of the athletic hero as a bastion of strength, fitness, and vitality contradicts the seemingly impossible tragedy of an athlete's unexpected death.

DEATH IN SPORT

"Death is an inevitable and accepted conclusion to life."[12] Many Christian traditions remind of the body's inescapable destination in liturgy: "Remember that you are dust, and to dust you shall return."[17] Despite a scientific or spiritual understanding of mortality, the sudden death of an athlete, particularly in youth, seems particularly tragic and often difficult to reconcile. The *Los Angeles Times* sports columnist Jim

Murray denotes it "the most unwelcome spectator"; the Roman poet Lucretius depicts it as "a pang among the flowers."[4,12] Although numerous population studies estimate athletic sudden death to be a rare event, the consequences of athletic sudden death "resound far beyond the individuals directly affected."[14,18–26] Because we are spectators, teammates, and coaches, athletic sudden death is often a witnessed death. Increased media coverage and the Internet allow the event to be readily accessible and reviewable.[14] Age, disease, or hospital walls cannot obscure sudden death in the athlete, which enhances its impact. In an attempt to better appreciate the somber effect of athletic sudden death and remember the lives that seem prematurely concluded by it, the following section reviews the literary subject of athletic sudden death and some of the athletes affected by it.

The Death of an Athlete in Literature

The association of sport and the risk of death was known to both modern and ancient authors.[27] Ernest Hemingway is generally attributed to using the relative risk of death to define sport itself: "There are only three sports: bullfighting, motor racing, and mountaineering; all the rest are merely games."[28] He expounded on the first event in his aptly named book *Death in the Afternoon*.[29] Another master of the short story, Edgar Allen Poe, wrote "A Tale of the Ragged Mountains", inspired by his wanderings in the countryside surrounding Charlottesville during his time at the University of Virginia.[30,31] This obscure tale vividly captures the phenotypic description of Marfan syndrome, which is known to carry risk of sudden death during exertion by aortic dissection.[31–33] Although the protagonist's demise was notably iatrogenic rather than secondary to disease, the tale is medically noteworthy for the profoundly eloquent description of dolichostenomelia published 52 years before the first scientific description of the syndrome by Antoine Marfan in 1896.[31,34]

The English poet and classicist A.E. Housman captures the effect of the sudden death of a young athlete more directly than anywhere else in verse.[35] Straightaway, Housman shows the townspeople supporting the athlete, who is undoubtedly a community hero, first in victory and then in mourning. The poem then leads the reader through imagery of transient glory frozen by the athlete's death, preserving the honor rather than allowing its inevitable erosion by time, age, and future champions. Although steadfastly melancholy, the poem reconciles the life lost in creating a legend in memory, whose decline is never to be known.

> The time you won your town the race,
>   We chaired you through the market-place;
>   Man and boy stood cheering by,
>   And home we brought you shoulder-high.
>
> Today, the road all runners come,
>   Shoulder-high we bring you home,
>   And set you at your threshold down,
>   Townsman of a stiller town.
>
> Smart lad, to slip betimes away
>   From fields where glory does not stay
>   And early though the laurel grows
>   It withers quicker than the rose.
>
> Eyes the shady night has shut

Cannot see the record cut,
And silence sounds no worse than cheers
After earth has stopped the ears:

Now you will not swell the rout
  Of lads that wore their honours out,
  Runners whom renown outran
  And the name died before the man.

So set, before its echoes fade,
  The fleet foot on the sill of shade,
  And hold to the low lintel up
  The still-defended challenge-cup.

And round that early-laurelled head
  Will flock to gaze the strengthless dead,
  And find unwithered on its curls
  The garland briefer than a girl's.
                    —A.E. Housman, "To an Athlete Dying Young" (1896)[35]

The Death of an Athlete in Ancient Athletics

The most famous athlete sudden death in Greek antiquity was that of Pheidippides in 490 BC.[2] Pheidippides, an Athenian hemerodromos, or foot messenger, was dispatched by his generals to Sparta to ask for assistance against the invading Persians.[2,4] His athletic endeavor was 3-fold: running between 136 and 153 miles (218 and 246 km) over rugged terrain from Athens to Sparta in less than 2 days, fighting in the Battle of Marathon itself, and running "with his armor hot from battle" the famed 26.3 miles (42.3 km) back to Athens from Marathon.[2,4] On his return, he pronounced, "Be happy! We have won!," simultaneously collapsing and dying.[2] Herodotus, Plutarch, Lucian, and Pliny attributed these feats to several athletes, which were consolidated in legend to Philippides, a.k.a. Pheidippides. The feasibility of such feats has been questioned but has been proved individually: the 26.3 miles by countless marathoners and Ironman finishers, the 153-mile run from Athens to Sparta by a British Royal Air Force officer in less than 36 hours in 1982, which has since germinated into the annual Spartathlon race.[4] Moreover, Pheidippides, employed as a hemerodromos, inherently covered long distances on foot regularly and likely would complement the methodology of renowned running coach Arthur Lydiard in emphasis of a strong aerobic foundation.[2,36,37] Indeed, Herodotus noted that Pheidippides was chosen by his generals because he "was used to doing this sort of thing."[2,4]

Most athlete deaths in the ancient games were traumatic and leave less speculation to etiology. Primary accounts note the death of a pankratiast by strangulation, a boxer by open chest trauma, and a youth by impalement of a javelin.[2] While these are rather extreme and gruesome examples of athlete death, the Greeks recognized a very real risk of death in athletics, concluding the reliably bloody day of chariot races with a ceremonial sacrifice over the burial mound of the mythological hero Pelops.[4]

Sudden Cardiac Death in Modern Athletics

Sudden death persists in modern athletics despite advances in medical knowledge and safety precautions. When the sad tragedy of an athlete death occurs, medicine and the sport's governing body should analyze, if possible, factors contributing to the death and consider approaches to prevent similar events in the future. Hank Gathers, a standout division I college basketball player for Loyola Marymount, was the second player in NCAA history to lead the nation in scoring and rebounding and played a critical role in the performance and aspirations of the school in the 1989 to 1990 season.[14,38–40] Gathers fainted on the court in December, 1989, causing him to miss 3 games.[14,39] During the initial evaluation, exercise-induced ventricular dysrhythmias were documented and believed to be secondary to underlying myocarditis.[14,39] His prescribed propranolol was purportedly taken intermittently because of its limiting effects on his exercise capacity.[14,39,40] Under what was undoubtedly intense pressure for Gathers to compete, he was medically cleared with the presence of an external defibrillator at courtside.[39,40] On March 4, 1990, Gathers collapsed during competition; he was brought outside the gym before application of the external defibrillator. Defibrillation and cardiopulmonary resuscitation (CPR) were not effective at resolving his pulseless arrest, and he was declared dead after more than an hour of resuscitation at a nearby emergency room.[39,40] The legacy of Gathers's death remains a sad and sore mark in recent sports history. The eerily similar story of professional basketball player and captain of the Boston Celtics Reggie Lewis followed just 3 years later, with its ominous warnings clear in hindsight.[41,42] Lewis experienced multiple episodes of exertional dizziness, and a team of prominent cardiologists recommended placement of an internal cardiac defibrillator and immediate end to his basketball career.[41,42] With understandable shock and denial, he transferred his care to another hospital and physician, who cleared him to play under medical supervision.[41,42] Two months later, he died suddenly, not in vigorous competition, but in casual shooting drills with the team.[41,42] The controversy, legal disputes, and medical discussion that followed Gathers's and Lewis's death has significantly changed sports cardiology's methodology regarding the approach, clearance, and liability associated with the medical management of elite athletes.[39,40,43]

The extent of those with athletic achievements and contributions to sport prematurely concluded stretches far beyond the basketball court. Fran Crippen, an elite swimmer and NCAA All-American while at the University of Virginia, died during open water competition in the United Arab Emirates, where air temperature was 100°F and water temperature was 87°F.[44–46] Several other competitors were hospitalized from heat stroke, and the controversial safety measures of the race have resulted in competition guideline reform.[44,45] Andy Palmer, an elite marathoner, coach, doctorate of sports psychology, and cofounder of ZAP Fitness Foundation, died unexpectedly from a myocardial infarction during a training run in 2002 at 48 years of age.[47–49] Jeff Drenth, an elite distance runner, died in 1994 at age 24 years from arrhythmia.[50] Flo Hyman, an Olympic volleyball player with Marfan syndrome, died of aortic dissection in 1986.[14] National Basketball Association star and Louisiana State University basketball legend Pete Maravich died after the conclusion of his competitive career during a pick-up basketball game; he was found to have a single coronary artery.[14,51] Tom Simpson died at 29 years of age on the ascent of Mont Ventoux during the 1967 Tour de France, likely secondary to amphetamine use.[52,53] Cameroon footballer Marc-Vivien Foe died during competition at 28 years of age from hypertrophic cardiomyopathy.[54] Many other athletes have died unexpectedly, including Jason Collier (basketball), Sergei Grinkov (ice skating), and Thomas Herrion (football).[14]

PROTECTING THE ATHLETE: STUDYING, DISCUSSING, SCREENING, AND PREVENTING SUDDEN CARDIAC DEATH

Development of Rule and Safety Organizations to Protect the Game and the Athlete

The advent of current sports governing associations generally followed tragedies that highlighted a need for safer play and consistent rules. The 1905 college football season, during which 18 deaths and more than 100 major injuries occurred, raised concerns to the national level, including the then President of the United States Theodore Roosevelt.[55,56] Football was still evolving significantly at that time, only recently differentiating itself from rugby and varying greatly from today's rules of play.[1] Roosevelt loved vigorous physical activity, particularly "rough sports which call for pluck, endurance, and physical address," recognizing its educational merits through the development of strength and courage, and noting the need for increased safety.[56] The combined effort from President Roosevelt and university leaders resulted in the formation of the Intercollegiate Athletic Association, which was renamed the NCAA in 1910.[55] The NCAA now governs 23 sports at more than 1000 institutions.[13]

Epidemiology of Athlete Death

In modern athletics, cardiac disease is responsible for most athlete deaths at multiple age and competitive levels.[18–26] In young athletes overall, the incidence ranges from 0.20 to 2.30 deaths/100,000 person-years; in high school athletes, from 0.20 to 1.14; in US College Athletes, from 1.20 to 2.28; and 13 in military recruits (**Table 1**).[18–26] The incidence of death among young athletes varied greatly with nationality and the population studied.[19,25,26] The incidence of death increased among competitive collegiate athletes and is particularly high in the African American population.[22,23] In the largest US study, by Maron and colleagues,[19] when sudden cardiac death was the confirmed cause of death (690 cases), the most common causes included hypertrophic cardiomyopathy (HCM), 251 deaths (36%); coronary artery abnormality, 119 deaths (17%); myocarditis, 41 deaths (6%); and arrhythmogenic right ventricular cardiomyopathy (ARVC), 30 deaths (4%). Contrastingly, ARVC was the most common cardiac cause of sudden athlete death in the European population.[25,26] Sudden cardiac death is exceeded by suicide, drug overdose, and accidents, which play a major role in overall causes of mortality in US college athletes.[22,23]

Primary Prevention: Athlete Screening and Challenges

The approach to screening athletes for conditions associated with sudden death varies greatly by country, competition level, and physician opinion, but the goal is uniform. The reasoning for screening includes prevention of athletic sudden death during training or competition by all reasonable measures; detection of undiagnosed congenital or acquired heart disease that could affect health, performance, and longevity; and detection of inheritable conditions that could lead to evaluation and treatment in family members.[57] The fourth edition of the *Preparticipation Physical Evaluation* (PPE-4) is the current athlete screening approach endorsed by the American Heart Association.[58–60] PPE-4 consists of an athlete history, family history, and physical examination, with concerns prompting additional evaluation such as electrocardiography (ECG) or echocardiography.[58]

Challenges in Decision Making: Cost, Cardiac Adaptations, and Consequences

PPE-4 is limited only to those athletes who present with symptoms or who have symptomatic family members. Although relatively uncommon, many dangerous

Table 1
Incidence of sudden death in athletes in recent studies

Title	Study Characteristics						Athlete Deaths	
	First Author	Publication Year	Years Studied	Country	Group Type	Age Range (y)	Number	Incidence of Death (per 100,000 Person-Years)
Sudden deaths in young competitive athletes: analysis of 1866 deaths in the United States, 1980–2006[19]	Maron	2009	1980–2006	United States	Young athletes	8–39	1866	0.61
Exercise and the risk of sudden cardiac death[25]	Corrado	2006	1979–1999	Italy	Young athletes	12–35	55	2.30
Incidence and etiology of sports-related sudden cardiac death in Denmark[26]	Holst	2011	2000–2006	Denmark	Young athletes	12–35	15	1.21
Incidence of sudden cardiac arrest in high school student athletes on school campus[21]	Toresdahl	2014	2009–2011	United States	High school students	—	18	1.14
Prevalence of sudden cardiac death during competitive sports activities in Minnesota high school athletes[20]	Maron	1998	1985–1997	United States	High school students	13–19	3	0.20
Incidence of sudden cardiac death in National Collegiate Athletic Association athletes[23]	Harmon	2011	2004–2008	United States	College athletes	17–23	80 (medical)	2.28
Sudden death in college athletes[22]	Maron	2014	2002–2011	United States	College athletes	17–26	64 (medical)	1.20
Sudden death in young adults: a 25-year review of autopsies in military recruits[24]	Eckart	2004	1977–2001	United States	Military recruits	18–35	126	13.00

cardiovascular conditions may be asymptomatic and go undetected by PPE-4.[14,61–65] Some life-threatening conditions which may be asymptomatic before arrest include: HCM, ARVC, congenital long QT, Brugada syndromes, ventricular preexcitation (Wolff-Parkinson-White), and an anomalous coronary artery.[14,61–65] Some countries and sports organizations follow a more detailed evaluation, including ECG or transthoracic echocardiography. For more than 25 years, Italy has subsidized a national ECG screening program, wherein all potential competitive athletes are screened with a 12-lead ECG.[66] The implementation has yielded a decrease in the incidence of sudden athlete death in Italy, and some have advocated for a similar program across Europe and in America.[66–68] The United States does not currently endorse a universal ECG program, mainly because of impracticality, excessive cost, and population differences.[69,70] Although the debate on additional screening techniques continues, the extent of screening and in which athletes screening is indicated cannot be answered definitively, and continued research has been called for in lieu of persistent controversy.[71]

The adaptation of an athlete's heart to the rigors of exercise is known to cause dilation, hypertrophy, and ECG changes; these changes vary greatly by gender, ethnicity, training intensity, and sport.[72–86] Cardiac changes as a result of exercise were noted as early as 1899 in Nordic skiers and Harvard rowers.[87,88] A major challenge of accurate athlete screening is the gray zone between normal adaptation to exercise and true disease.[18] The interpretation of an athlete's ECG and echocardiogram has also been a subject of discussion and evolution. The initial large consensus regarding interpretation of athlete ECGs was published by the European Society of Cardiology in 2010.[89] Although momentous in helping support physician decision making, it was subject to an excessively high false-positive rate, particularly in those of Afro-Caribbean descent, and is likely impractical in countries with a diverse ethnic background such as the United States.[89–91] The Seattle criteria of athlete ECG evaluation greatly enhanced specificity in 2012, which was further enhanced by the refined criteria by Sharma and colleagues in 2014.[91,92] The refined criteria are also noteworthy for their comparison of all 3 criteria with a population of trained athletes and a population of athletes with known HCM.[91]

Additional concerns have been raised about the reasoning behind some trends in athlete disqualification, particularly because the risk of some conditions may not statistically justify absolute disqualification.[93] Moreover, only competitive sports are limitable by physicians, and recreational activities, which are generally unsupervised by any trained medical personnel, are out of the physician's control. Because the absolute risk of sudden death is not fully understood in many conditions, limiting athletics may be detrimental to the athlete beyond decreasing risk of athletic sudden death.[14,93] Patients with congenital heart disease have been shown to have improved quality of life when participating in organized athletics, even when they participate in sports against the 36th Bethesda recommendations.[94] Participation is likely best assessed on an individual basis when possible. Some have advocated involving the athlete and the athlete's family in the decision-making process of whether and how to participate, similar in approach to most other medical decisions, by educating the athlete on the known and unknown risks, allowing a degree of "individual assumption of risk."[95]

Secondary Prevention: Defibrillator and Education

Many instances of sudden death occur without warning or indications of increased risk.[62–65] Automated external defibrillators (AEDs) and first-responder CPR will always have a role in averting sudden cardiac death. AEDs are common in schools and are often readily accessible in areas of training and competition.[96] Social media has allowed the long but ultimately successful resuscitation of footballer Fabrice Muamba from cardiac arrest during competition a very public example of AED and first responder capability.[97] Multiple studies have shown education to increase AED use, and CPR improves survival in athletic arrest, with the additional benefit of possible resuscitation of a spectator.[21,96,98–102] Perhaps more than any particular screening measure, appropriate AED use alongside spectator and physician education may allow organized sports to be the safest venue for exertional activity.

SUMMARY

The athlete is often a hero of our families, communities, and nations. The paradox of heroic fitness and sudden occurrence of an athlete's death increases the magnitude of the tragedy within and beyond the athlete's community. Sport and competition are heralded for their positive health effects and character development. In this article, athlete sudden death is analyzed from a historical and literary perspective and the development of modern initiatives to protect athletes from sudden death is reviewed, in the hope that the reader might better appreciate the significance of sudden death in the athlete population as well as the dramatic impact of an individual's death on that athlete's community.

REFERENCES

1. Scambler G. Sport and society: history, power and culture. New York: Open University Press; 2005 [Imprint].
2. Miller SG. Arete : Greek sports from ancient sources. 3rd edition. Berkeley (CA): University of California Press; 2004.
3. Golden M. Sport and society in ancient Greece. New York: Cambridge University Press; 1998.
4. Perrottet T. The naked Olympics: the true story of the ancient games. New York: Random House; 2004.
5. Homer. The Iliad. Reissue Edition. Toronto, Canada: Penguin; 1998.
6. Gardiner EN. Athletics of the ancient world. Amsterdam: J.C. Gieben; 1930. p. x–246.
7. Boutros L. Phoenician sport: its influence on the origin of the Olympic games. Amsterdam: J.C. Gieben; 1981.
8. Pollitt JJ. Art in the Hellenistic age. New York: Cambridge University Press; 1986. p. 1–329.
9. Pollitt JJ. Art and experience in classical Greece. New York: Cambridge University Press; 1972. p. xiv–205.
10. Lexicon Iconographicum Mythologiae Classicae (LIMC). Zurich: Artemis Verlag; 1988. IV(2). p. 444–559.
11. Lexicon Iconographicum Mythologiae Classicae (LIMC). Zurich: Artemis Verlag; 1990. IV(2). p. 6–188.
12. Williams RA. The athlete and heart disease. Philadelphia: Springhouse; 1999.
13. National Collegiate Athletics Association. Student-athlete participation: 1981-82-2013-14 [Internet]. 1–294. 2014. Available at: http://www.ncaapublications.com/p-4368-2013-14-ncaa-sports-sponsorship-and-participation-rates-report.aspx?CategoryID=0&SectionID=0&ManufacturerID=0&DistributorID=0&GenreID=0&VectorID=0&. Accessed December 28, 2014.
14. Battle RW, Mistry DJ, Baggish AL. Cardiovascular care and evaluation of the elite athlete. In: Miller M, editor. Delee & Drez's orthopaedic sports medicine. 4th edition. Elsevier; 2014. p. 185–201.

15. Roosevelt T. Citizenship in a Republic [Internet]. 1910. Available from: http://design.caltech.edu/erik/Misc/Citizenship_in_a_Republic.pdf. Accessed December 28, 2014.
16. Phillip Yancey, Tim Stafford. Niv student bible compact. Grand Rapids (MI): Zondervan; 2007.
17. The Episcopal Church. The book of common prayer. New York: Church Publishing Incorporated; 2011.
18. Maron BJ. Sudden death in young athletes. N Engl J Med 2003;349:1064–75.
19. Maron BJ, Doerer JJ, Haas TS, et al. Sudden deaths in young competitive athletes: analysis of 1866 deaths in the United States, 1980–2006. Circulation 2009;119:1085–92.
20. Maron BJ, Gohman TE, Aeppli D. Prevalence of sudden cardiac death during competitive sports activities in Minnesota high school athletes. J Am Coll Cardiol 1998;32:1881–4.
21. Toresdahl BG, Rao AL, Harmon KG, et al. Incidence of sudden cardiac arrest in high school student athletes on school campus. Heart Rhythm 2014;11: 1190–4.
22. Maron BJ, Haas TS, Murphy CJ, et al. Incidence and causes of sudden death in US College athletes. J Am Coll Cardiol 2014;63:1636–43.
23. Harmon KG, Asif IM, Klossner D, et al. Incidence of sudden cardiac death in National Collegiate Athletic Association Athletes. Circulation 2011;123:1594–600.
24. Eckart RE, Scoville SL, Campbell CL, et al. Sudden death in young adults: a 25-year review of autopsies in military recruits. Ann Intern Med 2004;141: 829–34.
25. Corrado D, Migliore F, Basso C, et al. Exercise and the risk of sudden cardiac death. Herz 2006;31:553–8.
26. Holst AG, Winkel BG, Theilade J, et al. Incidence and etiology of sports-related sudden cardiac death in Denmark–implications for preparticipation screening. Heart Rhythm 2010;7:1365–71.
27. Turner S. In cold blood: dead athletes in classical Athens. World Archaeol 2012; 44:217–33.
28. Ernest Hemingway FAQ [Internet]. Timelesshemingway.com. Available at: http://www.timelesshemingway.com/faq. Accessed December 23, 2014.
29. Hemingway E. Death in the afternoon. London: Simon and Schuster; 2014.
30. Poe EA. The essential tales and poems of Edgar Allan Poe. New York: Barnes & Noble Classics; 2004.
31. Battle RW. Edgar Allan Poe: a case description of the Marfan syndrome in an obscure short story. Am J Cardiol 2011;108:148–9.
32. Maron BJ, Ackerman MJ, Nishimura RA, et al. Task Force 4: HCM and other cardiomyopathies, mitral valve prolapse, myocarditis, and Marfan syndrome. J Am Coll Cardiol 2005;45:1340–5.
33. Chen HC, Kao FY, Huang SK. Epidemiological profile of Marfan syndrome in a general population: a national database study. Mayo Clin Proc 2014;89: 34–42.
34. Marfan AB. Un cas de déformation congénital des quatre members plus pronouncée aux extrémitiés charactérisée par l'allongement des os avec un certain degré d'amonassesment. Bull Mém Soc Méd Hôp 1896;13:220–6 [in French].
35. Housman AE. The works of A. E. Housman. Ware (United Kingdom): Wordsworth Editions; 1994.
36. Lydiard A. Running to the top. 3rd edition. Lansing (MI): Meyer and Meyer Sport; 2011.

37. Training the Lydiard way: 28 weeks to a PR. 2000. Available at: http://www. runnersworld.com/race-training/training-lydiard-way-28-weeks-pr?page=single. Accessed December 28, 2014.
38. Pond M, editor. Official 1990 NCAA Basketball Records. Overland Park (KS): 1991.
39. Maron BJ. Sudden death in young athletes. Lessons from the Hank Gathers affair. N Engl J Med 1993;329:55–7.
40. Hank Gathers collapses, dies of a heart condition [Internet]. ESPN. Available at: http://sports.espn.go.com/espn/espn25/story?page=moments/62. Accessed December 28, 2014.
41. Preston K. Doctor had Lewis family convinced he would be fine. The Reggie Lewis tragedy: a year later [Internet]. Baltimore Sun; 1994. Available at: http:// articles.baltimoresun.com/1994-09-11/sports/1994254130_1_mudge-reggie-lewis-clinical-cardiology. Accessed December 28, 2014.
42. Reggie Lewis's death, 20 years ago, one of the worst moments in Boston sports history–The Boston Globe. 2013. Available at: http://www.bostonglobe.com/ sports/2013/07/27/reggie-lewis-death-years-ago-one-worst-moments-boston-sports-history/pEK5MyYp7hXYf2ZGsU7kbN/story.html. Accessed December 28, 2014.
43. Hudson MA. A legacy on court, in court. Los Angeles Times 1992;A1.
44. James SD. Fran Crippen death: likely heat stroke or heart. 2010. Available at: http:// abcnews.go.com/Health/Wellness/fran-crippen-death-heat-stroke-heart-problems/ story?id=11967179. Accessed December 28, 2014.
45. Ford B. Crippen's memory still fuels reform fight [Internet]. ESPN. Available at: http://espn.go.com/olympics/swimming/story/_/id/7131352/one-year-fran-crippen-death-fight-change-continues. Accessed December 28, 2014.
46. About Fran Crippen [Internet]. Fran Crippen Elevation Foundation. Available at: http://francrippen.org/about-fran/. Accessed December 28, 2014.
47. Karu C. Giving back: paying it forward. Zika and Andy Palmer's ZAP fitness center [Internet]. Running Times; 2004. Available at: http://www.runnersworld.com/ rt-columns/giving-back-paying-it-forward?page=single. Accessed October 1, 2014.
48. Andy Palmer–ZAP fitness [Internet]. Available at: http://zapfitness.com/athletes/ andy-palmer/. Accessed December 28, 2014.
49. Classic Corner–Andy Palmer–a Tribute. Available at: http://www. billrodgersrunningcenter.com/clcoanpatr.html. Accessed December 28, 2014.
50. Runner, 24, dies after training. 1986. Available at: http://www.nytimes.com/1986/ 06/04/sports/runner-24-dies-after-training.html. Accessed December 28, 2014.
51. "Pistol" Pete Maravich–career recap. 2014. Available at: http://www.lsusports. net/ViewArticle.dbml?ATCLID=177319. Accessed December 28, 2014.
52. From the archive, 14 July 1967: Simpson dies after collapse on Tour. 1992; A1. Available at: http://www.theguardian.com/theguardian/2012/jul/14/archive-1967-simpson-death-tour-de-france. Accessed December 28, 2014.
53. Remebering a Sensation. Bbc.co.uk. 2004. Available at: http://www.bbc.co.uk/ insideout/northeast/series6/cycling.shtml. Acccessed April 10, 2015.
54. Cameroon star Foe dies [Internet]. bbc.co.uk. 2003 [cited 2015 Apr 10]; Available at: http://news.bbc.co.uk/sport2/hi/football/3024360.stm. Accessed April 10, 2015.
55. Smith RK. A brief history of the National Collegiate Athletic Association's role in regulating intercollegiate athletics. Marq Sports L Rev 2000;11:9–22.
56. Lewis GM. Theodore Roosevelt's role in the 1905 football controversy. Res Q 1965;40:717–24.

57. Battle RW, Mistry DJ, Malhotra R, et al. Cardiovascular screening and the elite athlete: advances, concepts, controversies, and a view of the future. Clin Sports Med 2011;30:503–24.
58. Bernhardt DT, Roberts WO. PPE: preparticipation physical evaluation. American Academy of Pediatrics; 2010.
59. Maron BJ, Thompson PD, Puffer JC, et al. Cardiovascular preparticipation screening of competitive athletes. A statement for health professionals from the Sudden Death Committee (clinical cardiology) and Congenital Cardiac Defects Committee (cardiovascular disease in the young), American Heart Association. Circulation 1996;94:850–6.
60. Maron BJ, Douglas PS, Graham TP, et al. Task force 1: preparticipation screening and diagnosis of cardiovascular disease in athletes. J Am Coll Cardiol 2005;45:1322–6.
61. Klein GJ, Bashore TM, Sellers TD, et al. Ventricular fibrillation in the Wolff-Parkinson-White syndrome. N Engl J Med 1979;301:1080–5.
62. Timmermans C, Smeets JL, Rodriguez LM, et al. Aborted sudden death in the Wolff-Parkinson-White syndrome. Am J Cardiol 1995;76:492–4.
63. Bromberg BI, Lindsay BD, Cain ME, et al. Impact of clinical history and electrophysiologic characterization of accessory pathways on management strategies to reduce sudden death among children with Wolff-Parkinson-White syndrome. J Am Coll Cardiol 1996;27:690–5.
64. Maron BJ, Roberts WC, Epstein SE. Sudden death in hypertrophic cardiomyopathy: a profile of 78 patients. Circulation 1982;65:1388–94.
65. Maron BJ, Olivotto I, Spirito P, et al. Epidemiology of hypertrophic cardiomyopathy-related death: revisited in a large non-referral-based patient population. Circulation 2000;102:858–64.
66. Corrado D, Basso C, Pavei A, et al. Trends in sudden cardiovascular death in young competitive athletes after implementation of a preparticipation screening program. JAMA 2006;296:1593–601.
67. Corrado D. Cardiovascular pre-participation screening of young competitive athletes for prevention of sudden death: proposal for a common European protocol: consensus statement of the Study Group of Sport Cardiology of the Working Group of Cardiac Rehabilitation and Exercise Physiology and the Working Group of Myocardial and Pericardial Diseases of the European Society of Cardiology. Eur Heart J 2004;26:516–24.
68. Myerburg RJ, Vetter VL. Electrocardiograms should be included in preparticipation screening of athletes. Circulation 2007;116:2616–26 [discussion: 2626].
69. Maron BJ. National electrocardiography screening for competitive athletes: feasible in the United States? Ann Intern Med 2010;152:324–6.
70. Chaitman BR. An electrocardiogram should not be included in routine preparticipation screening of young athletes. Circulation 2007;116:2610–5.
71. Levine BD. Research in sports and exercise cardiology: challenges, opportunities, future directions. Presented at the meeting of 2014 ACC Sports Cardiology Summit. Indianapolis (IN): 2014.
72. Fagard R. Athlete's heart. Heart 2003;89:1455–61.
73. Huston TP, Puffer JC, Rodney WM. The athletic heart syndrome. N Engl J Med 1985;313:24–32.
74. Weiner RB, Baggish AL. Exercise-induced cardiac remodeling. Prog Cardiovasc Dis 2012;54:380–6.
75. Pluim BM, Zwinderman AH, van der Laarse A, et al. The athlete's heart: a meta-analysis of cardiac structure and function. Circulation 2000;101:336–44.

76. Pelliccia A, Maron BJ, Spataro A, et al. The upper limit of physiologic cardiac hypertrophy in highly trained elite athletes. N Engl J Med 1991;324:295–301.
77. Morganroth J, Maron BJ, Henry WL, et al. Comparative left ventricular dimensions in trained athletes. Ann Intern Med 1975;82:521–4.
78. Scharhag J, Schneider G, Urhausen A, et al. Athlete's heart: right and left ventricular mass and function in male endurance athletes and untrained individuals determined by magnetic resonance imaging. J Am Coll Cardiol 2002;40: 1856–63.
79. Puffer JC. Overview of the athletic heart syndrome. In: Paul D. Thompson, editor. Exercise and sports cardiology. New York: McGraw-Hill; 2001. p. 30–42.
80. Marron BJ. Structural features of the athlete heart as defined by echocardiography. J Am Coll Cardiol 1986;7:190–203.
81. Utomi V, Oxborough D, Whyte GP, et al. Systematic review and meta-analysis of training mode, imaging modality and body size influences on the morphology and function of the male athlete's heart. Heart 2013;99:1727–33.
82. Barbier J, Ville N, Kervio G, et al. Sports-specific features of athlete's heart and their relation to echocardiographic parameters. Herz 2006;31:531–43.
83. Baggish AL, Wang F, Weiner RB, et al. Training-specific changes in cardiac structure and function: a prospective and longitudinal assessment of competitive athletes. J Appl Physiol (1985) 2008;104:1121–8.
84. Nagashima J, Musha H, Takada H, et al. New upper limit of physiologic cardiac hypertrophy in Japanese participants in the 100-km ultramarathon. J Am Coll Cardiol 2003;42:1617–23.
85. Thompson PD. Cardiovascular adaptations to marathon running: the marathoner's heart. Sports Med 2007;37:444–7.
86. George KP, Batterham AM, Jones B. Echocardiographic evidence of concentric left ventricular enlargement in female weight lifters. Eur J Appl Physiol Occup Physiol 1998;79:88–92.
87. Henschen SE. Mitteilungen aus der medizinischen Klinik zu Upsala. 1899. [in German].
88. Darling EA. The effects of training: a study of the Harvard University crews. Boston Med Surg J 1899;161:229–33.
89. Corrado D, Pelliccia A, Heidbuchel H, et al, Sections of Sports Cardiology of the European Association of Cardiovascular Prevention and Rehabilitation. Recommendations for interpretation of 12-lead electrocardiogram in the athlete. Eur Heart J 2010;31:243–59.
90. Gati S, Sheikh N, Ghani S, et al. Should axis deviation or atrial enlargement be categorised as abnormal in young athletes? The athlete's electrocardiogram: time for re-appraisal of markers of pathology. Eur Heart J 2013;34: 3641–8.
91. Sheikh N, Papadakis M, Ghani S, et al. Comparison of electrocardiographic criteria for the detection of cardiac abnormalities in elite black and white athletes. Circulation 2014;129:1637–49.
92. Drezner JA, Ackerman MJ, Anderson J, et al. Electrocardiographic interpretation in athletes: the 'Seattle criteria'. Br J Sports Med 2013;47:122–4.
93. Vaseghi M, Ackerman MJ, Mandapati R. Restricting sports for athletes with heart disease: are we saving lives, avoiding lawsuits, or just promoting obesity and sedentary living? Pediatr Cardiol 2012;33:407–16.
94. Dean PN, Gillespie CW, Greene EA, et al. Sports participation and quality of life in adolescents and young adults with congenital heart disease. Congenit Heart Dis 2014. [Epub ahead of print].

95. Levine BD, Stray-Gundersen J. The medical care of competitive athletes: the role of the physician and individual assumption of risk. Med Sci Sports Exerc 1994;26:1190–2.
96. Vetter VL, Haley DM. Secondary prevention of sudden cardiac death. Curr Opin Cardiol 2014;29:68–75.
97. Fabrice Muamba recalls the day he "died" and tells how grateful he is to the people who brought him back. 2012; Available at: http://www.telegraph.co.uk/ sport/football/9665055/Fabrice-Muamba-recalls-the-day-he-died-and-tells-how-grateful-he-is-to-the-people-who-brought-him-back.html. Accessed April 10, 2015.
98. Drezner JA, Toresdahl BG, Rao AL, et al. Outcomes from sudden cardiac arrest in US high schools: a 2-year prospective study from the National Registry for AED Use in Sports. Br J Sports Med 2013;47:1179–83.
99. Lawless CE, Asplund C, Asif EM, et al. Protecting the heart of the American athlete: proceedings of the American College of Cardiology sports and exercise cardiology think tank October 18, 2012, Washington, DC. J Am Coll Cardiol 2014;64:2146–71.
100. Drezner JA, Rao AL, Heistand J, et al. Effectiveness of emergency response planning for sudden cardiac arrest in United States high schools with automated external defibrillators. Circulation 2009;120:518–25.
101. Maron BJ, Haas TS, Ahluwalia A, et al. Increasing survival rate from commotio cordis. Heart Rhythm 2013;10:219–23.
102. Sharma S, Papadakis M. Improved survival rates from commotio cordis: a case for automatic external defibrillator provision during high-risk sports. Heart Rhythm 2013;10:224–5.

Index

Note: Page numbers of article titles are in **boldface** type.

Clin Sports Med 34 (2015) 587–593
http://dx.doi.org/10.1016/S0278-5919(15)00040-X
0278-5919/15/$ – see front matter © 2015 Elsevier Inc. All rights reserved.

sportsmed.theclinics.com

Moving?

Make sure your subscription moves with you!

To notify us of your new address, find your **Clinics Account Number** (located on your mailing label above your name), and contact customer service at:

Email: journalscustomerservice-usa@elsevier.com

800-654-2452 (subscribers in the U.S. & Canada)
314-447-8871 (subscribers outside of the U.S. & Canada)

Fax number: 314-447-8029

Elsevier Health Sciences Division
Subscription Customer Service
3251 Riverport Lane
Maryland Heights, MO 63043

*To ensure uninterrupted delivery of your subscription, please notify us at least 4 weeks in advance of move.

Printed and bound by CPI Group (UK) Ltd, Croydon, CR0 4YY

03/10/2024

01040488-0004